# MASTER TECHNIQUES IN ORTHOPAEDIC SURGERY

■

# THE WRIST

*Second Edition*

# MASTER TECHNIQUES IN ORTHOPAEDIC SURGERY

## Series Editor
## Roby C. Thompson, Jr., M.D.

### Volume Editors

## THE FOOT AND ANKLE
Second Edition: Harold B. Kitaoka, M.D.
First Edition: Kenneth A. Johnson, M.D.

## RECONSTRUCTIVE KNEE SURGERY
Douglas W. Jackson, M.D.

## KNEE ARTHROPLASTY
Second Edition: Paul A. Lotke, M.D. and Jess H. Lonner, M.D.
First Edition: Paul A. Lotke, M.D.

## THE HIP
Clement B. Sledge, M.D.

## THE SPINE
Second Edition: David S. Bradford, M.D. and Thomas A. Zdeblick, M.D.
First Edition: David S. Bradford, M.D.

## THE SHOULDER
Edward V. Craig, M.D.

## THE ELBOW
Bernard F. Morrey, M.D.

## THE WRIST
Richard H. Gelberman, M.D.

## THE HAND
Second Edition: James W. Strickland, M.D. and Thomas J. Graham, M.D.
James W. Strickland, M.D.

## FRACTURES
Donald A. Wiss, M.D.

# THE WRIST

## Second Edition

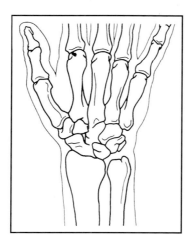

## Editor

### RICHARD H. GELBERMAN, M.D.

**Professor and Chairman**
**Department of Orthopaedic Surgery**
**Barnes-Jewish Hospital at Washington University**
**Saint Louis, Missouri**

## Illustrators

**Joel Herring, Oceanside, New York**

**Kate Sweeney, Seattle, Washington**

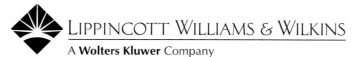

LIPPINCOTT WILLIAMS & WILKINS

A **Wolters Kluwer** Company

Philadelphia · Baltimore · New York · London
Buenos Aires · Hong Kong · Sydney · Tokyo

*Acquisitions Editor*: James Merritt
*Developmental Editor*: Lloyd Unverferth
*Supervising Editor*: Mary Ann McLaughlin
*Production Editor*: Sophia Elaine Battaglia, Silverchair Science + Communications
*Manufacturing Manager*: Benjamin Rivera
*Compositor*: Silverchair Science + Communications
Produced by Phoenix Offset
*Series Designer*: QT Design

**© 2002 by LIPPINCOTT WILLIAMS & WILKINS**
**530 Walnut Street**
**Philadelphia, PA 19106 USA**
**LWW.com**

Printed in China

**Library of Congress Cataloging-in-Publication Data**

The wrist / editor, Richard H. Gelberman ; illustrators, Joel Herring, Kate Sweeney.-- 2nd ed.
        p. ; cm. -- (Master techniques in orthopaedic surgery ; [v. 2])
    Includes bibliographical references and index.
    ISBN 0-7817-2372-8
    1. Wrist--Surgery.  I. Gelberman, Richard H. II. Master techniques in orthopaedic
surgery (2nd ed.) ; [v. 2].
    [DNLM: 1. Wrist--surgery.  2. Orthopedics. WE 168 M423 2001 v.2]
    RD559 .W74 2002
    617.5'74--dc21
                                                                    2001038741

Care has been taken to confirm the accuracy of the information presented and to describe generally accepted practices. However, the authors, editors, and publisher are not responsible for errors or omissions or for any consequences from application of the information in this book and make no warranty, expressed or implied, with respect to the currency, completeness, or accuracy of the contents of the publication. Application of this information in a particular situation remains the professional responsibility of the practitioner.

The authors, editors, and publisher have exerted every effort to ensure that drug selection and dosage set forth in this text are in accordance with current recommendations and practice at the time of publication. However, in view of ongoing research, changes in government regulations, and the constant flow of information relating to drug therapy and drug reactions, the reader is urged to check the package insert for each drug for any change in indications and dosage and for added warnings and precautions. This is particularly important when the recommended agent is a new or infrequently employed drug.

Some drugs and medical devices presented in this publication have Food and Drug Administration (FDA) clearance for limited use in restricted research settings. It is the responsibility of health care providers to ascertain the FDA status of each drug or device planned for use in their clinical practice.

10 9 8 7 6 5 4 3 2 1

For Diane Kasow—whose strength and courage I admire

■

# CONTENTS

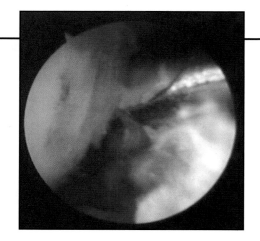

# PART IV   NONUNIONS OF THE DISTAL RADIUS

# PART V   SCAPHOID FRACTURES

# PART VI   SCAPHOID NONUNIONS

# PART VII   CARPAL INSTABILITY

# PART VIII  OSTEOARTHRITIS

# PART IX  DISTAL RADIOULNAR JOINT INSTABILITY

*Deceased.

# CONTRIBUTING AUTHORS

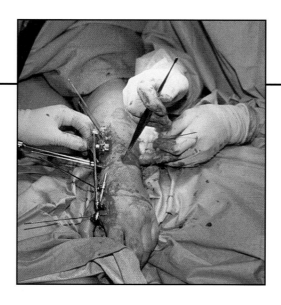

**A. Herbert Alexander, M.D.**
*Professor, Department of Surgery, Uniformed Services University of the Health Sciences F. Edward Hébert School of Medicine, Bethesda, Maryland*

**Charlotte E. Alexander, M.D.**
*Sun Valley Sports Medicine, Ketchum, Indiana*

**Duffield Ashmead IV, M.D.**
*Assistant Clinical Professor, Departments of Plastic Surgery and Orthopedics, University of Connecticut School of Medicine, Farmington, Connecticut*

**Terry S. Axelrod, M.D., M.Sc., F.R.C.S. (C.)**
*Associate Professor, Department of Surgery, University of Toronto Faculty of Medicine, Toronto, Ontario, Canada; Chief, Division of Orthopaedic Surgery, Sunnybrook Hospital, Toronto, Ontario, Canada*

**Robert D. Beckenbaugh, M.D.**
*Professor, Department of Orthopedics, Hand Division, Mayo Clinic, Rochester, Minnesota*

**Richard A. Berger, M.D., PH.D.**
*Professor, Departments of Orthopedic Surgery and Anatomy, Mayo Clinic/Mayo Foundation, Rochester, Minnesota*

**Allen Thorpe Bishop, M.D.**
*Professor, Department of Orthopedic Surgery, Mayo Medical School, Rochester, Minnesota; Consultant in Orthopedic Surgery and Surgery of the Hand, Department of Orthopedic Surgery, Mayo Clinic/Mayo Foundation, Rochester, Minnesota*

**Michael J. Botte, M.D.**
*Clinical Professor, Department of Orthopaedic Surgery, University of California, San Diego, School of Medicine, San Diego, California*

**C. Vaughan A. Bowen, M.D., F.R.C.S. (C.), M.B., C.h.B**
*Clinical Professor, Department of Surgery (Orthopaedics), University of Calgary Faculty of Medicine, Calgary, Alberta, Canada*

**William H. Bowers, M.S., M.D.**
*Associate Clinical Professor of Hand Surgery, Department of Surgery, Medical College of Virginia, Richmond, Virginia; Hand Surgery Specialists Ltd., Richmond, Virginia*

**Martin I. Boyer, M.D., F.R.C.S. (C.)**
*Assistant Professor, Department of Orthopaedic Surgery, Barnes-Jewish Hospital at Washington University, St. Louis, Missouri*

**James H. Calandruccio, M.D.**
*Assistant Professor, Department of Orthopaedics, University of Tennessee, Memphis, College of Medicine, Memphis, Tennessee; Campbell Clinic, Germantown, Tennessee*

**Charles Cassidy, M.D.**
*Assistant Professor, Department of Orthopaedic Surgery, Tufts University School of Medicine, New England Medical Center, Boston, Massachusetts*

**Paul Feldon, M.D.**
*Associate Clinical Professor, Department of Orthopaedic Surgery, Tufts University School of Medicine, Boston, Massachusetts*

**Colin W. Fennell, M.D.**
*Clinical Associate Professor, Department of Surgery, University of North Dakota School of Medicine and Health Sciences, Grand Forks, North Dakota*

**Larry D. Field, M.D.**
*Mississippi Sports Medicine and Orthopaedic Center, Jackson, Mississippi*

**Richard H. Gelberman, M.D.**
*Professor and Chairman, Department of Orthopaedic Surgery, Barnes-Jewish Hospital at Washington University, Saint Louis, Missouri*

**Charles A. Goldfarb, M.D.**
*Mary S. Stern Hand Surgery Fellow, Department of Orthopaedic Surgery, University of Cincinnati College of Medicine, Cincinnati, Ohio*

**David P. Green, M.D.**
*Clinical Professor, Department of Orthopaedics, University of Texas Health Science Center at San Antonio, San Antonio, Texas*

**Jeffrey A. Greenberg, M.S., M.D.**
*Clinical Assistant Professor, Department of Orthopaedics, Indiana University School of Medicine, Indianapolis, Indiana; Partner and Attending Physician, Indiana Hand Center, Indianapolis, Indiana*

**Timothy J. Herbert, M.B.B.S, F.R.C.S., F.R.A.C.S.**
*Honorary Consultant, Department of Hand Surgery, University of Sydney, Sydney and St. Luke's Hospitals, Sydney, Australia*

**Erich E. Hornbach, M.D.**
*Department of Orthopedic Surgery, Edward W. Sparrow Medical Center, Lansing, Michigan*

**James H. House, M.D., M.S.**
*Professor Emeritus, Department of Orthopaedic Surgery, University of Minnesota Medical School—Minneapolis, Minneapolis, Minnesota*

**Jesse B. Jupiter, M.D.**
*Professor, Department of Orthopaedic Surgery, Harvard University Medical School, Boston, Massachusetts; Director, Orthopaedic Hand Service, Massachusetts General Hospital, Boston, Massachusetts*

**Adalbert I. Kapandji, M.D.**
*Orthopaedist and Hand Surgeon, Clinique de l'Yvette, Longjumeau, France; International Member of the A.A.S.H.; Member and Past President (1997–1998) of the French Society for Surgery of the Hand; Member of the Italian Society for Surgery of the Hand; Correspondant Member of La Associaion Argentina de Ortopedia y Traumatologia*

**William B. Kleinman, M.D.**
*Clinical Professor, Department of Orthopaedic Surgery, Indiana University School of Medicine, The Indiana Hand Center, Indianapolis, Indiana*

**Hermann Krimmer, M.D.**
*Associate Professor, University of Würzburg, Würzburg, Germany; Hand Center Bad Neustadt, Bad Neustadt, Germany*

**Tung B. Le, M.D.**
*Attending Surgeon, Department of Orthopaedics/Hand Surgery, Kaiser Permanente Medical Center, Santa Clara, California*

**Fraser J. Leversedge, M.D.**
*Department of Orthopaedic Surgery, Barnes-Jewish Hospital at Washington University, St. Louis, Missouri*

**David M. Lichtman, M.D.**
*Chairman, Department of Orthopaedic Surgery, John Peter Smith Health Network, Fort Worth, Texas*

**Ronald L. Linscheid, M.D.**
*Professor Emeritus, Department of Orthopedic Surgery, Mayo Clinic, Rochester, Minnesota*

**Lewis H. Millender, M.D.***
*Clinical Professor, Department of Orthopaedic Surgery, Tufts University School of Medicine, Boston, Massachusetts; Assistant Chief, Hand Surgery Service, New England Baptist Hospital, Boston, Massachusetts*

**Craig C. Newland, M.D.**
*Liberty Orthopaedics, Liberty, Missouri*

**A. Lee Osterman, M.D.**
*Professor, Orthopedic and Hand Surgery, Jefferson Medical College of Thomas Jefferson University, Philadelphia, Pennsylvania; Director, The Philadelphia Hand Center and Fellowship Program, King of Prussia, Pennsylvania*

**Gary G. Poehling, M.D.**
*Professor and Chairman, Department of Orthopaedic Surgery, Wake Forest University School of Medicine, Wake Forest University Medical Center, Winston-Salem, North Carolina*

**Robin R. Richards, M.D., F.R.C.S.C.**
*Professor, Department of Surgery, University of Toronto Faculty of Medicine, Toronto, Ontario, Canada; Surgeon-in-Chief, Sunnybrook and Women's College Health Sciences Centre, Toronto, Ontario, Canada*

**Leonard K. Ruby, M.D.**
*Professor, Department of Orthopaedics, Division of Hand Surgery, Tufts University School of Medicine, New England Medical Center, Boston, Massachusetts*

**Felix H. Savoie III, M.D.**
*Mississippi Sports Medicine and Orthopaedic Center, Jackson, Mississippi*

---

*Deceased.

**Gary S. Shapiro, M.D.**

*Orthopaedics Fellow, Hospital for Special Surgery, New York, New York*

**Robert M. Szabo, M.D., M.P.H.**

*Professor of Orthopaedics and Plastic Surgery, Department of Orthopaedics, University of California, Davis, School of Medicine, Sacramento, California*

**Julio Taleisnik, M.D.**

*Clinical Professor, Department of Orthopaedics, University of California, Irvine, College of Medicine, Irvine, California*

**Andrew L. Terrono, M.D.**

*Associate Clinical Professor, Department of Orthopaedic Surgery, Tufts University School of Medicine, New England Baptist Bone and Joint Institute, Hand Surgical Associates, Inc., New England Baptist Hospital, Boston, Massachusetts*

**Marc E. Umlas, M.D.**

*Clinical Assistant Professor, Department of Orthopaedic Rehabilitation, University of Miami School of Medicine, Miami Beach, Florida*

**Ann E. Van Heest, M.D.**

*Associate Professor, Department of Orthopaedic Surgery, University of Minnesota Medical School—Minneapolis, Minneapolis, Minnesota*

**Steven F. Viegas, M.D.**

*Professor and Chief, Division of Hand Surgery, Department of Orthopaedic Surgery and Rehabilitation; Professor, Anatomy and Neurosciences; Professor, Preventative Medicine and Community Health, The University of Texas Medical Branch, Galveston, Texas*

**H. Kirk Watson, M.D.**

*Clinical Professor, Department of Orthopedic Surgery, University of Connecticut School of Medicine, Farmington, Connecticut; Director, Connecticut Combined Hand Surgery Fellowship, Hartford, Connecticut*

**Jeffry T. Watson, M.D.**

*Assistant Professor, Department of Orthopaedic Surgery, Vanderbilt University School of Medicine, Nashville, Tennessee*

**Andrew J. Weiland, M.D.**

*Professor of Surgery (Orthopaedic and Plastic Surgery), Department of Orthopaedics, Hospital for Special Surgery, New York, New York*

**Jeffrey Weinzweig, M.D.**

*Assistant Professor of Surgery, Department of Plastic Surgery, Brown University School of Medicine, Rhode Island Hospital, Hasbro Children's Hospital, Providence, Rhode Island*

**Rafael M. M. Williams, M.D.**

*Hand Surgery Fellow, Hand Surgery Specialists, Cincinnati, Ohio*

# SERIES PREFACE

The first volume of the series *Master Techniques in Orthopaedic Surgery* was published in 1994. Our goal in assembling the series was to create easy-to-follow descriptions of operative techniques that would help orthopaedists through the challenges of daily practice. The books were intended to be more than just technical manuals; they were designed to impart the personal experience of the "master orthopaedic surgeons."

*Master Techniques in Orthopaedic Surgery* has become precisely what we hoped for—books that are used again and again, and are found at home and in the offices of practicing orthopaedists and residents in training. Most important, they are recommended by orthopaedists who look to them for practical advice and suggestions concerning the difficult but common problems they encounter.

The series is now entering its second edition phase. You will again find recognized leaders as volume editors, known for their contributions to research, education, and the advancement of the surgical state of the art. Chapter authors have been selected for their experience, operative skills, and recognized expertise with a particular technique. The classic procedures are still included: some techniques have changed as new technology has been incorporated, and new procedures that have been popularized during the last several years have been added.

We are maintaining the same user-friendly format that was so well-received when the series was first introduced—a standardized presentation of information replete with tips and pearls gained through years of experience, with abundant color photographs and drawings to guide you step-by-step through the procedures.

With this new edition, we again invite you into the operating room to peer over the shoulder of the surgeon at work. It is our goal to offer the orthopaedic surgeon seeking an improved proficiency in practice access to the maximum confidence in selecting and executing the appropriate surgery for the individual patient.

*Roby C. Thompson, Jr., M.D.*
*Series Editor*

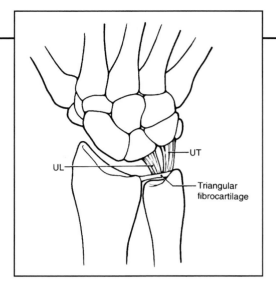

# PREFACE TO THE FIRST EDITION

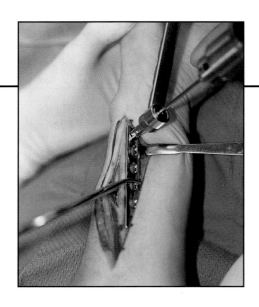

Because of the wide range of innovative concepts introduced over the past 15 years, wrist surgery has become an area of special interest among orthopaedists, hand surgeons, and traumatologists. As a result, it has become increasingly important for wrist surgeons to have a resource that provides systematic accounts of commonly performed operative procedures. This text is designed primarily to describe the indications and contraindications, as well as the operative techniques and pitfalls associated with the use of selected surgical approaches to clinical problems involving the wrist. Moreover, it is constructed to provide a detailed step-by-step account of the technical details that are required to carry out procedures that are used commonly, in an accomplished manner.

Contributors were carefully chosen for this volume. Not only are they leaders in research and clinical care in wrist surgery, but they are responsible for having either described or popularized the surgical approaches they depict. Each has accrued vast hands-on experience, allowing for the construction of uniquely detailed accounts of the most well-accepted operative methods. While the techniques described here are not the only ones that are used for specific clinical problems, I know of few techniques currently performed that are more soundly established in both principle and practice. Overall, it is the objective of this text to elevate the practice of wrist surgery to a plane that will see improved clinical outcomes with a reduced incidence of operative morbidity.

*Richard H. Gelberman, M.D.*

# PREFACE TO THE SECOND EDITION

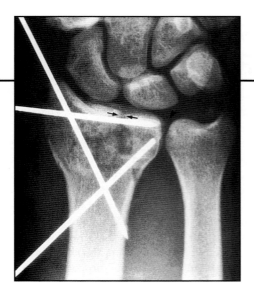

The second edition of this practical, popular text includes many important new chapters for the wrist surgeon. Four new chapters cover the treatment of distal radius fractures: limited open reduction and internal fixation, intrafocal arum pinning, fixation using SRS bone cement, and nonunion treatment using the LoCon T plate. For scaphoid nonunions, a new chapter describes open reduction internal fixation (ORIF) using a dorsal approach for small pole fragments. For treatment of the scaphoid-lunate advanced collapse (SLAC) wrist, I have added a chapter covering capitolunate fusion with scaphoid and triquetrum excision. New chapters for arthroscopic repair of the triangular fibrocartilage complex, ulnar shortening osteotomy, salvage of the failed Darrach procedure, and matched ulnar resection arthroplasty enhance the procedures for distal radioulnar joint instability.

To complement the new chapters, the original chapters have been updated thoroughly to include any changes since publication of the first edition, as these surgeons continue to refine their surgical technique. Although there is much content that is new in this second edition, the goals of this text have not changed, so the preface to the first edition is included.

*Richard H. Gelberman, M.D.*

# MASTER TECHNIQUES IN ORTHOPAEDIC SURGERY

# THE WRIST

## Second Edition

# PART I

# Utilitarian Operative Approaches

# 1

# Operative Exposure

Jeffry T. Watson, Richard H. Gelberman, and Martin I. Boyer

## EXTERNAL FIXATION FOR DISTAL RADIUS FRACTURES

External fixation is a well-established method of treatment for fractures of the distal radius. Several different systems are available, but all use bony fixation points in the shaft of the radius and in the index metacarpal. The fixator is placed along the dorsoradial plane of the radius. The ideal interval from proximal pin placement is the space between the extensor carpi radialis longus and the brachioradialis tendons.

The superficial branch of the radial nerve is at risk of injury in this procedure because it lies deep to the brachioradialis muscle, emerging to the brachioradialis tendon approximately 6 cm proximal to the radial styloid. Additionally, terminal branches of the lateral antebrachial cutaneous nerve lie subcutaneously in this region and are vulnerable to injury. Percutaneous placement of external fixator pins in the radius is ill advised because it carries the risk of painful neuroma formation and irreversible loss of sensation distally.

We prefer an open approach to the radial shaft for the placement of the proximal fixator pins. This allows the superficial radial nerve to be identified directly. Make a longitudinal incision on the lateral side of the radial shaft, approximately 5 cm proximal to the fracture (Fig. 1). Identify branches of the lateral antebrachial cutaneous nerve during subcutaneous dissection down to the forearm fascia, and retract them. Identify the tendons of brachioradialis and extensor carpi radialis longus (the extensor carpi radialis longus can be differentiated from the brachioradialis by observing its excursion with wrist flexion and extension).

Open the fascia overlying the interval and identify the superficial radial nerve as it lies deep or immediately radial to the tendon of brachioradialis (Fig. 2). Dissect the superficial radial nerve free throughout the length of the incision, and retract it. Use Hohmann or right-angle retractors to retract the soft tissues, and place the fixator pins in the radius under direct visualization.

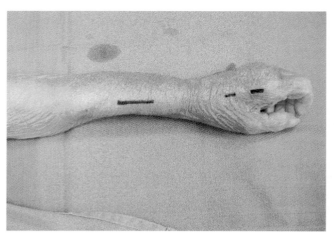

**FIGURE 1.** Incisions made for approach to the distal radial shaft and the second metacarpal.

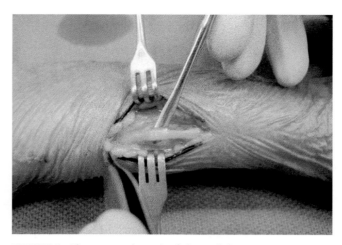

**FIGURE 2.** The sensory branch of the radial nerve.

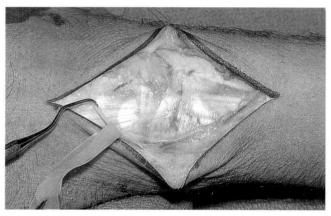

**FIGURE 3.** The dorsal longitudinal approach for wrist arthrodesis begins proximally at the junction of the radial diaphysis and metaphysis. The incision extends distally to the long finger metacarpal. In the distal portion of the incision, the dorsal sensory branch of the ulnar nerve is identified and protected with a rubber drain.

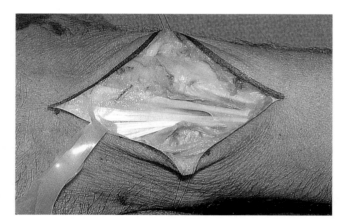

**FIGURE 4.** The extensor retinaculum is incised longitudinally, exposing the extensor digitorum communis tendons and the extensor indicis proprius tendon.

Either one or two incisions may be used along the dorsolateral or lateral aspect of the index metacarpal for placement of the two distal pins of the external fixator. Because it is possible to encounter terminal branches of the superficial radial nerve, we recommend direct visualization of the index metacarpal for the placement of both distal pins. Identify the metacarpal shaft immediately dorsal to the origin of the first dorsal interosseous muscle. Carry out placement of the fixator pins into the bone under direct visualization. Close all skin incisions before assembling the fixator apparatus.

## DORSAL APPROACHES

### Dorsal Longitudinal Approach

The dorsal longitudinal approach provides access to the entire dorsal aspect of the distal radius, distal radioulnar joint, and ulnar head, as well as the radiocarpal and ulnocarpal joints and the carpal bones. We use this approach most commonly for the treatment of acute fractures of the distal radius or osteotomy of the distal radius, treatment of disorders of the triangular fibrocartilage complex and distal

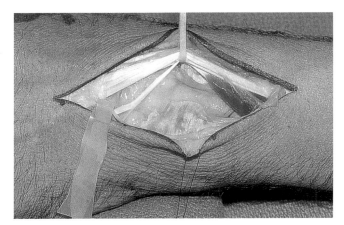

**FIGURE 5.** The extensor tendons are retracted radially, exposing the dorsal capsule of the radiocarpal joint. The muscular portion of the extensor indicis proprius is seen in the proximal limb of the incision.

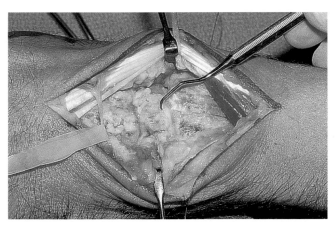

**FIGURE 6.** The infratendinous retinaculum and dorsal capsule are incised longitudinally, and full-thickness radial and ulnar flaps are dissected from the carpal bones and distal radius. The anatomy probe identifies the lunate.

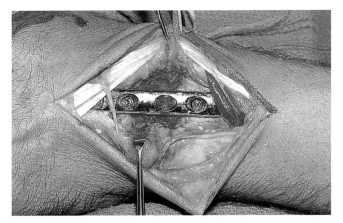

**FIGURE 7.** Following decortication, a dorsal plate is applied from the long finger metacarpal to the radius.

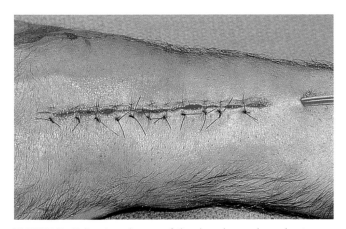

**FIGURE 8.** Following closure of the dorsal capsule and extensor retinaculum, the skin is closed with horizontal mattress sutures over a closed suction drain.

radioulnar joint, ligament reconstruction of the carpus, intercarpal arthrodesis, total wrist arthrodesis, and total wrist arthroplasty. This approach is extensile proximally, to expose the dorsal aspect of the distal radial diaphysis, and distally, to expose the metacarpal bones (Figs. 3–8).

Because the areolar tissue along the dorsal aspect of the wrist is loose, longitudinal scar contracture is of minimal consequence and does not limit wrist flexion. Start the utilitarian straight dorsal incision proximally over the central portion of the distal radius, proximal to Lister's dorsal radial tubercle. Continue the incision distally in line with the radius and the long-finger metacarpal (Fig. 9). Spread the subcutaneous tissue bluntly, and raise full-thickness skin flaps, exposing the extensor retinaculum (Fig. 10).

Familiarity with the location of the sensory branches of both the radial and the ulnar nerves on the dorsal wrist will aid in early identification of these structures after the skin is incised (Fig. 11). The sensory branch of the radial nerve becomes subcutaneous 5 to 10 cm proximal to the radial styloid, in the interval between the brachioradialis and extensor carpi radialis longus tendons. It bifurcates into two main branches before reaching the radiocarpal joint. The dorsal branch passes within 1 to 3 cm of the radial side of Lister's tubercle and continues distally to supply the first and second web spaces.

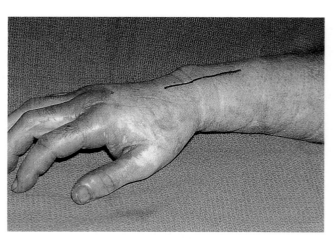

**FIGURE 9.** The dorsal longitudinal approach is ideal for the treatment of distal radius fractures with significant dorsal comminution, dorsal angulation, or articular incongruity. The incision is centered over the distal radius and extended from the diaphyseal-metaphyseal junction to the radiocarpal joint immediately ulnar to Lister's dorsal tubercle.

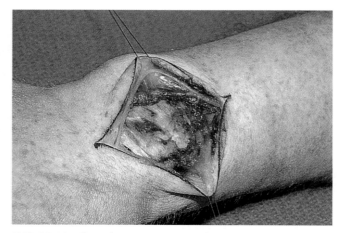

**FIGURE 10.** The subcutaneous tissue has been spread bluntly, exposing the dorsal aspect of the extensor retinaculum.

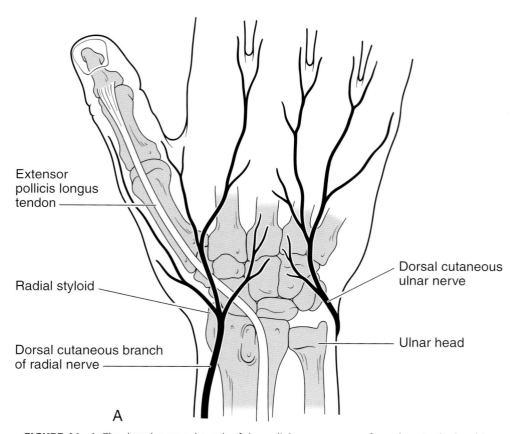

Extensor pollicis longus tendon

Radial styloid

Dorsal cutaneous branch of radial nerve

Dorsal cutaneous ulnar nerve

Ulnar head

A

**FIGURE 11.** **A:** The dorsal sensory branch of the radial nerve emerges from deep to the brachioradialis tendon approximately 6 cm proximal to the radial styloid. It travels distally in the superficial areolar tissue and branches into several fibers, crossing the extensor pollicis longus tendon (lying directly on it) at approximately the level of the scapho-trapezoid joint. The dorsal cutaneous branch of the ulnar nerve crosses from dorsal to volar just distal to the ulnar styloid at an angle of approximately 45° to the long axis of the extremity. The nerve may be palpated before skin incision by feeling directly over the dorsal triquetrum and triquetro-hamate articulation. (*continued.*)

The palmar branch passes within 2 cm of the first dorsal compartment and provides sensory innervation to the dorsolateral aspect of the thumb after passing directly over the extensor pollicis longus tendon. The dorsal cutaneous branch of the ulnar nerve arises from the ulnar nerve deep to the flexor carpi ulnaris tendon and becomes subcutaneous on the ulnar border of the forearm, approximately 5 cm from the proximal border of the pisiform. Branching of the nerve can begin proximal or distal to the ulnar head, and the nerve usually passes directly over its medial aspect, as well as the dorsal aspect of the triquetrum and hamate. Anatomic dissections have identified communicating branches between the ulnar and radial dorsal sensory branches.

Surgical procedures involving tenosynovectomy or tendon transfer involving the digital extensor tendons are best approached directly through the fourth dorsal compartment. Procedures involving the distal radioulnar joint or the triangular fibrocartilage complex are most effectively approached through the fifth dorsal compartment. The majority of other surgical procedures carried out on the distal radius and carpus are conveniently approached through the third dorsal compartment.

With passive motion of the thumb and the fingers, identify the interval between the extensor pollicis longus (third compartment) and the extensor digitorum communis (fourth compartment), and sharply incise the retinaculum directly overlying the third compartment. Mobilize the extensor pollicis longus tendon proximally and distally, and retract it radially. Then dissect the infratendinous retinaculum of the fourth dorsal compartment either from the underlying dorsal wrist capsule as a separate layer, or subperiosteally, along with the dorsal capsule, as a combined layer (Figs. 12–15).

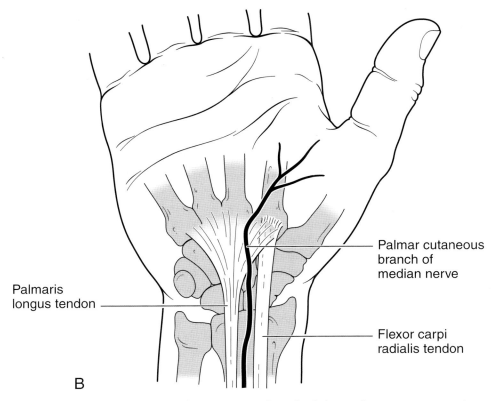

Palmar cutaneous branch of median nerve

Palmaris longus tendon

Flexor carpi radialis tendon

B

**FIGURE 11. (*continued.*) B:** The palmar cutaneous branch of the median nerve emerges from the volar-radial aspect of the median nerve approximately 5.4 cm proximal to the wrist crease and travels distally with the median nerve for 2.5 cm. It enters the palm in the superficial volar layer of adipose tissue in the interval between the tendons of palmaris longus and flexor carpi radialis.

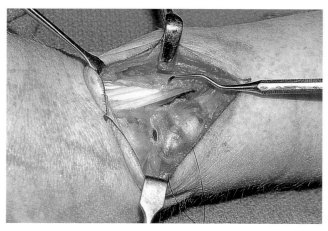

**FIGURE 12.** In this case, the extensor retinaculum has been incised longitudinally over the fourth dorsal compartment, exposing the tendons of the extensor digitorum communis and extensor indicis proprius. The probe is pointing to the dorsal aspect of the extensor retinaculum.

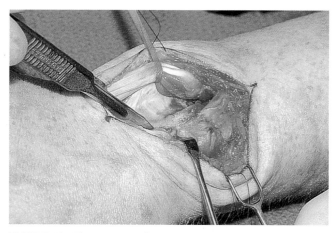

**FIGURE 13.** The extensor digitorum communis tendons and the extensor indicis proprius tendon are retracted ulnarly with a moistened umbilical tape, exposing the infratendinous retinaculum. The distal radial metaphysis is exposed, subperiosteally dissecting the infratendinous retinaculum and periosteum as one continuous layer.

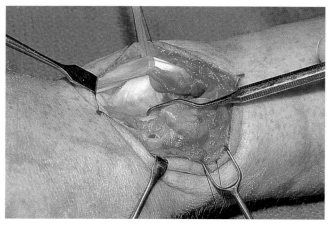

**FIGURE 14.** After dissection of the distal radius, the dorsal radiocarpal ligament is exposed distally. It is demonstrated here under the anatomy probe.

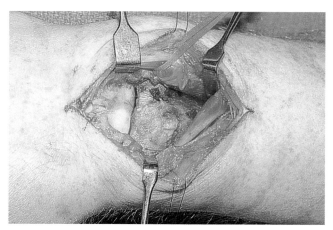

**FIGURE 15.** A longitudinal incision through the dorsal radiocarpal ligament exposes the proximal carpal row, the radiocarpal joint, and the distal radius.

Continue dissection subperiosteally to expose the distal radius radially as far as the tip of the radial styloid, and ulnarly to the dorsal capsule of the distal radioulnar joint. Preserve the dorsal distal radioulnar ligaments to prevent subsequent instability. Incise the dorsal capsule longitudinally over the carpal bones to elevate full-thickness capsular flaps medially and laterally. Take care to avoid injury to the dorsal aspects of the scapholunate and lunotriquetral interosseous ligaments during the elevation of the dorsal capsular flaps. Identify the extensor carpi radialis tendon distally as it sits on the dorsal proximal base of the long-finger metacarpal, and retract it radially with the capsular flap. Do not detach it from its insertion (Figs. 16, 17).

On completion of the surgical procedure, close the wound in anatomical layers. Close the dorsal wrist joint capsule with 2–0 braided nonabsorbable suture material, using interrupted figure-of-eight sutures. The extensor pollicis longus tendon is not replaced within its sheath and lies transposed radially deep to the subcutaneous tissue. In our experience, this situation does not lead to postoperative loss of thumb extension. Close the subcutaneous tissue with 4–0 absorbable suture and the skin with interrupted horizontal mattress sutures of 4–0 or 5–0 monofilament (Figs. 18, 19).

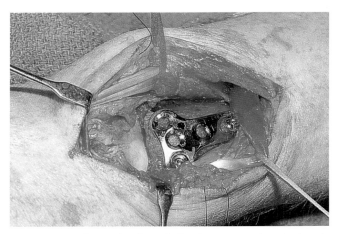

**FIGURE 16.** After reduction of the fracture, a dorsal plate is applied. The extensor pollicis longus tendon is retracted radially, whereas the extensor digitorum communis tendons and extensor indicis proprius tendon are retracted ulnarly.

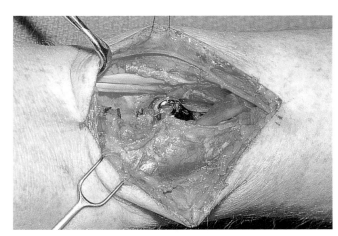

**FIGURE 17.** The dorsal radiocarpal ligament and infratendinous retinaculum are repaired with interrupted, nonabsorbable braided suture.

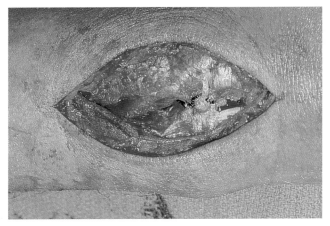

**FIGURE 18.** The dorsal aspect of the retinaculum is closed with interrupted sutures, incorporating the tendons of the extensor digitorum communis and extensor pollicis longus.

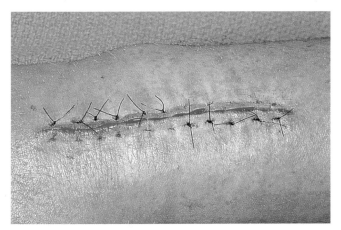

**FIGURE 19.** Horizontal mattress sutures have been used to close the skin because significant swelling is anticipated.

Extensor tenosynovectomy or tendon reconstruction requires entry into the fourth compartment. To isolate proximal and distal retinacular flaps, make transverse incisions along the distal and proximal borders of the extensor retinaculum, taking care not to damage the tendons underneath. Carry out exposure of the digital extensor tendons by elevating the distal portion of the extensor retinaculum as a radially based flap and the proximal portion as an ulnarly based flap. This technique facilitates retinacular closure when tenosynovectomy or tendon reconstruction is completed. If a smooth gliding surface must be restored deep to the extensor tendons, one flap of the extensor retinaculum may be passed deep to the tendons during closure (Figs. 20–27).

Procedures limited to the triangular fibrocartilage complex (TFCC) or the distal radioulnar joint should be approached through the floor of the fifth compartment; such techniques include TFCC repair or reconstruction and resection arthroplasty of the distal ulna. The dorsal approach offers visualization of the dorsal half of the ulnar head, the ulnocarpal joint, the entire TFCC, and the distal radioulnar joint.

Identify, preserve, and retract the dorsal cutaneous branch of the ulnar nerve in the distal portion of the incision. If an additional variable branch of the dorsal sensory branch of the ulnar nerve at the level of the distal radioulnar joint is present, take care not to transect it and thereby risk subsequent formation of a neuroma.

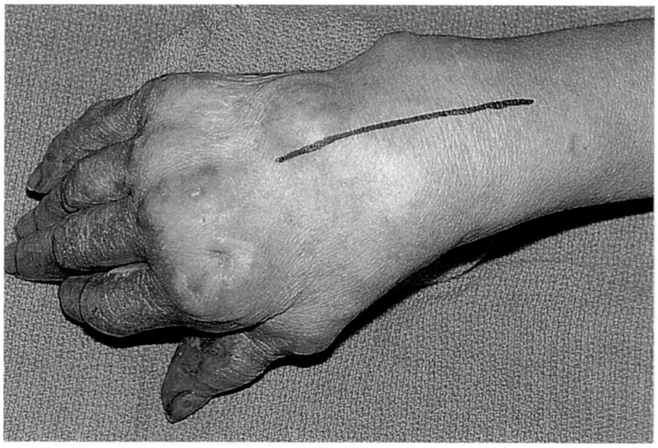

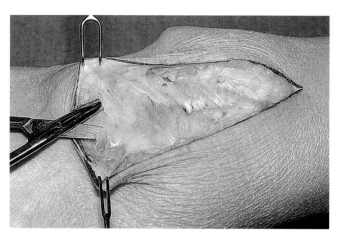

**FIGURE 20.** The skin incision for the dorsal longitudinal approach is centered over the fourth dorsal compartment. It extends from the midmetacarpal level distally and to the radial metaphysis proximally.

**FIGURE 21.** The subcutaneous tissue is spread bluntly with tenotomy scissors, exposing the dorsal aspect of the extensor retinaculum. When the extensor tendons are severely involved with inflammatory synovium, the extensor retinaculum is frequently covered with inflammatory tissue, and it may be difficult to discern from the surrounding tissue.

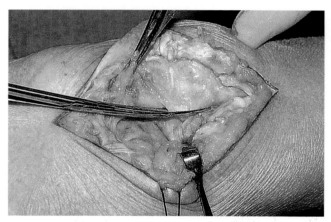

**FIGURE 22.** A straight incision is made through the extensor retinaculum using blunt tenotomy scissors to avoid injury to the underlying extensor tendons.

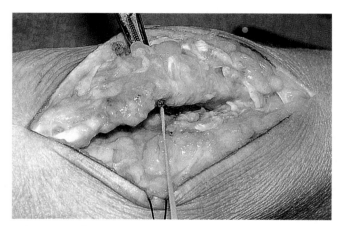

**FIGURE 23.** The extensor tendons are isolated and retracted with a moistened umbilical tape.

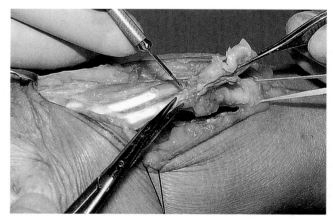

**FIGURE 24.** Using tenotomy scissors or a scalpel blade, the synovium is dissected from the extensor tendons. The synovium is firmly adherent to the tendons and must be removed sharply.

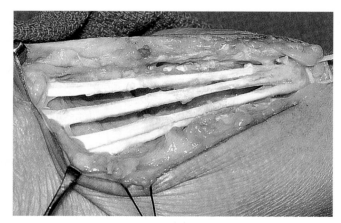

**FIGURE 25.** The synovium must be excised completely from the edge of the synovial sheath distally to the musculotendinous junction proximally.

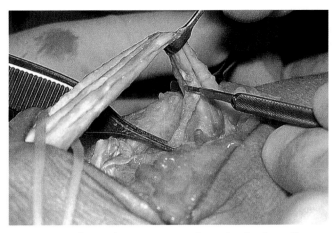

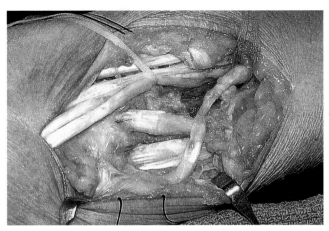

**FIGURE 26.** The palmar tenosynovium is firmly adherent between the extensor tendons and the dorsal wrist joint capsule. With severe inflammatory disease, the synovium of the wrist joint may be contiguous with that of the extensor tendons.

**FIGURE 27.** Following complete synovectomy, the tendons of the extensor digiti minimi, extensor digitorum communis, extensor indicis, proprius, extensor pollicis, longus, extensor carpi radialis brevis, and extensor carpi radialis longus are clearly identifiable.

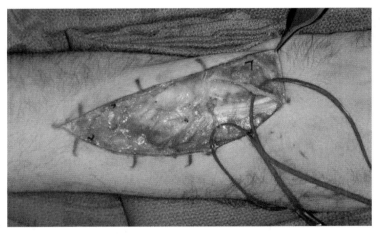

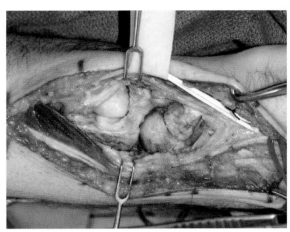

A                                                                                                          B

**FIGURE 28. A:** This figure shows the initial longitudinal dorsal approach with skin incision overlying the fifth dorsal extensor compartment and the distal radioulnar joint (DRUJ), illustrating the isolation of the two branches of the dorsal cutaneous branch of the ulnar nerve (the main branch traveling distally and the side branch to the skin overlying the DRUJ). **B:** A longitudinal incision over the fifth dorsal compartment and DRUJ is made, followed by the immediate identification of the dorsal cutaneous branch of the ulnar nerve located over the ulnar carpus (held by orange vessel loop). The tendon of EDQ is identified and retracted ulnarly (held by a Penrose drain). The dorsal capsule is lifted off the dorsal triangular fibrocartilage and is retraced ulnarly (capsule held by the double-prong skin hook overlying the Penrose drain). The dorsal radio-ulnar ligament and the triangular fibrocartilage may be seen clearly after DRUJ and ulnocarpal arthrotomies are completed. In this photograph, the LT ligament has been resected and the lunate and triquetral articular surfaces prepared for arthrodesis.

Sharply incise the retinaculum overlying the fifth dorsal compartment. Retract the extensor digiti quinti tendon radially. Raise an ulnarly based capsular flap off the distal ulna. Take care not to separate the TFCC or the dorsal radioulnar ligaments from the attachment to the dorsal aspect of the distal radius, as the undersurface of the TFCC is approached from below.

Expose the ulnocarpal joint by a direct longitudinal incision extending proximally from the lunotriquetral joint, and visualize the superficial aspect of the TFCC. Separate the ulnar-based flap of tissue from the dorsal TFCC by scalpel dissection (Fig. 28).

On completion of the surgical procedure, close the wound in anatomical layers. Close the dorsal capsule using 2–0 braided nonabsorbable suture material and figure-of-eight sutures. The extensor digiti minimi tendon is not replaced within its sheath and lies superficially within the subcutaneous tissue. In our experience, this arrangement does not lead to postoperative loss of small-finger extension. Close the subcutaneous tissue with 4–0 absorbable suture and the skin with interrupted horizontal mattress sutures of 4–0 or 5–0 monofilament nylon.

## PALMAR APPROACH TO THE WRIST

Palmar approaches to the wrist are used for treatment of distal radius and scaphoid fractures, malunions or nonunions, and decompression of the carpal tunnel and Guyon's canal. They are also useful in the harvesting of distal radius cancellous bone graft, ligamentous reconstruction of the carpus, drainage of wrist joint infections that have ruptured into Parona's quadrilateral space, flexor tenosynovectomy, and silhouette capsulectomy of the distal radioulnar joint.

Several approaches to the volar aspect of the wrist are available to carry out these procedures. Each is designed to allow for both direct and extensile exposure of the desired structures, as well as to minimize risk of injury to adjacent neurovascular structures. The radial artery, volar carpal branch of the radial artery, median nerve, palmar cutaneous branch of the median nerve, and ulnar nerve and artery are at risk of injury in carrying out volar surgical approaches to the wrist. It is important for the surgeon to have a firm grasp of the anatomic locations and courses of these structures for safe, efficient dissection and exposure. The surgeon must also understand the anatomic constraints for potential extension of a given exposure.

### Palmar-Radial Approach to the Distal Radius

The palmar-radial approach may be used to treat the entire distal radius, the radiocarpal joint, and the scaphoid. We have found it most valuable in the treatment of distal radius fractures with palmar comminution or subluxation of the carpus, for osteotomy of the distal radius (such as for Madelung's deformity), and for the harvest of distal radius bone graft. The approach is extensile distally to expose the scaphoid and proximally to expose the entire radius, the radial artery, the median nerve, and the flexor muscles of the forearm. It should not extend so far distally that it exposes the median nerve in the carpal tunnel, because the subcutaneous position of the palmar cutaneous branch of the median nerve limits exposure to the ulnar border of the flexor carpi radialis tendon. The palmar cutaneous branch of the median nerve reaches the undersurface of the antebrachial fascia approximately 1 to 2 cm proximal to the transverse carpal ligament, in the interval between the tendons of the flexor carpi radialis and palmaris longus. From that point it travels distally to innervate the skin over the thenar eminence.

Make the incision from the distal transverse wrist crease distally to the region over the flexor carpi radialis tendon proximally (Fig. 29). Spread the subcutaneous tissue bluntly to expose the flexor carpi radialis tendon sheath and incise the sheath longitudinally directly over the tendon (Fig. 30). Retract the tendon radially to expose the deep aspect of the flexor carpi radialis tendon sheath. It is prudent at this point to identify the radial artery and its two venae comitantes, which lie in the soft tissue directly radial to the tendon sheath (Figs. 31, 32).

Once the vascular structures are identified and protected, incise the tendon sheath sharply. This sheath lies directly over the flexor digitorum superficialis tendon to the index finger, which is retracted ulnarly. Identify the flexor pollicis longus tendon in the deep portion of the wound and retract it radially to expose the insertion of the pronator quadratus muscle on the distal radius (Fig. 33). Incise the insertion sharply from distal to proximal, leaving a 5-mm cuff of muscle and investing fascia for subsequent repair (Fig. 34). Reflect the pronator quadratus muscle subperiosteally from the distal radius, thus exposing the entire distal radial epiphysis, metaphysis, and distal diaphysis (Figs. 35, 36).

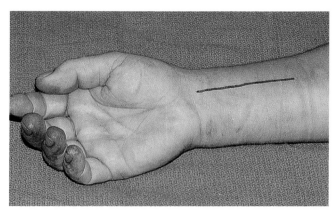

**FIGURE 29.** A longitudinal palmar approach provides excellent exposure of the distal radius for fixation of distal radius fractures or radial osteotomy, and for harvesting distal radial bone graft. The incision begins at the junction of the distal transverse wrist crease and flexor carpi radialis tendon and extends proximally along the radial shaft.

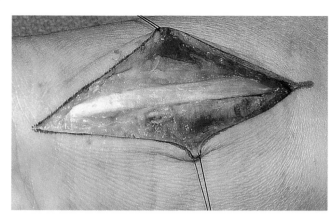

**FIGURE 30.** The subcutaneous tissue is spread bluntly directly over the flexor carpi radialis tendon. The tendon sheath is incised longitudinally.

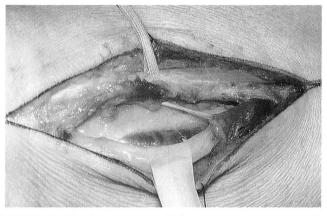

**FIGURE 31.** The flexor carpi radialis tendon is retracted radially with a moistened umbilical tape, and the median nerve and palmar cutaneous branch are identified in the ulnar portion of the incision. A soft rubber drain is placed around the median nerve to protect it from injury during the operative procedure.

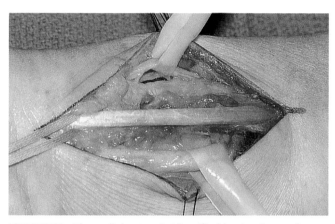

**FIGURE 32.** The radial artery is identified in the deep subcutaneous tissue on the radial side of the flexor carpi radialis tendon. It should be retracted with a soft rubber drain. A longitudinal incision in the dorsal aspect of the flexor carpi radialis tendon sheath exposes the flexor pollicis longus tendon.

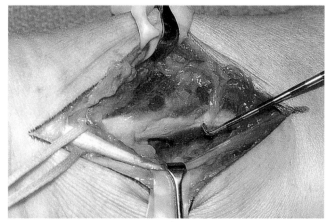

**FIGURE 33.** The flexor pollicis longus tendon is bluntly dissected and separated from the flexor digitorum superficialis tendons ulnarly.

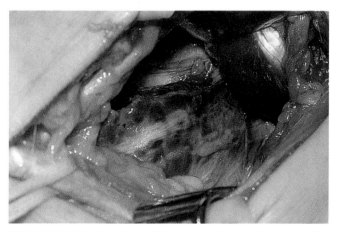

**FIGURE 34.** The insertion of the pronator quadratus on the distal radius is identified and incised longitudinally 5 mm from its insertion on the lateral edge of the distal radial metaphysis. The pronator quadratus is then dissected from the distal radius subperiosteally, reflecting it ulnarly.

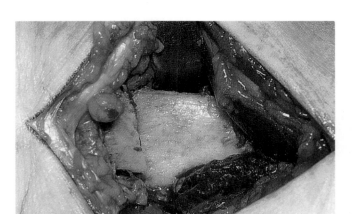

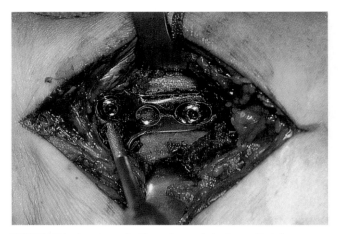

**FIGURE 35.** The distal radial fracture is isolated and the fragments reduced. Blood clots and bone debris must be removed for accurate fracture reduction.

**FIGURE 36.** A palmar buttress-type plate is applied for secure fracture reduction. The plate is held with cortical bone screws proximally in the diaphysis and cancellous bone screws in the metaphysis and epiphysis.

Following treatment of the fracture or osteotomy, or harvesting of the bone graft, repair the pronator quadratus back to its tendinous insertion, using interrupted 2–0 absorbable suture. Repair the dorsal sheath of the flexor carpi radialis tendon using 2–0 absorbable suture, but leave the palmar sheath open. The tourniquet may be deflated prior to wound closure to assess the flow in the radial artery and to ensure adequate hemostasis. Close the subcutaneous tissue with 4–0 absorbable suture, and the skin with interrupted horizontal mattress sutures of 4–0 or 5–0 monofilament.

### Palmar Approach to the Scaphoid

The palmar approach to the scaphoid is ideal for the treatment of nonunions, malunions, and acute fractures without associated intercarpal ligament tears. Anatomically, the waist of the scaphoid lies at the junction of the flexor carpi radialis tendon and the proximal transverse wrist crease.

Start the incision radially at the base of the thumb metacarpal, and extend it proximally to the junction of the distal transverse wrist crease and the flexor carpi radialis tendon. Continue the incision proximally over the flexor carpi radialis tendon (Fig. 37). Raise a laterally based skin flap and place a skin retraction suture through the apex of the flap. Identify the radial artery proximal in the wound and dissect it distally. Incise the flexor carpi radialis tendon sheath proximally (Fig. 38).

In the distal portion of the incision, the flexor carpi radialis tendon passes through a tunnel adjacent to the trapezium. Incise the fibrous roof of this tunnel longitudinally, using a scalpel. Retract the tendon ulnarly to expose the palmar carpal ligaments. The palmar branch of the radial artery is routinely found in this portion of the incision, and may be safely ligated.

Make a straight longitudinal incision through the palmar radiocarpal ligaments and the wrist capsule. Raise full-thickness radial and ulnar capsular flaps by incising Sharpey's fibers from their attachments to the scaphoid and the capsular attachments to the distal radius. Elevate the proximal radial aspect of the thenar musculature to further expose the wrist capsule overlying the scaphoid and trapezium. To expose the scaphotrapezial joint, perform a transverse capsulotomy at the distal margin of the capsular incision at the distal pole of the scaphoid. Wrist extension and ulnar deviation aid in visualization of the entire scaphoid. The exposure may be extended proximally to obtain bone graft from the distal radius (Figs. 39–43).

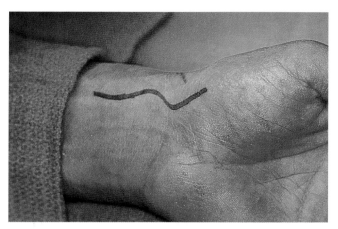

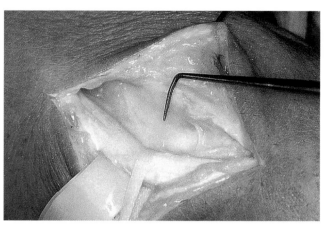

**FIGURE 37.** The palmar approach to the scaphoid is ideal for treating scaphoid fractures and scaphoid nonunions. Complete exposure of the palmar surface of the scaphoid is possible through this approach; it also exposes the distal radius for harvesting bone graft. A 5-cm curvilinear incision begins over the thenar eminence and extends proximally just radial to the flexor carpi radialis tendon. The incision is carried no farther medially than the flexor carpi radialis tendon to avoid injury to the palmar cutaneous branch of the median nerve, which courses in the interval between the palmaris longus and the flexor carpi radialis tendons.

**FIGURE 38.** The flexor carpi radialis tendon is isolated and tagged with an umbilical tape, and the sheath of the flexor carpi radialis is isolated. The waist of the scaphoid is located at the intersection of the proximal wrist crease and the flexor carpi radialis tendon.

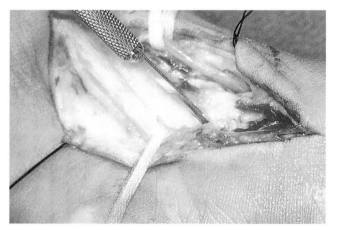

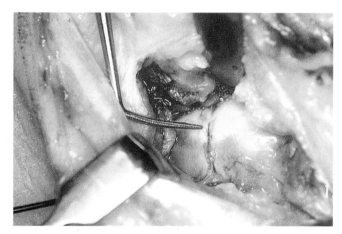

**FIGURE 39.** A sharp incision is made to bone through the floor of the carpi radialis tendon sheath, incising the palmar wrist capsule and ligaments.

**FIGURE 40.** The scaphoid fracture site is isolated and the scaphoid cleared radially and ulnarly of soft tissue.

Close the incision in anatomical layers. Repair the combined layer of palmar wrist capsule and palmar radiocarpal ligaments using figure-of-eight sutures of nonabsorbable 2–0 braided suture. Close the sheath of the flexor carpi radialis tendon dorsally using 2–0 absorbable suture. Close the subcutaneous tissue using 4–0 absorbable suture, and the skin using interrupted horizontal mattress sutures of 4–0 or 5–0 monofilament.

## Central Palmar Approach

The central palmar approach, most commonly used for release of the transverse carpal ligament, is useful for ligamentous reconstruction of the wrist joint, drainage of wrist joint infections that have ruptured into Parona's space, and flexor tendon tenosynovectomy. It is good for exposure of the palmar portion of the distal

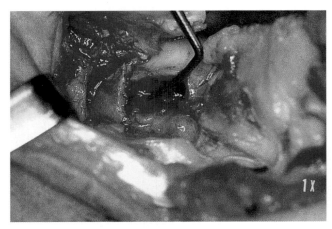

**FIGURE 41.** A 3 mm × 13 mm trough is created in the palmar surface of the scaphoid if a Russe graft is planned.

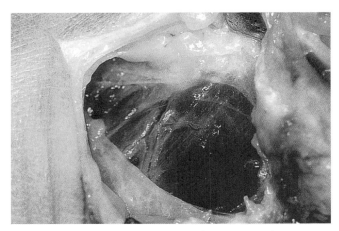

**FIGURE 42.** In the proximal portion of the incision, the pronator quadratus is isolated and incised sharply along its radial margin.

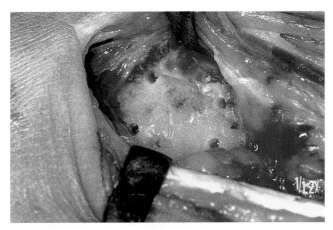

**FIGURE 43.** The pronator quadratus muscle is elevated ulnarly. The metaphysis of the distal radius is isolated and drill holes made, marking the site for later bone grafting.

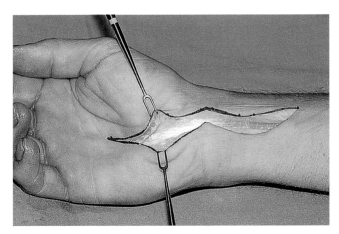

**FIGURE 44.** The extensile palmar approach to the wrist joint, palmar capsule and ligaments, and the carpal tunnel. The incision begins distally in line with the ring finger metacarpal, approximately 1 cm proximal to the distal palmar crease. The incision extends proximally parallel to the thenar crease. At the distal transverse wrist crease, the incision curves slightly radially and crosses the wrist crease obliquely. The incision extends proximally in the mid-third of the distal forearm. The subcutaneous tissue is spread bluntly to expose the palmar fascia and the palmaris longus tendon.

radioulnar joint and for direct visualization of distal radius fractures involving depression of the palmar lunate facet. It also is useful for the treatment of palmar dislocations of the carpus, in which the lunate is incarcerated within the carpal canal.

Start the incision distally at the junction of Kaplan's cardinal line, which is drawn by extending the line along the distal edge of the abducted thumb across to the hook of hamate and the axis of the ring finger ray, approximately 0.5 to 1 cm radial to the palpable hook of the hamate (Fig. 44). Extend it proximally parallel to the thenar crease, and curve it slightly radially as it approaches the distal transverse wrist crease. The incision does not cross the palmaris longus tendon; the palmar cutaneous branch of the median nerve lies subcutaneously immediately radial to the tendon.

Cross the distal wrist crease obliquely and then curve the incision ulnarly to create an ulnar-based flap. Extend the incision proximally for 3 to 4 cm and spread subcutaneous tissue bluntly, using tenotomy scissors. Retract the palmaris

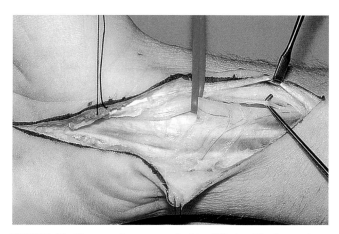

**FIGURE 45.** The median nerve is identified with the palmar cutaneous branch and protected with a rubber drain. The deep transverse carpal ligament is incised longitudinally, releasing the carpal tunnel.

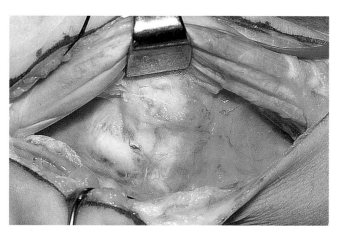

**FIGURE 46.** All of the flexor tendons are retracted radially, exposing the floor of the carpal tunnel, the palmar wrist capsule, and ligaments.

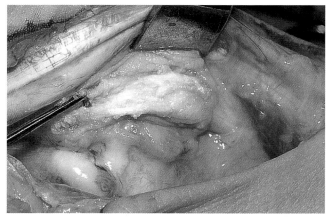

**FIGURE 47.** In this patient with a chronic palmar dislocation of the lunate, erosion of the flexor digitorum profundus tendon of the index finger is demonstrated.

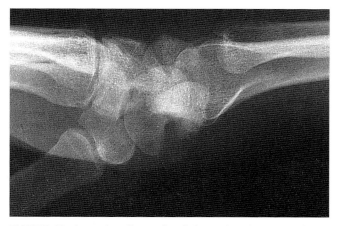

**FIGURE 48.** Lateral radiograph of the wrist, demonstrating a palmer dislocation of the lunate.

longus tendon radially to expose the distal palmar antebrachial fascia, and incise the fascia longitudinally to expose the flexor digitorum superficialis tendons.

Expose the median nerve in the proximal portion of the incision as it emerges from deep to the flexor digitorum superficialis tendon to the third finger. Identify the palmar cutaneous branch of the median nerve and protect it as it separates from the palmar ulnar aspect of the median nerve, approximately 5 to 6 cm proximal to the proximal transverse wrist crease. It travels with the median nerve for a variable distance to emerge subcutaneously between the flexor carpi radialis and palmaris longus tendons at the proximal transverse wrist crease (Fig. 45).

Incise the fibers of the palmar fascia sharply, and identify the superficial palmar vascular arch distally beneath the palmar fascia. Identify the proximal and distal aspects of the transverse carpal ligament and divide them under direct vision. Radially retract all the flexor tendons and the median nerve to expose the floor of the carpal tunnel and the tenosynovial tissue overlying the palmar carpal ligaments (Fig. 46). Make a longitudinal incision if needed, from the capitate to the distal radius, to expose the palmar aspect of the radiocarpal and midcarpal joints (Figs. 47, 48). Repair the capsule using figure-of-eight sutures of nonabsorbable 2–0 braided suture. Close the subcutaneous tissue with 4–0 absorbable suture, and the skin with interrupted horizontal mattress sutures of 4–0 or 5–0 monofilament.

## DIRECT ULNAR APPROACH

Direct ulnar approaches may be used for treatment of fractures or nonunions of the ulnar styloid. The Darrach distal ulnar resection also has been described through this exposure. Visualization beyond the ulnar aspect of the ulna is limited; volar or dorsal extensile approaches are more suitable for visualization of the distal radioulnar joint, TFCC, ulnar carpus, or the ulnar neurovascular bundle. Because the dorsal sensory branch of the ulnar nerve is vulnerable to injury during subcutaneous dissection, identification and protection of this nerve are recommended as the first steps in this approach.

Either a transverse or a longitudinal incision may be used. Center the transverse incision over the midportion of the ulnar styloid, and extend it from the dorsal to the palmar midaxial portions of the ulna. Spread subcutaneous tissue bluntly, and identify, protect, and retract the dorsal cutaneous branch of the ulnar nerve palmarward. Use blunt dissection to expose the ulnar styloid deep to the subcutaneous tissue. If fixation is to be attempted, carry out exposure of the base of the styloid and cancellous surface on the distal ulna so that fixation by tension band wire or screw may proceed. If excision of the styloid fragment is carried out, suture the ulnar aspect of the TFCC to the ulnar aspect of the distal ulna using nonabsorbable suture.

## DIRECT LATERAL APPROACH

The direct lateral approach may be used for the treatment of radial styloid fractures and for radial styloidectomy. This approach allows excellent visualization of the radial styloid, but because of the proximity of the superficial branch of the radial nerve, the radial artery, and the tendons of the first dorsal compartment at this level, exposure should be performed with caution.

Make a 3-cm transverse incision centered over the midaxial radial line, directly over the styloid process of the radius. Spread the subcutaneous tissue gently; identify branches of the superficial radial nerve and protect them by gentle retraction. Release the abductor pollicis longus and extensor pollicis brevis tendons by longitudinal incision over the dorsal aspect of the first dorsal compartment and retract them palmarly. Following excision or fixation of the radial styloid, return the tendons of the first dorsal compartment to their anatomic position. Close the skin using nonabsorbable monofilament suture.

## RECOMMENDED READING

1. Auerbach, D., Collins, E., et al.: The radial sensory nerve: an anatomic study. *Clin. Orthop.*, 308: 241–249, 1994.
2. Axelrod, T.: A prospective randomized trial of external fixation and plaster cast immobilization in the treatment of distal radial fractures. *J. Orthop. Trauma*, 5(1): 114–115, 1991.
3. Botte, M., Cohen, M., et al.: Dorsal branch of the ulnar nerve: an anatomic study. *J. Hand Surg.*, 15A(2): 603–607, 1990.
4. Catalano, L., Cole, R., et al.: Displaced intra-articular fractures of the distal aspect of the radius. Long-term results in young adults after open reduction and internal fixation. *J. Bone Joint Surg.*, 79A(9): 1290–1302, 1997.
5. Dellon, A., Mackinnon, S.: Susceptibility of the superficial sensory branch of the radial nerve to form painful neuromas. *J. Hand Surg. [Br]*, 9(1): 42–45, 1984.
6. Lourie, G., King, J., et al.: The transverse radioulnar branch from the dorsal sensory ulnar nerve: its clinical and anatomical significance further defined. *J. Hand Surg.*, 19(2): 241–245, 1994.
7. Mackinnon, S., Dellon, A.: The overlap pattern of the lateral antebrachial cutaneous nerve and the superficial branch of the radial nerve. *J. Hand Surg.*, 10(4): 522–526, 1985.
8. Matloub, H., Yan, J., et al.: The detailed anatomy of the palmar cutaneous nerves and its clinical implications. *J. Hand Surg. [Br]*, 23(3): 373–379, 1998.

# PART II

# Arthroscopy

# Diagnostic and Operative Arthroscopy

Felix H. Savoie III and Larry D. Field

Arthroscopy of the wrist has rapidly obtained acceptance, although its widespread use is a relatively recent phenomenon. Diagnostic and operative arthroscopy has advanced our knowledge of the anatomy and function of the wrist. It has also facilitated anatomically specific repair of previously unrecognized pathology.

## INDICATIONS/CONTRAINDICATIONS

Patients with wrist pain have a variety of symptoms, which generally are either mechanical or dystrophic. Mechanical symptoms include snapping, locking, crepitation, or grinding, as well as activity-related pain that decreases with rest. Mechanical symptoms usually are related to an injury and often are due to problems with ligaments, bone, or cartilage. They often can be successfully managed with arthroscopy.

Patients with dystrophic symptoms have a constant burning pain that is exacerbated by any activity or contact and is associated with nonspecific, nonanatomical neurovascular changes. Wrist arthroscopy is not usually helpful for these patients except during diagnostic scopes for exclusionary purposes.

Many patients have both mechanical and dystrophic symptoms. The examining physician must determine which category, or blend of categories, fits the patient's symptoms, and decide whether arthroscopy is indicated for that patient.

## PREOPERATIVE PLANNING

Begin by taking a meticulous history to focus on the etiology and on examination of findings related to pathology. It is especially important to note functional loss, the patient's ability to perform activities of daily living, and activities that exacerbate or lessen the problem.

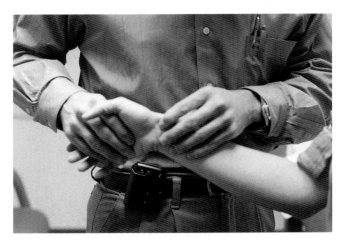

**FIGURE 1.** Watson's maneuver brings the wrist from ulnar to radial deviation with pressure over the tubercle of the scaphoid. If the scapholunate ligament is disrupted, pressure on the tubercle in ulnar deviation with the scaphoid dorsiflexed does not allow palmar flexion of the scaphoid with radial deviation and causes subluxation of the scaphoid dorsally out of the scaphoid fossa of the radius.

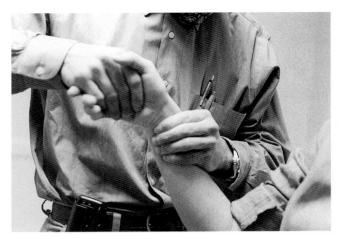

**FIGURE 2.** In the triangular fibrocartilage complex grind test, movement from flexion pronation to extension supination with ulnar deviation causes maximal stress to the ulnar side of the wrist, especially the triangular fibrocartilage and lunotriquetral ligament.

Physical examination is also important, including inspection, palpation, balloting, shifting, and grind tests such as a triangular fibrocartilage complex (TFCC) grind test. General areas of swelling, tenderness, or pain can lead the examiner to specific pathologic entities. Mechanical problems in the radioscapholunate area cause pain and swelling over the radiocarpal joint and often are associated with limitations of flexion and extension. Scapholunate ballottement, the Watson's test for scapholunate instability, and radiocarpal grind test are useful examinations in this area (Fig. 1).

Ulnar-sided pathology often manifests as an irritation or tendinitis of the extensor carpi ulnaris (ECU) or flexor carpi ulnaris tendons, with swelling along the ulnar side of the wrist. Pain with pronation and supination is common with ulnar-sided problems. Lunotriquetral ballottement, the TFCC grind test, and distal radial ulnar joint Shuck test in neutral, pronation, and supination may indicate pathology in this area (Fig. 2).

Midcarpal problems, such as instability and volar ganglion cysts, cause pain and swelling more distal in nature and located primarily over the triscaphe joint or ulnarly over the triquetral hamate articulation.

### Radiography

It is essential to take routine radiographs of all patients, including anteroposterior, lateral, and oblique views (Fig. 3). When indicated, pronation, supination, and posteroanterior radiographs, six-view motion studies with or without clinch view, and stress radiographs may be helpful.

### Specific Tests

Occasionally, the diagnosis remains unclear even after adequate history, physical examination, and routine radiographic studies have been completed. Such cases may warrant further diagnostic studies. Of the many different studies available, technetium bone scan, arthrograms, digital subtraction arthrograms, computed tomography arthrograms, magnetic resonance imaging scans, and magnetic resonance arthrograms are all useful in different cases. However, the most defini-

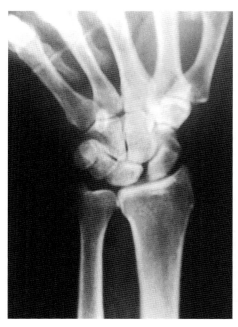
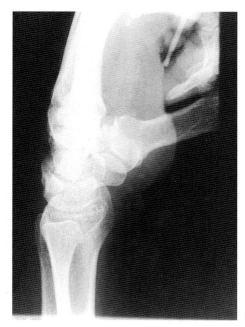

A                                                                              B

**FIGURE 3. A:** A standard anteroposterior radiograph of the wrist. **B:** A standard lateral radiograph of the wrist.

tive study available for diagnosing wrist pathology seems to be the magnetic resonance arthrogram, with a midcarpal injection followed by a distal radial ulnar joint injection (Fig. 4).

## SURGERY

Proper equipment, which is essential for accuracy of arthroscopy, begins with the basics: video arthroscope, shaver, TV monitor (with printer, to document the intraarticular findings), and hand-held instruments (Fig. 5). As arthroscopy has advanced, more specialized equipment has become available, allowing for more advanced surgical procedures. Advanced equipment, including TFCC repair kits, retrograde retrievers, ablation shrinkage devices, and fracture fixation systems, is necessary for advanced wrist arthroscopy procedures (Fig. 6).

### Portal Anatomy

Eleven access portals are currently used in the wrist. Radiocarpal portals include the 3–4, 4–5, 6R, 6U, and 1–2 portals. Midcarpal portals include the midcarpal radial (MCR), midcarpal ulnar, triquetral hamate, and triscaphe portals. Distal radioulnar joint portals include the proximal and distal radioulnar joint portals (Fig. 7).

**3–4 Portal.** The 3–4 portal is bordered on the radial side by the extensor pollicis longus and the extensor carpi radialis brevis, on the ulnar side by the extensor digitorum communis, on the proximal side by the distal radius, and on the distal side by the scapholunate ligament. The 3–4 portal is established 1 cm distal to Lister's tubercle. Its site is located by palpating the distal edge of the radius between the ulnar border of the extensor carpi radialis brevis and the radial margin of the common extensors.

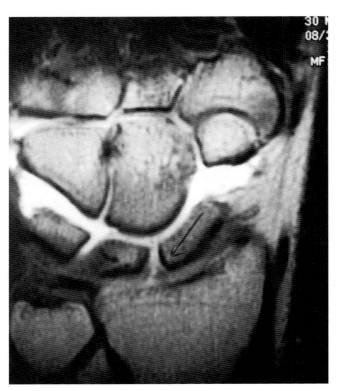

**FIGURE 4.** In this magnetic resonance arthrogram of the wrist, the dye was injected into the radiocarpal joint but also can be seen in the distal radioulnar and midcarpal joints (*arrow*), which suggests pathology in the triangular fibrocartilage and the interosseous ligaments.

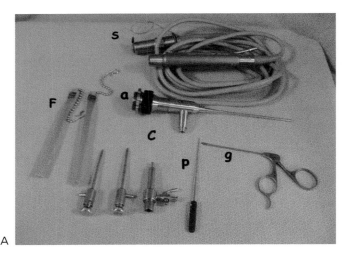

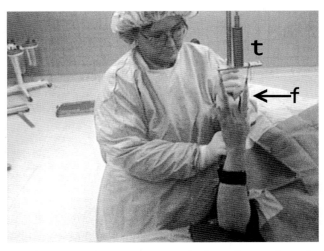

A                                                                                              B

**FIGURE 5. A:** Basic equipment used for wrist arthroscopy. **B:** More basic equipment for wrist arthroscopy. a, arthroscope and camera; c, cannula system; f, finger traps; g, grasper; p, probe; s, shaver and blades; t, traction tower.

**4–5 Portal.** The 4–5 portal is bordered on the radial side by the common extensors, on the ulnar side by the extensors, on the ulnar side by the extensor digiti minimi, on the proximal side by the attachment of the radius and the triangular fibrocartilage, and on the distal side by the lunate. This portal is established 1 cm directly ulnar to the 3–4 portal.

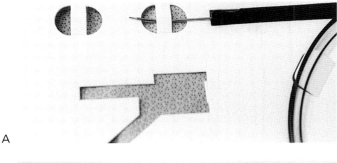

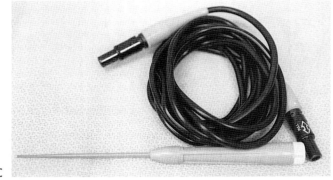

A

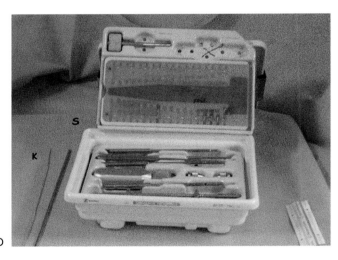

C

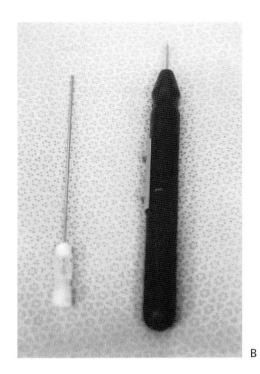

B

**FIGURE 6.** Equipment needed for an advanced arthroscopy includes: **(A)** laser; **(B)** triangular fibrocartilage complex repair kit; **(C)** radio-frequency probe; **(D)** wires (k) and Herbert-Whipple set (s).

D

**6R Portal.** The 6R portal is bordered radially by the extensor digiti quinti, ulnarly by the ECU, proximally by the triangular fibrocartilage, and distally by the lunotriquetral joint.

**6U Portal.** The 6U portal is established volar to the ECU tendon. The skin incision may be placed as far volar as the dorsal border of the ECU tendon. The portal enters the wrist joint distal to the TFCC, dorsal ulnar to the ulnotriquetral ligament and through the prestyloid recess.

**1–2 Portal.** The 1–2 portal can be established between the first and second extensor compartments 1 to 2 mm distal to the ulnar styloid.

**Midcarpal Radial Portal.** The MCR portal is bordered radially by the extensor carpi radialis brevis, ulnarly by the common extensors, proximally by the scapholunate ligament, and distally by the capitate. It should be established in alignment with the radial border of the third metacarpal, 1 cm distal to the 3–4 portal.

**Midcarpal Ulnar Portal.** The midcarpal ulnar portal is bordered radially by the common extensors, ulnarly by the extensor digiti quinti, proximally by the luno-

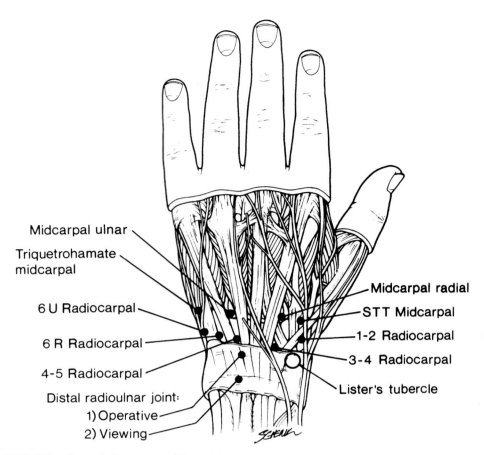

**FIGURE 7.** The portal anatomy of the wrist.

triquetral joint, and distally by the capitate hamate joint. It is in line with the center of the fourth metacarpal.

**Triquetrohamate Portal.** The triquetrohamate portal is established on the ulnar side of the wrist distal to the triquetrum and ulnar to the midcarpal ulnar portal. The extensor digiti quinti borders it on the radial side and the end of the ECU on its ulnar side.

**Triscaphe Portal.** The triscaphe portal is established radial to the extensor pollicis longus (EPL) distal to the distal pole of the scaphoid.

**Distal Radioulnar Joint Portal.** The distal radioulnar joint (DRUJ) is entered from a proximal portal at the base of the DRUJ. It is bounded by the radius and ulna. The distal DRUJ portal is placed in the same line, just proximal to the TFCC.

### Technique of Diagnostic Wrist Arthroscopy

Diagnostic wrist arthroscopy begins with a 3–4 portal. Palpation and testing of this portal with a spinal needle are essential. We do not usually inflate the joint before beginning this procedure because of the risk of altering the intraarticular anatomy.

Use only *blunt* trocars in establishing portals. Once a 3–4 portal is established, perform a diagnostic radiocarpal arthroscopy. First examine the radial styloid and radial capsule (Fig. 8). Examine the proximal borders of the scaphoid and distal border of the radial scaphoid facet, then examine the radio-

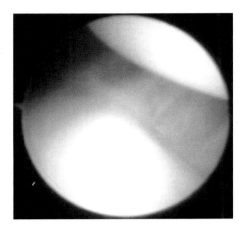

**FIGURE 8.** An arthroscopic view of the radial styloid and radial wrist capsule.

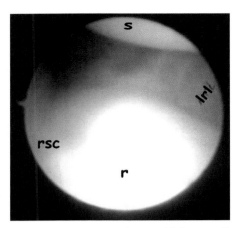

**FIGURE 9.** A 3–4 portal view. lrl, long radiolunate ligament; r, radius; rsc, radio scaphocapitate; s, scaphoid.

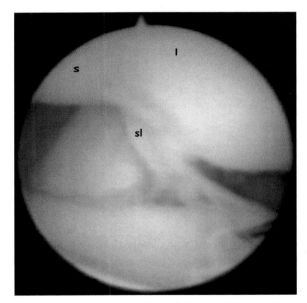

**FIGURE 10.** A 3–4 portal view of the scapholunate ligament indicates the scaphoid, lunate, and scapholunate ligaments. l, lunate; s, scaphoid; sl, scapholunate.

scaphocapitate and long radiolunate ligaments (Fig. 9). Evaluate the scapholunate interosseous ligament and the proximal surface of the lunate and the distal surface of the radius (Fig. 10). Evaluate the radial attachment of the triangle fibrocartilage and the volar and dorsal radioulnar ligaments (Fig. 11). Examine the ulnolunate and ulnotriquetral ligaments, as well as the lunotriquetral interosseous ligament, the prestyloid recess, and the peripheral attachment of the TFCC (Fig. 12).

Use the MCR portal to establish a diagnostic arthroscopy portal here. The scoping in this area begins at the scapholunate joint, which should be perfectly congruous (Fig. 13). Evaluate the distal surface of the lunate and the triquetrum, as well as the concave proximal surface of the hamate (Fig. 14). Evaluate the capitate in the capitohamate articulation distally to the triscaphe joint (Fig. 15) and the distal portals of the scaphoid in the proximal surface of the trapezium and trapezoid (Fig. 16). On completion of the diagnostic midcarpal arthroscopy, establish a proximal DRUJ portal and evaluate the ulnar surface of the radius, the radial

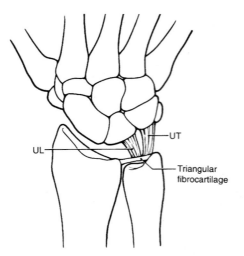

**FIGURE 11.** The triangular fibrocartilage complex. UL, ulnolunate; UT, ulnotriquetral.

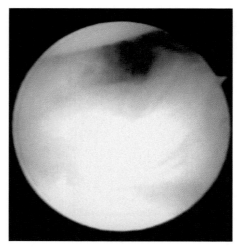

**FIGURE 12.** The peripheral aspect of the wrist.

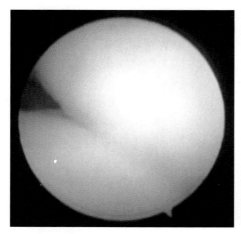

**FIGURE 13.** A midcarpal view of the scapholunate articulation.

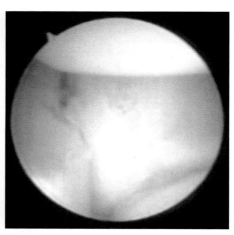

**FIGURE 14.** A midcarpal view of the lunotriquetral articulation.

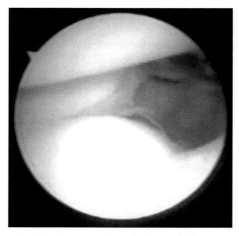

**FIGURE 15.** A midcarpal view of the capitolunate articulation.

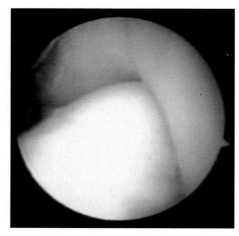

**FIGURE 16.** A midcarpal view of the triscaphe joint.

surface of the ulna, and the distal surface of the ulnar head, as well as the proximal surface of TFCC.

## ARTHROSCOPIC PROCEDURES

Arthroscopic procedures in the wrist may be divided into three major groups. The first group includes débridement and resection procedures, the second includes repairs, and the third includes fusions. Débridement resection procedures include débridement of the TFCC central disc, radial styloid resection, ulnar head resection, distal radial ulnar joint resection, resection of the dorsal ganglion, and resection of the volar ganglia. Repair procedures include peripheral TFCC repair, lunotriquetral plication, DRUJ stabilization with volar and dorsal capsular plication, scapholunate repair with pinning, ulnar capsular plication for midcarpal instability, and fracture fixation (including radius and scaphoid fractures). Fusion procedures include radiocarpal fusion and intercarpal fusion procedures.

### Group One: Resection

Resection of central perforations in the TFCC may be accomplished using a knife, burr, or thermal ablation device such as a laser or radiofrequency probe. The arthroscope is left in the 3–4 portal, and the 4–5 and 6U portals are used for instrument access. The central area is resected until a smooth rim remains. The dorsal or volar radioulnar ligament should not be penetrated, or instability will occur (Fig. 17).

The radial styloid may be resected arthroscopically by using a 1–2 radiocarpal portal. Leave the arthroscope in the 3–4 portal, and place the burr in the 1–2 portal, using it to resect the tip of the styloid. The bone may be resected until the radial attachment of the radio scaphocapitate ligament is encountered (Fig. 18).

The distal ulna and ulnar portions of the DRUJ may be resected. In cases in which the TFCC is torn, introduce the burr via the 6U portal and resect the ulnar by dorsal to volar planing. If necessary, this planing can continue through the defect until the entire distal ulna is resected (except for the styloid and ulnar cortex). Normally a 3- to

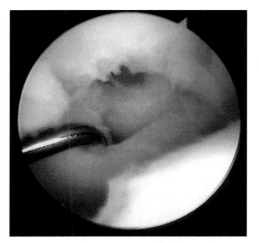

**FIGURE 17.** A central disc perforation of the triangular fibrocartilage complex is shown.

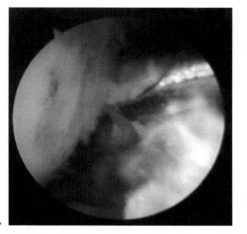
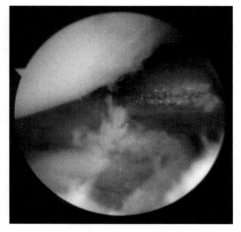

A                                                                                                B

**FIGURE 18.** Before **(A)** and after **(B)** an arthroscopic resection of the radial styloid.

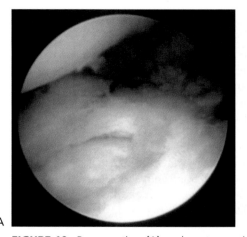
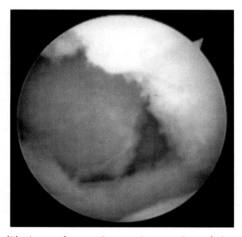

A                                                                                                B

**FIGURE 19.** Pre-resection **(A)** and post-resection **(B)** views of an arthroscopic resection of the distal ulna.

6-mm gap between the radius and ulna is sufficient to eliminate DRUJ impingement. In cases with an intact TFCC, resection is accomplished by introducing the arthroscope through a proximal DRUJ portal; insert the burr distally. Resection then occurs via medial-lateral planing (Fig. 19).

Both dorsal and volar ganglion may be resected using arthroscopic techniques. Osterman has pioneered the technique for dorsal ganglion excision. In these cases, introduce the arthroscope into the wrist via a 4–5 or 6R portal. Identify the scapholunate articulation and "track" it dorsally to the attachment of the capsule. The origin of the dorsal ganglion and the stalk arising from it can be seen at this location. Establish a 3–4 portal through the ganglion, and ablate the "bleb" of origin and stalk. A small hole is resected in the capsule and the walls of the cyst are resected as well (Fig. 20).

In resection of a volar ganglion, place the arthroscope in the MCR portal and the shaver in the triscaphe portal. The origin of the cyst, readily visualized, can be resected. Next, place a blunt probe through this site and out of the volar aspect of the wrist, penetrating the cyst. Introduce the shaver cannula and shaver into the wrist over this blunt probe, and resect the cyst. It is essential to be aware of the location of the radial nerve and artery during the procedure, and convert to open excision if the anatomy is distorted (Fig. 21).

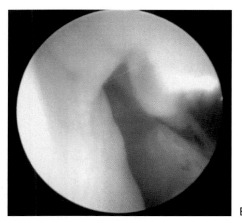

A                                                                                        B

**FIGURE 20.** Pre-resection **(A)** and post-resection **(B)** views of an arthroscopic resection of a dorsal ganglion. b, bleb; c, cyst; sl, scapholunate ligament.

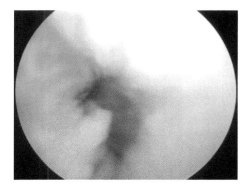

**FIGURE 21.** The origin of a volar ganglion.

### Group Two: Repairs

Repair of peripheral TFCC tear represents one of the most rewarding uses of arthroscopic wrist surgery. Visualize the tear with the scope in the 3–4 portal. Place instruments through the 6U and 6R portals. Place an 18-gauge spinal needle through the most volar aspect of the tear. Place a #2.0 PDS suture through the needle into the joints using a wire retriever or grasper. Retrieve the suture out of the 6R portal. This process continues until three or four sutures are placed. The sutures are then retrieved *under* the ECU tendon and tied over the capsule (Fig. 22).

Lunotriquetral instability may be repaired via arthroscopic techniques. Once the instability has been confined, introduce an 18-gauge spinal needle via a volar 6U portal across the volar aspect of both the ulnotriquetral and ulnolunate ligaments. Pass a suture through the spinal needle and hold it while the needle is removed. Then retrieve it back out of the 6U portal, creating a "lasso" and pulling together the ulnolunate and ulnotriquetral ligaments. Place a second suture in a similar fashion 3 to 4 mm distal to the first and, if necessary, followed by a third distal to the second. Use the last stitch to plicate the ulnar capsule. Then place the arthroscope into the metacarpal (MC) joint and place two K-wires across the L-T articulation (Fig. 23).

DRUJ stabilization is accomplished by combining the techniques for TFCC and L-T repairs. Arthroscopic pinning of S-L tears remains controversial. It is best used in conjunction with thermal tightening for dynamic instability and for acute

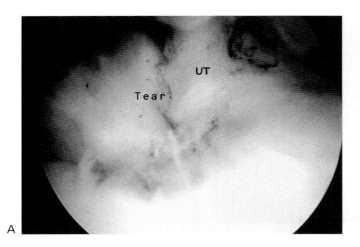

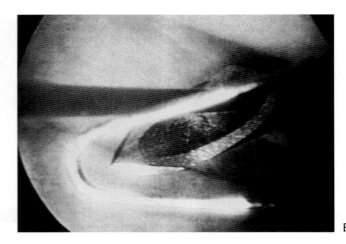

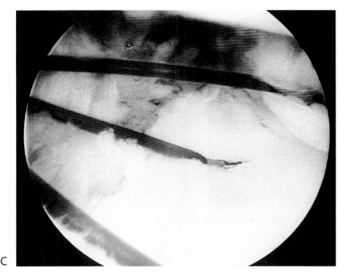

**FIGURE 22.** An arthroscopic triangular fibrocartilage complex repair is indicated in these figures. The figures show **(A)** tear, **(B)** suture placement, and **(C)** repaired lesion. UT, ulnotriquetral.

S-L tears. In chronic tears, it has not been useful except as a supplement to other repair techniques. In these instabilities, lightly abrade the opposing surfaces at the scaphoid and lunate. Preserve and tighten any remaining ligament using the thermal technique. Then place the arthroscope in the midcarpal ulnar portal and establish an MCR portal. A blunt probe or trocar often is sufficient to reduce the scaphoid to the lunate. Otherwise, a joystick wire may be placed into the scaphoid; use it to pull it out of volar flexion and reduce it to the dorsiflexed lunate. Then place K-wires across the scaphoid into the lunate. Both the reduction and the pin placement are monitored via fluoroscopy as well as with the arthroscope (Fig. 23).

Distal radius fracture fixation has been well described. Débride the joint of loose fragments and hematoma. Reduce the fragments using a combination of probes and joystick wires. Place K-wires into each, stabilizing the fracture (Fig. 24).

### Group Three: Arthrodesis

Arthroscopic arthrodesis may be accomplished in any area of the wrist. The basic principle is to abrade the opposing surfaces, then compress them. Finally, place cannulated screws across the area to be fused (Figs. 25, 26).

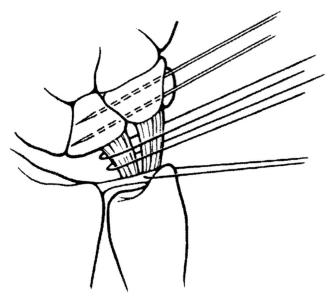

**FIGURE 23.** L-T plication is used as an arthroscopic technique to repair lunotriquetral instability.

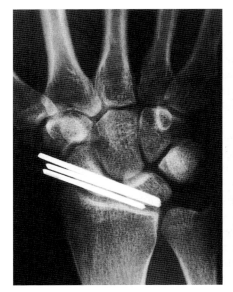

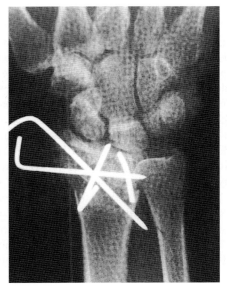

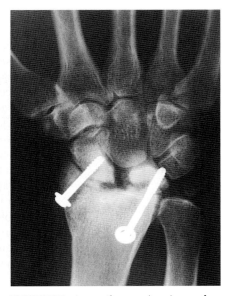

**FIGURE 24.** A radiograph of pins that lie across the S-L joint.

**FIGURE 25.** An arthroscopic fixation of a distal radial fracture.

**FIGURE 26.** An arthroscopic view of a radio scapholunate arthrodesis performed arthroscopically.

## POSTOPERATIVE TREATMENT

In all débridement and resection procedures, use a compressive wrap in the postoperative phase. Start range-of-motion exercises immediately and initiate other exercises 1 week after surgery. If necessary, start formal physical therapy 3 to 4 weeks out. Normal use is allowed as pain and strength dictate.

In repair procedures, we favor the use of a Muenster cast for approximately 6 weeks (Fig. 27). Place the wrist in slight dorsiflexion and neutral pronation/supination. This cast prevents pronation/supination of the forearm. Approximately 4 weeks after surgery, switch to a removable Muenster splint and start gentle range-

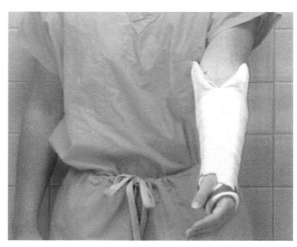

**FIGURE 27.** The Muenster cast for postoperative immobilization after reconstructive wrist surgery.

of-motion exercises. Discontinue use of the splint and begin other exercises in the sixth to eighth postoperative week. Full recovery takes 3 to 9 months.

## COMPLICATIONS

Excessive extravasation of fluid may occur in recently injured patients with torn capsules, or if the inflow cannula is placed extraarticularly. If extravasation occurs, it is recognized and the causative factor addressed, or the arthroscopic portion of the procedure is stopped. Even with significant extravasation of fluid, nothing more than elevating the extremity is necessary for correction; excessive pressure diminishes quickly when the inflow is halted.

Postoperative infection is extremely uncommon. If there is any evidence of superficial infection, broad-spectrum antibiotics are usually sufficient. If a deep intraarticular infection develops, irrigation, arthroscopic débridement, and intravenous antibiotic therapy are the best treatments.

For the patient who has dystrophic problems as well as intraarticular mechanical problems, we recommend treating the dystrophy first. Once the dystrophy has improved as much as can be expected, the mechanical problems can be addressed. Often the dystrophy is caused by a mechanical problem, and will become less bothersome for the patient when a smoothly functioning joint is restored.

Dystrophic problems are the most difficult cases to treat, and the results are guarded at best. Reflex sympathetic dystrophy may occur with irritation of the sensory branches of the dorsal aspect of the wrist. The most problematic areas are (a) between the first and second extensor compartments, with irritation of the dorsal sensory branch of the radial nerve, and (b) in the 6U portal, lying ulnar to the ECU, with irritation of the dorsal sensory branch of the ulnar nerve. If sutures need to be passed through either of these areas, we recommend a longitudinal incision with dissection down to the capsule, followed by separation and retraction of the subcutaneous tissue and the sensory nerves. This procedure diminishes the chances of nerve injury and subsequent dystrophy.

## ACKNOWLEDGMENTS

The authors gratefully acknowledge the contributions of G. G. Poehling, S. J. Chabon, and D. B. Siegel, who wrote the previous version of this chapter.

## RECOMMENDED READING

1. Blanchard, J., Ramamurthy, S., Walsh, N., Hoffman, J., Schoenfeld, L.: Intravenous regional sympatholysis: a double-blind comparison of guanethidine, reserpine, and normal saline. *J. Pain Sympt. Manag.*, 5: 357–361, 1990.

2. Brody, A.S., Ball, W.S., Towbin, R.B.: Computed arthrotomography as an adjunct to pediatric arthrography. *Radiology*, 170: 99–102, 1989.

3. Davis, K.D., Treede, R.D., Raja, S.N., Meyer, R.A., Campbell, J.N.: Topical application of clonidine relieves hyperalgesia in patients with sympathetically maintained pain. *Pain*, 47: 309–317, 1991.

4. Doi, K., Hattori, Y., Otsuka, K., Abe, Y., Yamamoto, H.: Intra-articular fractures of the distal aspect of the radius: arthroscopically assisted reduction compared with open reduction and internal fixation. *J. Bone Joint Surg.*, 8(1A): 1093–1102, 1999.

5. Duncan, K.H., Lewis, R.C. Jr., Racz, G., Nordyke, M.D.: Treatment of upper extremity reflex sympathetic dystrophy with joint stiffness using sympatholytic Bier blocks and manipulation. *Orthopedics*, 11: 883–886, 1988.

6. Gennant, H.K., Kozin, F., Bekerman, C., McCarty, D.J., Sims, J.: The reflex sympathetic dystrophy syndrome: a comprehensive analysis using fine-detail radiography, photon absorptiometry, and bone and joint scintigraphy. *Radiology*, 117: 21–32, 1975.

7. Ghostine, S.Y., Comair, Y.G., Turner, D.M., Kassell, N.F., Azar, C.G.: Phenoxybenzamine in the treatment of causalgia: report of 40 cases. *J. Neurosurg.*, 60: 1263–1268, 1984.

8. Hobelmann, C.F. Jr., Dellon, A.L.: Use of prolonged sympathetic blockade as an adjunct to surgery in the patient with sympathetic maintained pain. *Microsurgery*, 10: 151–153, 1989.

9. Koman, L.A., Mooney, J.F. III, Poehling, G.G.: Fractures and ligamentous injuries of the wrist. *Hand Clin.*, 6(3): 477–491, 1990.

10. Koman, L.A., Poehling, G.G.: Reflex sympathetic dystrophy, chap. 102. In: *Operative Nerve Repair and Reconstruction*, vol 2, edited by R.H. Gelberman, J.B. Lippincott, Philadelphia, pp. 1497–1523, 1991.

11. Koman, L.A., Poehling, G.G., Toby, E.B.: Chronic wrist pain: indications for wrist arthroscopy. *Arthroscopy*, 6: 116–119, 1990.

12. Mooney, J.F., Poehling, G.G.: Disruption of the ulnolunate ligament as a cause of chronic ulnar wrist pain. *J. Hand Surg.*, 16A: 347–349, 1991.

13. North, E.R., Meyer, S.: Wrist injuries: correlation of clinical and arthroscopic findings. *J. Hand Surg.*, 15A: 915–920, 1990.

14. Poehling, G.G., Roth, J., Wipple, T., et al.: Arthroscopic surgery of the wrist information manual, 1990.

15. Reinus, W.R., Hardy, D.C., Totty, W.G., Gilula, L.A.: Arthrographic evaluation of the carpal triangular fibrocartilage complex. *J. Hand Surg.*, 12A: 495–503, 1987.

16. Roth, J.H., Poehling, G.G., Whipple, T.L.: Hand instrumentation for small joint arthroscopy. *Arthroscopy*, 4: 125–128, 1988.

17. Tham, S., Coleman, S., Gilpin, D.: An anterior portal for wrist arthroscopy. *J. Hand Surg.*, 24B: 445–447, 1999.

18. Whipple, T.L., Marotta, J.J., Powell, J.H. III.: Techniques of wrist arthroscopy. *Arthroscopy*, 2: 244–252, 1986.

19. Zinberg, E.M., Palmer, A.K., Coren, A.B., Levinsohn, E.M.: The triple-injection wrist arthrogram. *J. Hand Surg.*, 13A: 803–809, 1988.

20. Zlatkin, M.B., Chao, P.C., Osterman, A.L., Schnall, M.D., Dalinka, M.K., Kressel, H.Y.: Chronic wrist pain: evaluation with high-resolution MR imaging. *Radiology*, 17(3): 723–729, 1989.

# PART III

## Distal Radius Fractures

# 3

# External Fixation

Martin I. Boyer, Fraser J. Leversedge,
and Terry S. Axelrod

## INDICATIONS/CONTRAINDICATIONS

Despite recent advances in imaging, operative treatment, and understanding of the natural history of distal radius fractures, management of these injuries remains a difficult challenge. Understanding the configuration of the fracture is more important for the distal radius than perhaps for any other body site.

To proceed with individualized treatment, the surgeon must investigate the components of the fracture itself and the limb in which the fracture has occurred. The patient's physiologic age, occupational and athletic demands, and hand dominance may dictate how aggressive the attempt at surgical restoration of bony anatomy should be. Additionally, the presence of associated injuries, such as acute compartment syndrome or carpal tunnel syndrome and fractures or dislocations of the hand, forearm, elbow, or humerus may necessitate a different type of fixation than a distal radius fracture considered in isolation. Finally, the fracture anatomy itself—extraarticular or intraarticular, involving the radiocarpal joint or distal radioulnar joint, the degree of comminution of the dorsal or volar metaphysis or of the articular surface, and whether there is volar or dorsal carpal subluxation— dictates which form of fixation should be considered.

Treatment of any distal radius fracture should begin with an attempt at closed reduction. If a satisfactory reduction can be obtained (but not maintained) by closed means, then external skeletal fixation alone may be an appropriate technique for fracture treatment, without the need for supplementary fixation or bone grafting. The use of additional techniques of fracture reduction and stabilization may be of benefit in certain fracture patterns. These techniques include the use of percutaneous pins or screws, supplemental bone graft or bone graft substitutes, and internal fixation with concurrent external fixator application.

However, if satisfactory reduction cannot be obtained by closed means, external fixation alone is likely to be insufficient for fracture treatment. Active infection at the site of pin placement may contraindicate placement of an external fixator, although in the presence of an unstable distal radius fracture it may be the only option available to the surgeon.

In open fractures of the distal radius, external fixation may be indicated to facilitate wound care. Advanced physiologic age is, by itself, not a contraindication for external fixation.

## Preoperative Planning

The initial patient evaluation includes discerning the mechanism of injury and medical and surgical history, as well as the patient's current use of medications, specific medication allergies, and social history. The presence of sickle cell disease should be considered, as it is relevant to the management of the pneumatic tourniquet during the surgical procedure.

Physical examination focuses on the vascular status of the hand, the sensory and motor function of the median and ulnar nerves, and the presence or absence of open wounds. Examination of posteroanterior and lateral radiographs of the distal radius and the elbow is carried out to define fracture pattern and associated injuries. Occasionally, in the presence of highly comminuted fractures, computed tomography scans are useful for the definition of articular fragments.

## Surgery

A standard set of surgical instruments is required, in addition to a portable fluoroscopy device and a radiolucent hand table. The fixator device consists of 2.5-mm, 3.0-mm, and 4.0-mm partially threaded half-pins, pin-to-bar and bar-to-bar connector clamps, steel or graphite connecting bars between 60 and 200 mm in length, and rubber caps to cover the pin ends (Figs. 1, 2).

The approach to the shaft of the radius proximal to the fracture site is described in Chapter 1. Once the site is exposed, use a 2.0-mm drill bit with a soft-tissue protector to predrill both near and far cortices of the radius to accept the fixation pin (Figs. 3–7).

Drill both holes approximately 3 cm apart. Make the drill hole at an angle between 65° and 70° to the long axis of the radius. The pins are, therefore, ori-

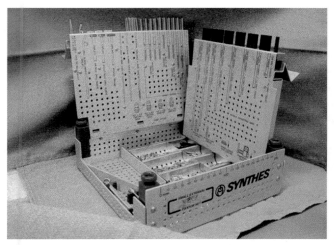

**FIGURE 1.** The small external fixator set (made by Synthes U.S.A, Monument, CO) is the set that is used commonly in our practice.

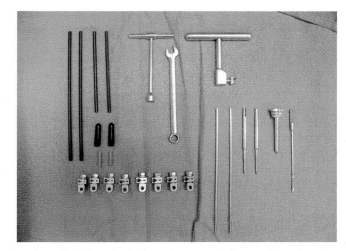

**FIGURE 2.** Before initiation of the surgical procedure, the necessary supplies should be arranged for easy access. Two long graphite bars and two short graphite bars, a closed and an open socket wrench, a T-handled wrench, two 2.5 and two 3.0 pins, in addition to a trocar, drill bit, and pin-bar and bar-bar couplers (two pin-bar and six bar-bar couplers) should be set up.

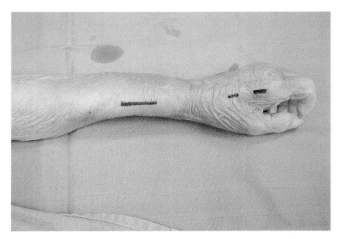

**FIGURE 3.** Incisions made for approach to the distal radial shaft and the second metacarpal.

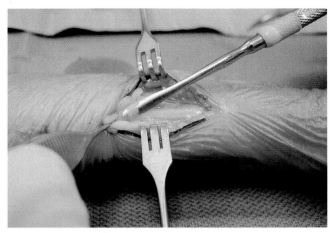

**FIGURE 4.** The dorsal sensory branch of the radial nerve is identified. The freer elevates a thin layer of fascia, which is directly divided under direct vision to expose the radial nerve.

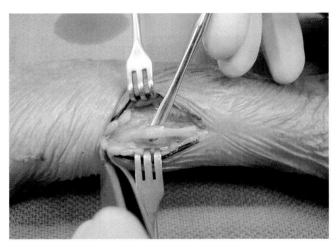

**FIGURE 5.** The sensory branch of the radial nerve.

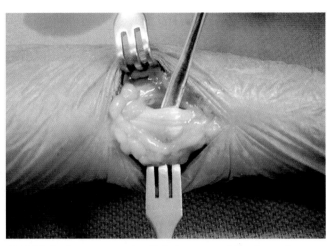

**FIGURE 6.** Extensor carpi radialis longus and brevis tendons are identified in the depth of the wound. Retraction allows for exposure of the radial shaft.

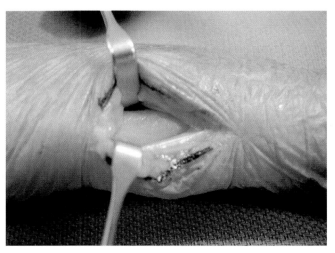

**FIGURE 7.** Exposure of the radial shaft.

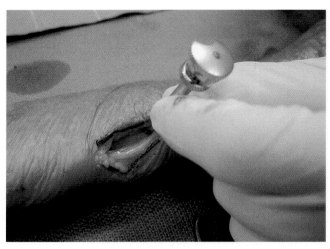

**FIGURE 8.** Placement of the trocar directly against the radial shaft while protecting the sensory branch of the radial nerve. The 2.0 drill bit is then used to drill both proximal and distal cortices of radius.

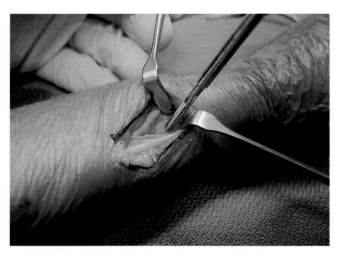

**FIGURE 9.** A 3.0 partially threaded pin is inserted into the radial shaft.

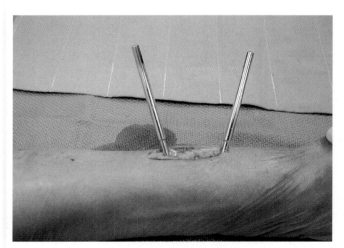

**FIGURE 10.** This is followed by insertion of the other 3.0mm pin at a 45° angle to the first. Pins engage both cortices.

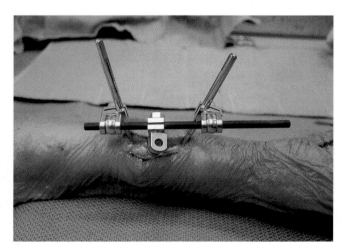

**FIGURE 11.** Assembly of the proximal portion of the external fixator apparatus, using three bar-bar clamps and a short graphite rod.

ented at approximately 45° with respect to one another, with their tips converging (Figs. 8–10).

Hand-drill a 2.5-mm partially threaded AO half-pin, or, in larger patients, a 3.0-mm partially threaded AO half-pin, into the radius to engage the far cortex. We reserve the 4.0-mm pins only for very large boned individuals; pins of this size rarely are necessary, and the chances of fracturing the radius with them are significant.

Place the second half-pin in a similar fashion, and close the wound with interrupted horizontal mattress sutures of 4–0-monofilament suture material. Confirm pin position by fluoroscopy. Place a connector bar joining the two half-pins such that it lies no more than 2 cm from the skin, with at least 3 cm of open bar extending past the distal half-pin. Place a bar-bar connecting coupler onto the connector bar between the couplers, attaching the bar to the two radial half-pins (Fig. 11).

Make one or two additional incisions over the dorsal-radial aspect of the second metacarpal as described in Chapter 1. In addition to clearing the peritendinous tis-

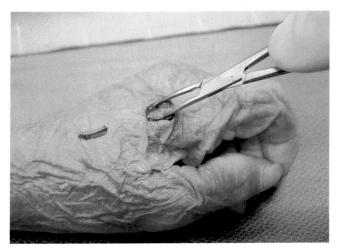

**FIGURE 12.** The incisions used for exposure of the second metacarpal.

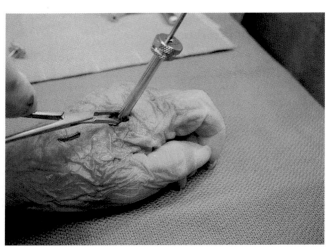

**FIGURE 13.** While protecting surrounding structures using a curved snap, the trocar and drill bit are placed and subsequently the index finger is flexed at the metacarpophalangeal joint to 90°.

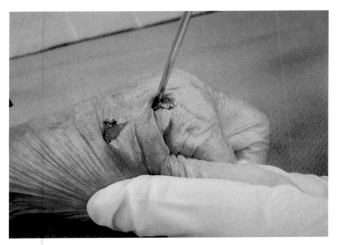

**FIGURE 14.** The 2.0-mm partially threaded pin is inserted.

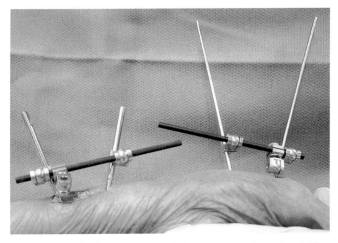

**FIGURE 15.** Final appearance of the metacarpal construct. The pins lie coplanar at 45° to one another. The construct consists of a short graphite bar, two pin-bar connectors, and one bar-bar connector.

sue and periosteum to expose the bone, hold the metacarpophalangeal joint of the index finger in flexion during insertion of the 2.5-mm AO partially threaded half-pin; this avoids a postoperative extension contracture due to tethering of the dorsal hood.

To add to the fixation in osteopenic individuals, it can be helpful to insert the proximal metacarpal pin more horizontally to engage the radial cortex of the base of the third metacarpal. Predrilling of the metacarpal is recommended as well, because sudden torque of the threaded pin within the metacarpal can cause a fracture that might necessitate placement of the fixation pins into the third metacarpal shaft (Figs. 12–14). Confirm pin position by fluoroscopy.

Place a connector bar joining the two half-pins so that it lies no more than 2 cm from the skin, with at least 3 cm of open bar extending proximal to the proximal half-pin. Place a bar-bar connecting coupler onto the connector bar between the couplers, joining the bar to the two metacarpal half-pins (Fig. 15).

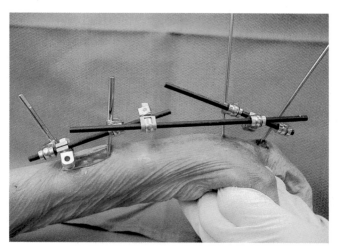

**FIGURE 16.** Closed reduction is performed. The long graphite rod is connected to the two short graphite rods as shown.

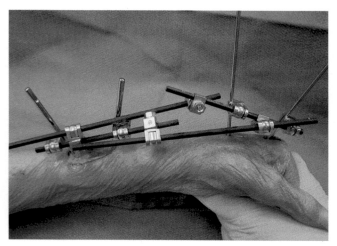

**FIGURE 17.** After tightening all connections and performing fluoroscopic examination of the reduction to check for restoration of radial tilt in the frontal and sagittal planes and for radial length, the second graphite rod is placed as shown. The radiograph is evaluated for radiocarpal and intercarpal distraction. If it is excessive, other modalities besides external fixation alone may be required.

Once the threaded half-pins have been positioned in the radius and metacarpal, couple a long connector bar loosely to the proximal portion of the connector bar joining the two metacarpal pins, and to the bar-bar coupler on the proximal connector bar situated between the two radial half-pins (Fig. 16). Carry out the closed reduction maneuver by longitudinal traction and manipulation of the hand and wrist into slight palmar flexion and ulnar deviation. Never use the fixator pins to exert additional manual distraction forces on the hand and wrist because of the risk of pullout or metacarpal fracture.

Once the reduction has been performed, tighten the proximal and distal bar-bar couplers. Carry out fluoroscopic examination of the fracture and confirm satisfactory reduction. Affix the second long connector bar using two bar-bar couplers to the distal portion of the short proximal connector bar, and the mid-portion of the distal short connector bar (Fig. 17). Tighten all couplers and cut and cap the pins.

Place heavy padding circumferentially around the frame to prevent sedated patients from injuring themselves. A plaster splint is not required. Take a final plain radiograph before the patient leaves the operating room. Evaluate fracture reduction in terms of radial length, inclination, and articular tilt, and note the amount of radiocarpal and midcarpal distraction; excessive traction has been associated with postoperative difficulty in regaining full digital flexion.

## Postoperative Management

Most patients return home the day of surgery. Have them begin immediate postoperative digital motion exercises with emphasis on metacarpophalangeal joint flexion to obviate extension contracture of these joints. Control edema by the use of elevation, ice, and circumferential wraps using compressive bandages. Encourage active, active-assisted, and passive digital motion.

Begin forearm pronation and supination at approximately 2 to 3 weeks postoperatively, and gradually increase them over time. Take radiographs weekly for the first 3 weeks after placement of the fixator, and prior to removal at 6 weeks. Tighten couplers at each postoperative clinic visit. We routinely dress all cutaneous pin sites with Betadine-soaked gauze; pin site care, however, is left to the discretion of the patient and surgeon.

External fixators are rarely left on longer than 6 weeks time, as wrist flexion-extension and radioulnar deviation motions are increasingly difficult to regain after this time period has elapsed. Splints are rarely required after fixator removal; most patients, however, benefit from outpatient therapy to regain wrist and forearm motion, especially extension and supination.

## Complications

Complications of external skeletal fixation of distal radius fractures may occur intraoperatively or perioperatively, or during the early or late postoperative periods. Perioperative complications include fracture of the metacarpal or shaft of the radius through a pin hole, possibly requiring immediate fixation of the radius or metacarpal and the use of different points of bony fixation, such as the third metacarpal shaft.

Traction injury to the superficial radial nerve in the proximal or the distal wounds, with associated hypoesthesia or paresthesia distally, requires early recognition. Excessive radiocarpal or intercarpal distraction diagnosed on placement of the fixator or during the immediate postoperative period necessitates release of the distraction force of the fixator; alternative or additional methods of fracture fixation may be required.

Early postoperative complications include pin site infections, loss of reduction, and pin breakage. Pin site infections are treated by local wound care, dressing changes, and oral antibiotics as long as the pin remains fixed solidly within the bone. Occasionally, intravenous antibiotics are required. Pin removal is rarely indicated; however, if a pin must be removed due to infection (or, if a pin breaks), the stability of the remaining fixator must be assessed and the need for placement of an additional threaded half-pin to maintain fracture reduction is evaluated.

If reduction is lost before 2 to 3 weeks have elapsed, consider remanipulation of the fracture under anesthesia. Late postoperative complications consist of digital stiffness (especially of the metacarpophalangeal joints), reflex sympathetic dystrophy and osteopenia secondary to over-distraction, adduction contracture of the thumb and first web space, and distal radioulnar joint volar capsular contracture. These sequelae necessitate sustained therapeutic intervention, and often require static and dynamic splinting and aggressive pain control measures, as well as tenolysis and capsulectomy to restore motion to hand, wrist, and forearm.

## RECOMMENDED READING

1. Ahlborg, H., Josefsson, P.: Pin-tract complications in external fixation of fractures of the distal radius. *Acta. Orthop. Scand.*, 70(2): 116–118, 1999.
2. Catalano, L., Cole, R., et al.: Displaced intra-articular fractures of the distal aspect of the radius. Long term results in young adults after open reduction and internal fixation. *J. Bone Joint Surg.*, 79A(9): 1290–1302, 1997.
3. Dunning, C., Bicknell, C.L., et al.: Supplemental pinning improves the stability of external fixation in distal radius fractures during simulated finger and forearm motion. *J. Hand Surg.*, 24A(5): 992–1000, 1999.
4. Goldfarb, C., Yin, Y., et al.: Wrist fractures: what the clinician wants to know. *Radiology*, 219(1): 11–28, 2001.
5. Herrera, M., Chapman, C., et al.: Treatment of unstable distal radius fractures with cancellous allograft and external fixation. *J. Hand Surg.*, 24A(6): 1269–1278, 1999.
6. Kaempffe, F.: External fixation for distal radius fractures: adverse effects of excess distraction. *Am. J. Orthop.*, 25(3): 205–209, 1996.

7. Trumble, T., Wagner, W., et al.: Intrafocal (Kapandji) pinning of distal radius fractures with and without external fixation. *J. Hand Surg.*, (3): 381–394, 1998

8. Vandersluis, R., Richards, R., et al.: Use of the external fixation apparatus for percutaneous insertion of pins in the distal one-third of the radius: an anatomic study. *Can. J. Surg.*, 36(6): 517–519, 1993.

9. Wolfe, S., Austin, G., et al.: A biomechanical comparison of different wrist external fixators with and without K-wire augmentation. *J. Hand Surg.*, 24A(3): 516–524, 1999.

# 4

# Open Reduction and Internal Fixation

Jesse B. Jupiter

## INDICATIONS/CONTRAINDICATIONS

The therapeutic approach to fractures of the distal end of the radius is still influenced today by the observations of Colles, who noted 178 years ago that "one consolation only remains, that the limb will at some remote period again enjoy perfect freedom in all its motions, and be completely exempt from pain; the deformity, however, will remain undiminished through life" (10). Although many still believe this to be the case, it has become increasingly apparent, particularly with those individuals who place a high demand on their wrists, that anatomy does correlate with function (7). This becomes of further importance when the fracture involves the radiocarpal articulation. It has become evident that articular fractures that unite with incongruity of 2 mm or greater will likely result in symptoms of pain, weakness, and radiographic evidence of posttraumatic arthrosis (6,8).

A number of treatment options have proved effective in the management of fractures of the distal radius. Whereas closed reduction and plaster immobilization remains the most common and appropriate method for so-called "stable fractures" or minimally displaced or impacted lesions, this is not the case with the unstable fracture patterns or fractures with associated soft tissue or ipsilateral skeletal injuries. Distal fractures associated with extreme initial displacement and comminution, either extraarticular or intraarticular or combined, do not do well with traditional methods of casting alone. If, however, acceptable metaphyseal or articular reduction is achieved following closed manipulation, the fracture can be effectively stabilized with "semi-constrained" methods such as percutaneous pins, external fixation, or pins and plaster techniques (13).

When, then, is operative treatment of the complex comminuted distal radius fracture appropriate? Operative exposure of the fracture becomes necessary if acceptable reduction cannot be achieved by closed means, or in those high-energy injuries in which extensive soft tissue or associated skeletal injury requires stable fixation of the distal radius (1–4,8,11,12). There are two basic types of fractures that ordinarily require open reduction and internal fixation. The first comprises the shearing fractures of the joint surface, which include Barton's, reverse Barton's, and radial styloid fractures (7,9). Although anatomical reduction can at times be achieved by closed means, these fractures are extremely unstable and represent radiocarpal fracture-dislocations. As these injuries often occur in younger adults with more substantial cortical and metaphyseal bone quality, buttress plate fixation is the approach of choice that will assure maintenance of the anatomic restoration.

The second group of fractures includes the compression fractures of the articular surface or combinations of injury patterns in which articular fragments are displaced, rotated, and not amenable to reduction even through a limited operative exposure (1–5,8,11,12).

Associated severe medical illnesses, patient unreliability, or a localized septic process would preclude a surgical approach to a distal radius fracture. In addition, massive soft tissue swelling, lack of basic equipment, or unfamiliarity with the surgical approaches would mandate a delay in a surgical treatment and call for either further reevaluation or additional expertise.

## PREOPERATIVE PLANNING

Decisions regarding the indications and surgical tactics for the operative treatment of comminuted fractures of the distal radius take into account the individual anatomy of the fracture, local factors such as the degree of soft tissue trauma or associated injuries, and specific patient considerations such as systemic injury or disease, reliability, and functional demands (7).

The complex radial fractures that tend to require operative intervention are often widely displaced on presentation. As such, routine radiographs or tomograms may be difficult to interpret. Longitudinal traction and temporary plaster splint support is recommended as an initial procedure in the emergency ward. At that point, anteroposterior, lateral, and oblique radiographs effectively reveal most extraarticular fracture patterns. Axial and coronal computed tomography, and, more recently, three-dimensional reconstructed tomography, are extremely important to define the specific nature of the articular disruption. The decision as to the specific surgical approach frequently will be dependent on the direction of displacement, which is often best revealed in the lateral tomogram.

Many complex articular fractures have the lunate facet of the distal radius disrupted by direct impaction of the lunate (Fig. 1). Restoration of this "medial complex" (as termed by Melone) is the foundation of any operative intervention (10) (Fig. 2). In my experience, the lateral tomogram reveals this injury most accurately. Although some have chosen computed axial tomography or even three-dimensional reconstructions from those studies, these more sophisticated studies are not necessary and are often more difficult to interpret.

With clear radiologic representation of the fracture pattern, the fracture is classified. This is critical not only to accurately reflect the morphologic complexity, but also the difficulty of treatment and prognosis. While a number of classifications have been developed, the most detailed to date has been the AO system, which is organized in order of increasing severity of the skeletal and articular lesions. The classification divides these fractures into extraarticular (type A), partial articular (type B), and complete articular (type C). Each type is subdivided into three subgroups; for example, simple articular and metaphyseal fractures ($C_1$), simple articular with complex metaphyseal ($C_2$), and complex articular and metaphyseal fractures ($C_3$). These in turn can be further subdivided by the complexity of the articular injury (10) (Fig. 3).

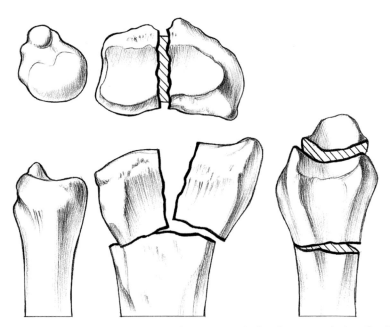

**FIGURE 1.** A common pattern of an intraarticular fracture of the distal radius involves the articular surface split into two major fragments.

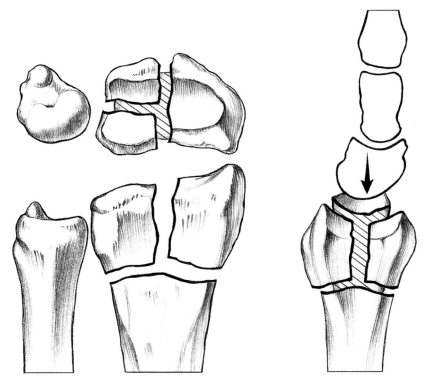

**FIGURE 2.** A four-part intraarticular distal radius fracture reflects the lunate into the lunate facet of the distal radius. The articular surface is split in both the coronal and sagittal planes (*arrow*).

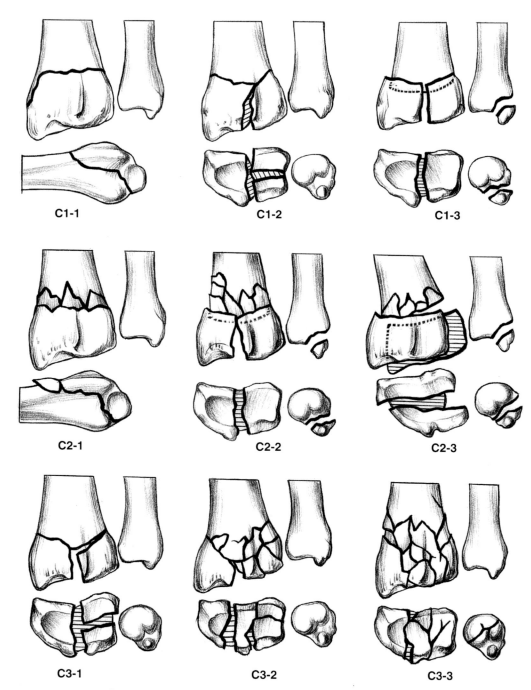

**FIGURE 3.** The AO classification of intraarticular fractures of the distal radius.

Finally, careful attention is paid to the carpal alignment, as many complex distal radial fractures have radiocarpal ligament injury.

Complex fractures often are associated with significant soft tissue trauma. Palmar compartment syndrome or dense median or ulnar sensory or motor deficit requires expeditious surgery. In the setting of soft tissue swelling alone it is advisable to allow for a few days of elevation to ultimately facilitate the operative approach and tension-free wound closure.

When faced with impacted subchondral metaphyseal bone or metaphyseal-diaphyseal comminution, one prepares for the possibility that autogenous cancellous graft will be required. Preoperative discussion, surgical consent, and appropriate anesthesia are required if iliac crest graft is utilized.

Although there has been little disagreement regarding the operative management of complex distal radius fractures in young adults, this approach has had a less enthusiastic following for patients who are older than 65 years of age or those with fewer demands on their wrists. It is important, however, to take a careful history of the patient's daily activity level, recreational interests, and lifestyle to carefully weigh the patient's needs on a physiological rather than chronological basis. By the same token, osteopenia and serious systemic medical conditions may argue against an enthusiastic operative approach.

## SURGERY

Axillary block or general anesthesia is ordinarily preferable, as the operative approach to these fractures can prove a lengthy and demanding procedure. As iliac crest bone graft may be needed, my preference has been for general anesthesia with sterile preparation of the iliac crest donor site.

The patient is placed in a supine position with the hand and arm on a hand table, preferably a radiolucent table capable of allowing fluoroscopic imaging. Provisional or definitive distraction with an external fixation device is extremely useful when approaching high-energy complex fractures. The extent of soft tissue trauma due to retraction or manipulation is minimized when this device is applied prior to the surgical incision. Additionally, in those fractures that are extremely comminuted or in osteopenic bone-negating stable fixation with plate and screws, the external fixation neutralizes the axial loading of the carpus in the reconstructed fracture. In those instances, intraoperative fluoroscopy with image intensifiers is useful at the onset of the procedure. Thus, preoperative notification of the radiology technician is extremely important.

### Technique

**Dorsal Approach.** The choice of surgical approach is dependent on type of fracture, direction of displacement, and associated soft tissue lesions (if any). Whereas many complex, dorsally displaced fractures can be managed by manipulative reduction, distraction fixation with an external fixation device, and percutaneous pinning and/or limited open reduction and articular elevation, shearing fracture-dislocations or complex dorsally displaced fractures seen after a few weeks require formal open reduction.

Under pneumatic tourniquet control, a straight longitudinal incision is marked out over the dorsal radius between the second and third dorsal extensor compartments, extending between 5 and 10 cm (Fig. 4). Care is taken to identify and preserve large dorsal veins rather than ligating or cauterizing them, which might subsequently add to the postoperative swelling (Fig. 5). The extensor retinaculum is opened between the second and third extensor compartments, with the extensor pollicis longus tendon mobilized proximally and distally to permit better access to the fracture site (Fig. 6). The fourth dorsal compartment is elevated subperiosteally, preserving the integrity of this compartment; this diminishes the problem of extensor tenosynovitis, which is often seen when the digital extensor tendons are left unprotected as they pass over a dorsal plate.

At this juncture, small Hohmann retractors are placed along the radial and ulnar margins of the radius and the fracture site identified and gently disimpacted with an elevator (Fig. 7). With displaced complex metaphyseal fractures or shearing dorsal fracture-dislocations, the dorsal wrist capsule can be preserved as the accuracy of the

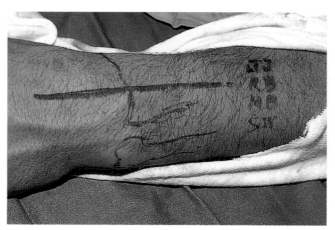

**FIGURE 4.** Mark out a straight longitudinal incision for a dorsal approach to the distal radius.

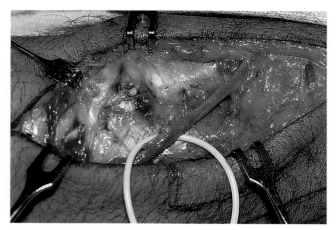

**FIGURE 5.** Large crossing veins are best identified and preserved rather than sacrificed.

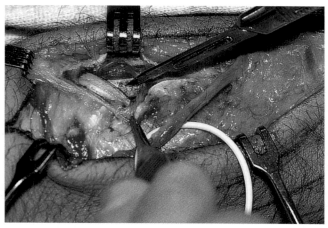

**FIGURE 6.** Open the extensor retinaculum between the second and third extensor compartments. Preserve the fourth compartment, elevating it in a subperiosteal fashion.

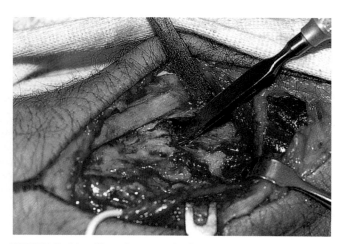

**FIGURE 7.** Identify and expose the fracture with small Hohmann retractors placed on either side of the distal radial shaft.

reduction is effectively judged by the interdigitation of the fracture lines and confirmed by radiographic control. In these instances, gentle fracture reduction is facilitated by the intraoperative placement of a small distractor. A 4.0-mm Schantz pin is drilled obliquely into the distal fragment and proximal radial diaphysis, and the distractor assembled on the pins (Fig. 8). Distraction is now performed by gently turning the distracting nut on the frame under direct vision until the fracture is disimpacted and the distal fragment brought out to length (Fig. 9). The distractor is then locked in place. This procedure must be performed slowly, and the distal pin in the cancellous metaphyseal bone monitored to avoid the pin "cutting" out of the bone. Grasping the radial diaphysis with a serrated bone-holding clamp is particularly helpful in assisting the reduction by applying direct countertraction, as the distal fragment and carpus require not only lengthening but also palmar displacement (Fig. 9).

With accurate reduction confirmed visually and radiographically, the stability of the reduction is assessed. If, in spite of the provisional hold of the distractor, it is unstable, a 0.062-in.-diameter smooth Kirschner wire is directed percutaneously from the tip of the radial styloid across the fracture site and into the cortex of the ulnar side of the radial diaphysis proximal to the fracture (Fig. 10). If a fracture gap is present at this juncture, autogenous iliac crest bone graft is harvested using trephines developed for iliac crest bone biopsy. This allows the graft to be obtained through small skin incisions with soft tissue dissection. The graft is compacted into the fracture gap.

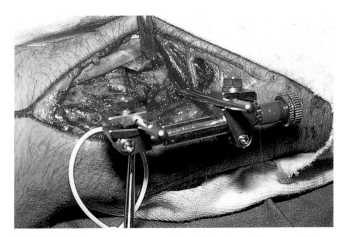

**FIGURE 8.** Place an intraoperative distractor with one 4.0-mm Schantz pin in the distal fragment and one in the radial diaphysis.

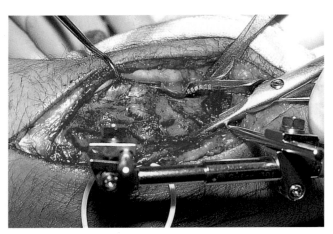

**FIGURE 9.** Under direct vision, disimpact the fracture and bring it to length with the distractor. Note the increased length between the Schantz pins. A serrated bone-holding clamp provides counter-traction on the proximal radius, while palmar reduction of the dorsally displaced distal fragment is manually accomplished.

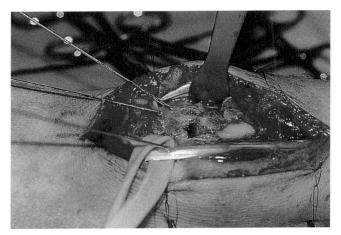

**FIGURE 10.** Provisional fixation can be achieved with Kirschner wires. Take care to place them from a distal direction to avoid interference with the placement of a plate. Note the defect that will be filled with autogenous iliac crest graft.

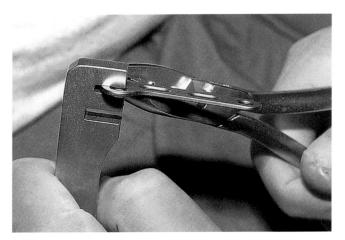

**FIGURE 11.** It is important to contour any implant to fit the anatomy of the dorsal aspect of the distal radius. Plate benders and pliers will effectively bend the tips of the titanium T plate.

Definitive fixation is achieved preferentially with an angled titanium T plate or a specially designed plate for the distal radius (the Pi plate). The radial and ulnar borders of the distal part of the plate are contoured to the dimensions of the distal radius (Fig. 11). This may also require removal of Lister's tubercle. Next, the plate is provisionally placed on the radius to assure its location both proximally and distally before screws are placed (Fig. 12).

Using a 2.5-mm drill bit and a 3.5-mm tap, the first screw is placed proximally but not completely tightened, to assure plate position. If acceptable, a 3.5-mm screw is placed through the middle hole of the distal T portion of the plate. In general, I do not tap the screw hole in metaphyseal bone. The remaining screws are placed and tightened, and intraoperative radiographs obtained to confirm both the fracture reduction and plate and screw placement. The distractor is now removed (Fig. 13).

In the case of complex impacted articular fragments, the dorsal wrist capsule is opened longitudinally and the fragments are reduced under direct vision and held with 0.035- or 0.045-in. Kirschner wires. Bone graft and plate fixation are accomplished as previously described. When using the Pi plate, the plate is contoured both proximally and distally; a plate cutter removes some unnecessary holes. Four

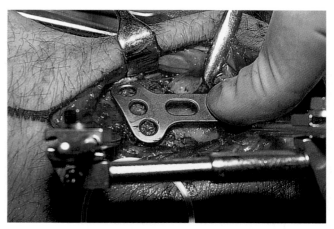

**FIGURE 12.** Place the plate provisionally on the distal radius by hand to ensure its location and contour.

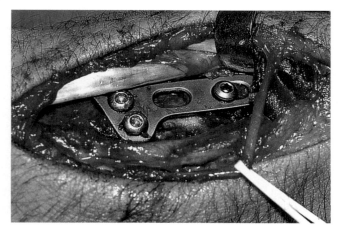

**FIGURE 13.** Secure the plate using 3.5-mm screws. Tap screw thread in the cortical diaphyseal bone but not in the distal metaphyseal fragment. The intraoperatively placed distractor can be removed at this point.

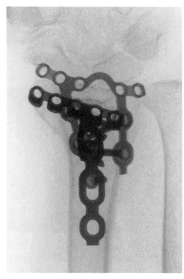

**FIGURE 14.** The Pi plate (Synthes, Paoli, PA) is one of a group of new plates designed specifically for application to the complex anatomy of the dorsal surface of the distal radius. Distally, the plate can be secured to the radius either with 2.4-mm screws or 1.8-mm smooth bolts, which screw into the plate.

screws usually are required proximally and two 2.4-mm screws or smooth 1.8-mm bolts distally (Fig. 14).

The extensor retinaculum is reapproximated with nonabsorbable suture, leaving the extensor pollicis longus above the retinaculum (Fig. 15), and the tourniquet released and hemostasis obtained. The skin is then closed with interrupted sutures over a suction drain. Dacron batting is wrapped around the wound (Fig. 16) and a palmar plaster splint incorporated into a nonelastic dressing (Fig. 17).

**Palmar Approach.** In contrast to the dorsal approach, in which the distal radial skeleton is relatively subcutaneous, the surgical approach to the anterior aspect of the distal radius must provide adequate exposure and yet respect the median and ulnar nerves, flexor tendons, and palmar capsular radiocarpal ligaments.

With palmar shearing two-part fracture-dislocations (Fig. 18), a surgical approach is taken between the flexor carpi radialis tendon and radial artery with detachment of the pronator quadratus (Fig. 19). Following removal of the fracture hematoma and exposure of the fracture surface, fracture reduction is simplified by hyperextending the wrist over a towel roll with the forearm in full supination. Fracture reduction is provisionally held with smooth 0.045-in. Kirschner wires placed through the radial styloid, with attention taken to prevent the interference of these wires with the placement of a T buttress plate. In contrast to the angled plate applied dorsally, this plate has a prebend to conform more closely to the palmar distal radius anatomy. The fracture reduction is confirmed with intraoperative radiographs.

The plate is contoured so that a small space will remain between the midportion of the plate and the area of the radius just proximal to the fracture site. The most proximal screw is inserted in the plate first. When the second screw is inserted, it compresses the plate against the radial shaft, obtaining a buttressing effect on the distal fragment (Fig. 20). This is sufficient for most two-part shearing fractures, and additional screw fixation usually is unnecessary. However, additional screws can be added if absolute stability is not gained effectively with the buttress effect of the plate (Fig. 21).

The surgeon does not extend this particular incision distally if release of the transverse carpal ligament is required, as the palmar cutaneous branch of the median nerve will be in jeopardy of being transected. Rather, the carpal tunnel is released through a separate incision on the ulnar side of the palm.

When faced with a more complex, palmarly displaced fracture, particularly with displacement of the medial complex, a different approach is chosen. An incision

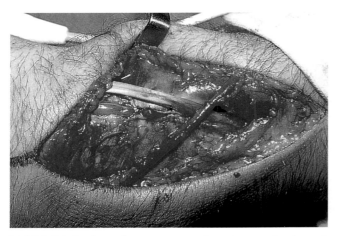

**FIGURE 15.** Replace the extensor retinaculum and suture it with nonabsorbable suture. Leave the extensor pollicis longus tendon outside the retinaculum to prevent ischemic rupture.

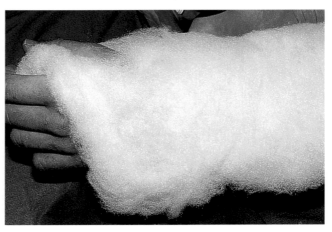

**FIGURE 16.** Wrap Dacron batting around the operative site as the primary dressing.

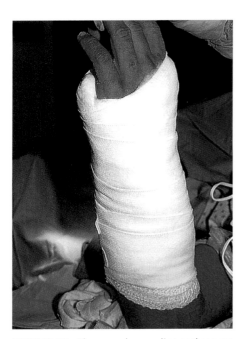

**FIGURE 17.** Place a palmar splint and secure it with nonelastic wrapping.

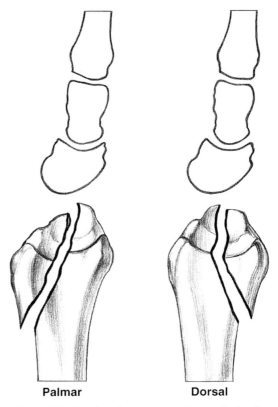

Palmar                    Dorsal

**FIGURE 18.** The shearing two-part intraarticular fractures are, in reality, fracture-dislocations of the radiocarpal joint.

is marked out to extend from the mid-palm obliquely crossing the wrist flexion crease and extending proximally for approximately 4 inches (Fig. 22). As with complex dorsally displaced fractures, an external fixator can be placed at this juncture (prior to elevation of the pneumatic tourniquet) to permit intraoperative distraction and to help support the hand and wrist, aiding in surgical exposure (Fig. 23).

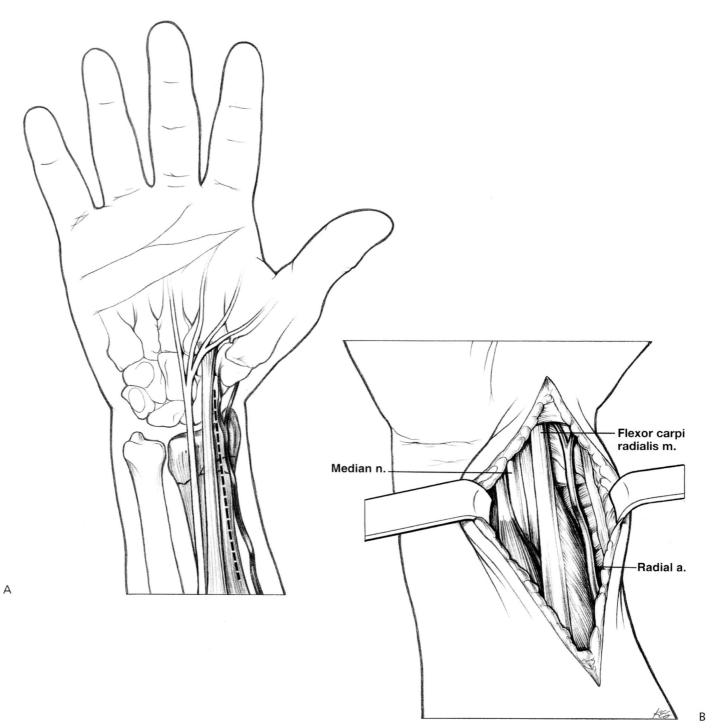

A

B

Flexor carpi
radialis m.

Median n.

Radial a.

**FIGURE 19.** The palmar approach to the shearing two-part fracture-dislocation. **A:** Make a straight longitudinal incision along the radial side of the distal forearm. **B:** Identify the radial artery, the flexor carpi radialis, and median nerve. (*continued.*)

As extensile exposure is required, the transverse carpal ligament is opened longitudinally in its central portion, which permits later closure with a Z-plasty. The plane between the ulnar neurovascular structures and flexor tendons is developed with retraction of the tendons, median nerve, and radial artery in a radial direction, exposing the pronator quadratus (Fig. 24). The muscle is elevated from its ulnar

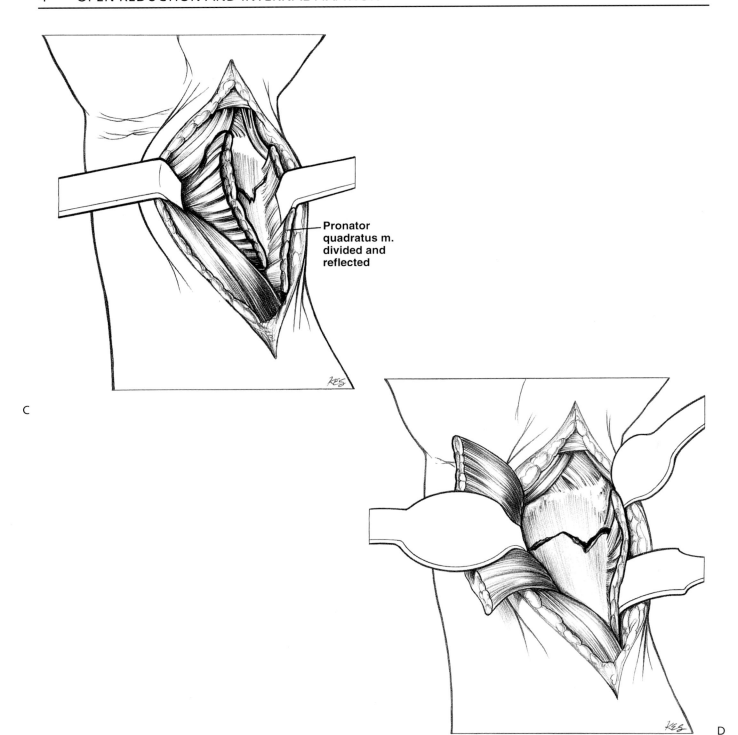

Pronator
quadratus m.
divided and
reflected

C

D

**FIGURE 19.** (*continued.*) **C:** Elevate the pronator quadratus muscle from its radial attachment
and use it to protect the median nerve and flexor tendons. **D:** Expose the palmar surface; identify
the fracture lines, and reduce them under direct vision.

attachment, allowing excellent exposure of the medial side of the radius as well as
serving to protect the median nerve and flexor tendons during retraction (Fig. 25).

Although there may be an associated palmar capsular ligamentous injury, it usually is not visible, as the external capsule ordinarily remains intact. The surgeon
should resist the temptation to cut across the wrist capsule to facilitate visualiza-

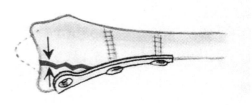

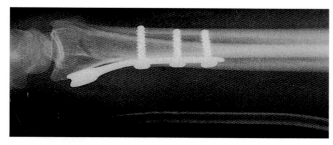

**FIGURE 20.** The placement of the palmar buttress T plate is such that a slight gap remains between the plate and radius just proximal to the reduced fracture (*arrows*). (From Müller ME, Allgöwer M, Scheider R, Willenegger H. *Manual of Internal Fixation,* 2nd ed. New York: Springer-Verlag, 1979:195, with permission.)

**FIGURE 21.** On the tightening of the second most proximal screw, the plate will further impact the distal fragment, adding to its "buttress" effect.

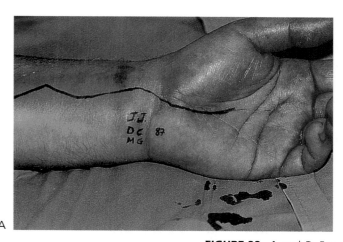

A

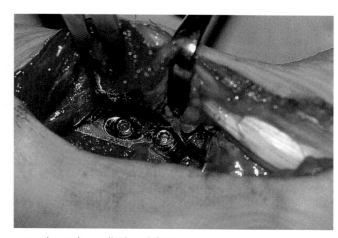

B

**FIGURE 22. A** and **B:** For more complex palmar displaced fractures, a more extensile surgical incision is required.

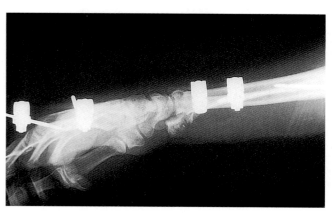

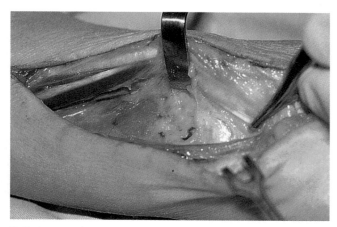

**FIGURE 23.** The placement of an external fixation device prior to fracture exposure greatly facilitates the surgical reduction and minimizes additional soft tissue trauma.

**FIGURE 24.** The interval between the ulnar neurovascular structures and flexor tendons provides access to the pronator quadratus. The transverse carpal ligament is released for later repair with a Z-plasty.

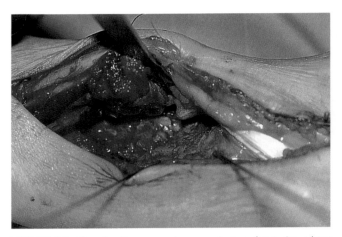

**FIGURE 25.** Elevate the pronator quadratus from its ulnar attachment, leaving a cuff for later repair. The muscle helps protect the flexor tendons and median nerves from excessive pressure with retraction.

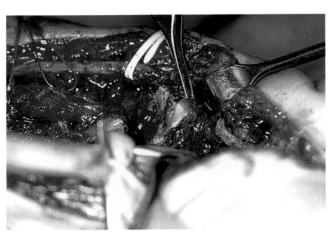

**FIGURE 26.** Intraoperative distraction helps pull the articular fragments apart. They can be opened like a book from the metaphyseal area; this avoids risking injury of the palmar capsular ligaments by incising them for exposure.

tion of the articular fragments. Rather, the metaphyseal fragments themselves should be opened like a book, exposing the articular injury from within the metaphyseal bone. Increased distraction with the external fixator helps pull the fragments apart (Fig. 26).

At this juncture, reduction of the fragments is carefully done and provisional fixation accomplished with 0.035- or 0.045-in. smooth Kirschner wires, carefully placed from a distal position to avoid interference with the placement of a plate. Autogenous iliac crest bone graft is almost always needed to fill in the areas of impacted metaphyseal bone, as well as for critical support of the articular fragments.

As with the two-part shearing fractures, a palmar buttress T plate is preferred to support the articular reconstructions. A full inventory of small and minifragment plates must be available because some fractures require two plates to completely buttress the fracture. The newer volar plate of the Pi plate system (Synthes, Paoli, PA) offers wider versatility for the complex fractures and has become my personal preference.

Two situations may arise that can add to the complexity of the internal fixation. First, if the radial styloid is fractured and displaced, one should avoid added dissection without knowledge of the location of the palmar cutaneous branch of the median nerve (Fig. 27). It is preferable to manipulate the styloid using a large pointed reduction clamp with the point placed percutaneously into the styloid, fixing it to the proximal radius with a 0.062-in.–diameter smooth Kirschner wire (Fig. 28). The second situation involves disruption of the medial complex of the radius, with displacement in both a dorsal and ulnar direction (Fig. 29). In this case, it may be exceedingly difficult to achieve accurate reduction with a second incision made dorsally with reduction of the dorsally displaced fragment of the lunate facet performed initially, which provides a template on which the palmar fragment can be more accurately reduced (Fig. 30).

The closure of the palmar approach includes replacement of the transverse carpal ligament with a Z-plasty. This is recommended not only for later functional considerations, but also to help prevent palmar subluxation of the flexor tendons, which potentially could develop adherence in the surgical site. The pronator quadratus is reapproximated with resorbable suture and the skin is closed over a suction drain.

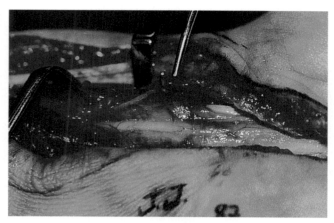

**FIGURE 27.** Knowledge of the location of the palmar cutaneous branch of the median nerve is essential if surgical exposure of the radial styloid is necessary.

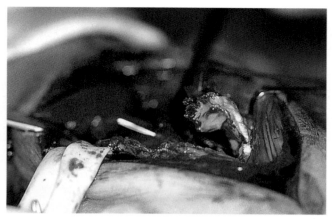

**FIGURE 29.** There are occasions in which a dorsal and palmar incision is required to support a displaced medial complex. In this instance, the dorsal fragment is held attached by the dorsal radioulnar ligaments.

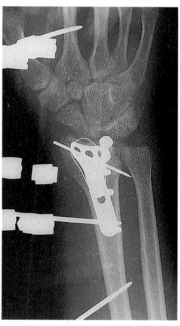

**FIGURE 28.** It may not be possible to buttress the radial styloid with a plate. Therefore, a 0.062-in.–diameter Kirschner wire can support the styloid reduction.

## POSTOPERATIVE MANAGEMENT

Unless complications develop, the dressing and suction drain are removed on the first postoperative day. A palmar orthoplast splint is made that the patient is encouraged to remove for active wrist motion. Coban is wrapped over each digit and thumb, and extended up the forearm to minimize postoperative edema. Digital exercises are also encouraged.

Rehabilitation is initiated with postoperative active digital and wrist exercises and continued on an outpatient basis. The patient is also given a series of upper extremity mobility exercises to prevent shoulder or forearm problems.

The palmar splint is to be discontinued by 2 weeks postoperatively if the wound and fracture healing progresses satisfactorily.

Grip-strengthening exercises are begun 3 weeks postoperatively and increased with resistive exercises by 6 weeks postoperatively—again, all based on the progress of healing as demonstrated by serial radiographs.

Our experience, as well as that in the literature, suggests that if articular anatomy is restored and maintained, the outcome is favorable (1–4,7,8,11,12). In fact, one can expect between two-thirds and three-fourths of patients to have good to excellent results, although it may take between 12 to 18 months to reach an end result. Wrist extension and flexion are likely to have residual impairment, but one can expect a 75% return of this motion. Forearm rotation is likely to return to full or nearly full motion, unless there was an associated disruption of the distal radioulnar joint. The patient is likely to have residual discomfort for at least 6 months and perhaps as long as 12 to 18 months. Grip strength returns progressively and can be expected to return to 75% to 90% of normal.

If anatomy cannot be accurately restored or surgical dissection is excessive, leading to peritendinous adhesions or periarticular fibrosis, the results are far less encouraging, and in fact there may be considerable disability. This is the case particularly with those high-velocity injuries associated with excessive periarticular comminution. A word of caution is extended prior to embarking on the surgical management of these cases, as the outcome is likely to be compromised even with the best of surgical execution. The patient and family are counseled prior to the initiation of surgery.

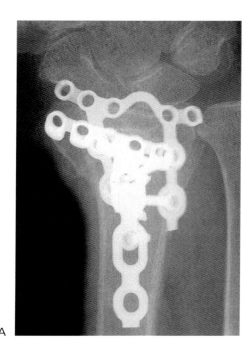

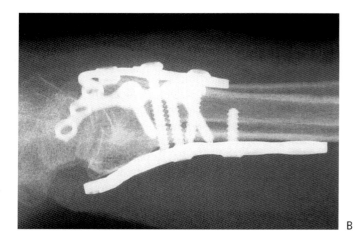

A

B

**FIGURE 30. A** and **B:** The medial complex was split, requiring dorsal and palmar incisions; the placement of plates on either side secured the anatomic reduction.

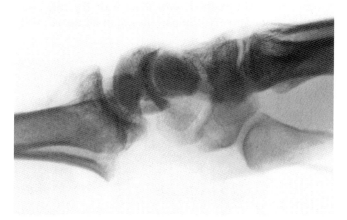

**FIGURE 31.** Radiograph of a 20-year-old college ice hockey player demonstrates a displaced distal radius fracture with an impacted articular surface. The radiographic appearance of the lunate suggests a palmar tilt.

## COMPLICATIONS

*Wound necrosis*: Caution is exercised not to proceed with the surgery until the soft tissues recover from the initial trauma. In addition, wounds are not closed under tension. Rather, skin graft or temporary biologic dressing offsets a wound breakdown. Once this occurs, débridement of devitalized tissue and expedient coverage minimizes long-term complications.

*Neurologic*: Prolonged surgery with continuous retraction on the median nerve can result in sensory or motor dysfunction. In addition to the surgical exposures outlined above, care is taken to limit retraction on the nerves and to move retractors frequently.

*Unstable internal fixation*: The complexity of some fractures precludes effective internal fixation. In these cases, the external fixator offsets the tendency of the carpus to displace the fracture and should be left in place for at least 3 weeks. Liberal use of autogenous bone graft also supports the articular fragments and facilitates healing.

*Loss of reduction or fixation*: This potential problem is associated with any operative approach to articular fractures. Management must be individualized, but some general principles can be offered. First, the patient should be informed of the problem. Next, should consultation be considered, it is best arranged expeditiously. Repeat surgery after 4 to 6 weeks may not be feasible, thus surgical salvage is considered early. Finally, of the articular surfaces remaining in place, one option is to allow healing of the fracture and consider an extraarticular osteotomy at a later stage.

*Peritendinous adhesions*: Following dorsal or palmar surgery, the possibility of limited digital mobility is considered. Early and persistent intervention with a therapist may prevent this from occurring. However, the surgeon discusses and monitors this program to ensure that the internal fixation remains stable.

## ILLUSTRATIVE CASE FOR TECHNIQUE

A 20-year-old college ice hockey player fell and sustained an impacted articular fracture of the distal radius (Fig. 31). Through a dorsal approach, the fracture was disimpacted, lengthened with a mini-distractor, and stabilized with a dorsal Pi plate. Postoperatively, the patient regained nearly full mobility (Fig. 32).

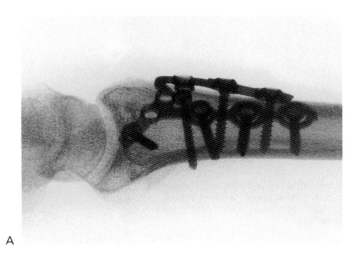

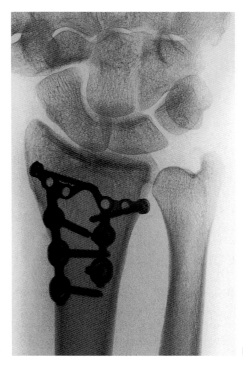

**FIGURE 32.** **A** and **B:** Follow-up radiographs show an anatomic restoration of the radius. Nearly full function was regained.

A

B

## RECOMMENDED READING

1. Axelrod, T.S., McMurty, R.Y.: Open reduction and internal fixation of comminuted intraarticular fractures of the distal radius. *J. Hand Surg.*, 15A: 1–11, 1990.
2. Axelrod, T.S., Paley, D., Green, J., McMurtry, R.Y.: Limited open reduction of the lunate facet in comminuted intraarticular fractures of the distal radius. *J. Hand Surg.*, 13A: 372–377, 1988.
3. Bradway, J., Amadio, P.C., Cooney, W.P. III.: Open reduction and internal fixation of displaced, comminuted intraarticular fractures of the distal end of the radius. *J. Bone Joint Surg.*, 71A: 839–847, 1989.
4. Fernandez, D.L., Geissler, W.G.: Treatment of displaced fractures of the radius. *J. Hand Surg.*, 16A: 375–384, 1991.
5. Fernandez, D.L., Jupiter, J.B.: *Fractures of the Distal Radius*. Springer-Verlag, New York, 1995.
6. Jupiter, J.B.: Current concepts review. Fractures of the distal end of the radius. *J. Bone Joint Surg.*, 7: 461–469, 1991.
7. Jupiter, J.B., Lipton, H.A.: Operative treatment of intraarticular fractures of the distal radius: the upper extremity pilon fracture. *Clinch Orthop. Rel. Res.*, 292: 1–14, 1993.
8. Knirk, J.L., Jupiter. J.B.: Intraarticular fractures of the distal end of the radius in young adults. *J. Bone Joint Surg.*, 68A: 647–659, 1986.
9. McMurtry, R.Y., Jupiter, J.B. Fractures of the distal radius. In: *Skeletal Trauma*, edited by B. Browner, J. Jupiter, A. Levine, P. Trafton, W.B. Saunders, Philadelphia, pp. 1063–1094, 1991.
10. Melone, C.P. Jr.: Open treatment for displaced articular fractures of the distal radius. *Clinch Orthop. Rel. Res.*, 202: 103–111, 1986.
11. Missakian, M.L., Cooney, W.P. III, Amadio, P.C., Glidewell, H.L.: Open reduction and internal fixation for distal radius fractures. *J. Hand Surg.*, 17A: 745–755, 1992.
12. Pattee, G.A., Thompson, G.H.: Anterior and posterior marginal fracture-dislocation of the distal radius. *Clinch Orthop. Rel. Res.*, 231: 183–195, 1988.
13. Weber, S.C., Szabo, R.M.: Severely comminuted distal radius fractures as an isolated problem: complications associated with external fixation and pins and plaster techniques. *J. Hand Surg.*, 11A: 157–165, 1986.

# 5

# Limited Open Reduction and Internal Fixation

Terry S. Axelrod

Orthopaedists have expressed a great deal of interest in the management of distal radius fractures, particularly fractures in young, active individuals, as the many publications, ideas, and directions on the management of these sometimes complex fractures attest. There is clearly no "one way" to manage all of these fractures.

Some patients do well with simple closed treatment with a closed reduction and a cast; in others more intervention is necessary to provide additional stability to the fracture or to manipulate fracture fragments. Often, external fixation or percutaneous pinning can afford the additional stability many fractures require, but these methods may not be fully adequate to reduce and maintain an intraarticular displaced fracture. Open reduction and internal fixation using a buttress plate or similar configuration are the best means to manage joint-shearing fractures.

Formal open reduction and internal fixation of complex joint depression or combined distal radius fractures is a challenging undertaking, one that, in many cases, should be undertaken only by the experienced wrist trauma surgeon. The surgeon who engages in the management of distal radius fractures needs to be comfortable with performing one of many different techniques to afford the best surgical results and outcomes for the patients being treated.

The fracture that continues to create substantial controversy in management is the type III or joint compression type in the Fernandez Classification (1). This fracture pattern involves the depression of the dorsal portion of the lunate facet as a separate fragment isolated from the scaphoid facet of the distal radial articular margin.

Publications by Jupiter et al., Axelrod et al., and others indicate the need to strive to restore congruence to the joint to within 2 mm or less in active, young individuals with a distal radius fracture (2–4). Failure to do so will result in a significantly higher degree of posttraumatic osteoarthritis at 7-year follow-up.

Several authors have explored the means to achieve this reduction. Axelrod and McMurtry have indicated that it is possible to achieve a congruent joint through open reduction and internal fixation, at the cost of substantial complications (3). A later publication introduced the role of percutaneous or limited open reduction to achieve a level joint without the need to go to formal open reduction and internal fixation (5).

More recently, Fernandez has compared the results to be expected when the joint can be restored either by open or percutaneous means (6). In a series of 40 patients, Fernandez demonstrated that if the joint surface is restored to within 2 mm of congruence, the results in the intermediate term remain the same, whichever technique (open or limited open) is used.

A technique that provides an intermediate degree of help in the management of displaced intraarticular joint compression is the limited open reduction or the percutaneous open manipulation and pinning of the articular segments. This more limited exposure may help to reduce the morbidity of the extensive exposures, as well as the difficulties of small-fragment fixation associated with formal open reduction and internal fixation (3,5,7–9).

## INDICATIONS

As mentioned, this technique lends itself only to a specific subset of distal radius fractures; for this reason, patient selection is critical. The ideal patient is a young, active individual with a type III or joint depression type of fracture. This "die-punch" type of fracture may not reduce by simple ligamentotaxis, owing to a lack of adequate soft tissue attachments or severe impacting into the metaphysis (11) (Fig. 1).

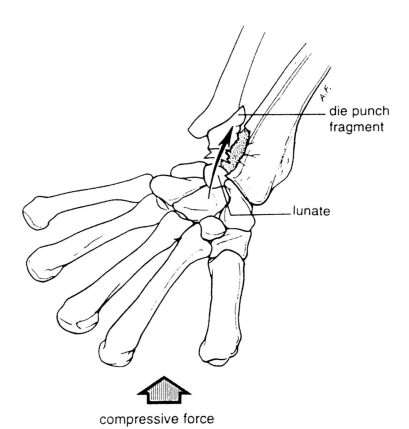

**FIGURE 1.** The mechanism of force transmission resulting in the type III joint depression fracture. The impacted dorsal segment of the lunate facet is commonly known as the "die punch" fragment. (From Scheck, M.: Long-term follow-up of treatment of comminuted fractures of the distal end of the radius by transfixation with Kirschner wires and cast. *J. Bone Joint Surg.*, 44A: 337–351, 1962, with permission.)

In the elderly or low-demand individual, a joint step-off of 2 mm or greater may not have any long-term consequence, and often can be left unreduced. In young, active individuals this lack of congruency must be addressed. A joint depression of the lunate or, rarely, of the scaphoid facet, needs to be elevated directly. The cutoff in my opinion is 2 mm, as per Jupiter et al. Usually the depression is greater than 2 mm.

Some other fractures may be amenable to this limited open technique. Specifically, a shearing fracture of the scaphoid facet (commonly known as the *chauffeur's fracture*) may also require a small amount of percutaneous manipulation to reduce it to perfect joint alignment.

## PREOPERATIVE PLANNING

This technique does not require much "on paper" preoperative planning; it is usually a sequential add-on to the closed reduction and external fixation, if the joint cannot be reduced perfectly.

Have the appropriate equipment available, specifically the mini-C arm, a small elevator, and a K-wire driver with some 1.6-mm Kirschner wires.

Carefully analyze the x-rays to define the size and location of the depressed fragment. Pay attention to the degree of associated dorsal comminution as it pertains to the need for cancellous bone grafting or bone substitute material. A computed tomography scan with two- or three-dimensional reconstruction can greatly facilitate the understanding of the fracture pattern and displacement.

Bone graft, if required, can easily be obtained from the olecranon as an alternative to the iliac crest. Use of this site significantly reduces the morbidity of the procedure and makes it possible to do the operation under regional anesthesia, even as an outpatient procedure. At our center, we do not have much experience with bone graft substitute materials; the costs of such materials are currently prohibitive to widespread use in a government-funded health-care system.

## SURGERY

Position the patient supine on the operating room table. Use a radiolucent hand table or two thin arm boards side by side to support the affected limb. Use a tourniquet.

A mini-C arm is ideal for this surgery. As an alternative, the large fluoroscope can be used, although it is awkward, needs a technician, and exposes the team to a larger amount of both direct and scatter radiation. Live imaging is essential; plain static x-rays can be used to confirm reduction. If an image intensifier is not available, reschedule the surgery (Fig. 2A–D).

Anesthesia can be general or regional. Preparation and draping should be proximal enough to allow access to the elbow for potential bone graft material, if necessary.

Begin the procedure with the application of a simple external fixation frame in whatever configuration is recommended by the manufacturer. Dorsal access to the wrist must be preserved in assembling the fixator. Imaging, both posteroanterior (PA) and lateral, must be possible with the frame in place.

If using a multi-bar external fixator, it is worthwhile at first simply to link the terminally threaded pins with a single bar, reducing the bulk of the fixator and the blocks to imaging until the limited open reduction is complete. Complete the frame with whichever bars are needed.

As described in Chapter 3, manipulate the wrist as needed to effect the best overall reduction of the distal segment. Following reduction, lock the frame in a fairly neutral position. It is essential to avoid excess distraction of the radiocarpal

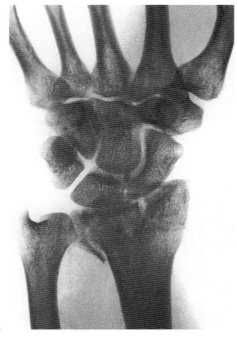

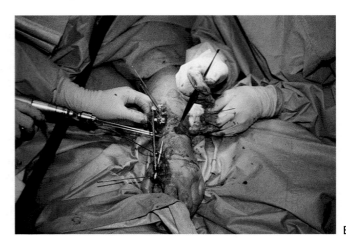

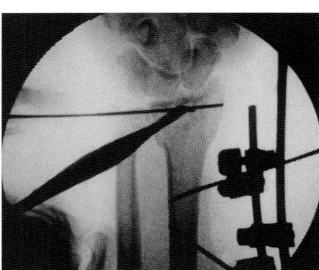

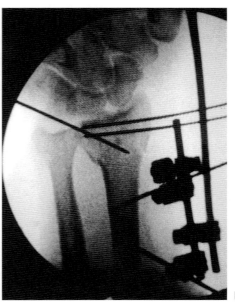

**FIGURE 2. A:** Posteroanterior x-ray of the wrist of a 28-year-old male with a type III joint compression fracture. The impacted lunate facet failed to reduce with simple ligamentotaxis with the application of an external fixation frame and limited traction. **B:** The intraoperative setup: The external fixator has been applied. The hand rests on the surface of the image intensifier. A small dorsal incision is present, and a Howarth elevator has been inserted into the proximal end of the fracture line. **C:** Image-guided reduction of the lunate facet with the elevator. The fragment has been initially stabilized with a single Kirschner wire supporting the subchondral bone. **D:** Final construct with two subchondral Kirschner wires supporting the joint surface and an optional third wire providing some extra support to the lunate facet.

joint. It is not advisable to pull the remaining rim fragments into position through overdistraction of the joint, which is associated with an increased incidence of severe wrist stiffness following external fixation. Flexion of the distal segment is best obtained by applying palmar translation force through the external fixation frame, in combination with flexion of no more than 10° of the wrist.

Use the fixator to obtain overall alignment of the fracture—that is, length and radial inclination. If the joint surface—in particular, the lunate facet fragment—

does not reduce anatomically, the next step is to attempt the limited open reduction technique.

Localize the central portion of the distal radial metaphysis and the proximal extent of the fracture line of the depressed fragment with the mini-C arm. Make a small, 1 cm to 2 cm longitudinal incision 1 cm from the proximal extent of the fracture line to allow for entry of the elevator on the appropriate angle. The entry point for the procedure usually is just proximal to and ulnar to Lister's tubercle. Once the skin incision is made, the subcutaneous tissues are spread with a small snap, avoiding injury to any local cutaneous nerve branches. This technique allows the tendons to be mobilized without damage.

Insert a small elevator—either a Howarth, a Freer, or a small curved bone punch—directly through the incision, twist it down onto the bone, and slide it distally until you feel the edge of the fracture line. Using the image intensifier to control this portion of the surgery, slide the elevator into the fracture line and direct it distally until it engages the central portion of the depressed fracture fragment, just below the subchondral cortical bone.

Direct manipulation of the fragment now takes place. Using the mini-C arm, under direct PA visualization, disimpact the impacted fragment and gently elevate it until it is anatomically reduced. Generally, it is better to slightly overreduce the fragment, as it will tend to settle when load is placed across the wrist joint. Check the reduction with the image intensifier in all planes. An acceptable reduction is one in which the subchondral line of the articular surface is smooth, showing less than a 2-mm step-off on the PA projection. It is usually easy to obtain a near perfect reduction of the joint surface.

In doing this reduction, the surgeon often will note that the palmar tilt of the distal segment is improved. The impaction of the lunate facet fragment is dorsal, the limited technique is dorsal, and the manipulation will tend to reduce the dorsal rim preferentially, thus improving the palmar tilt.

Once you are satisfied with the reduction, internal fixation is needed to maintain the reduction. This may be complemented with bone graft or substitute to further support the surface (Fig. 3).

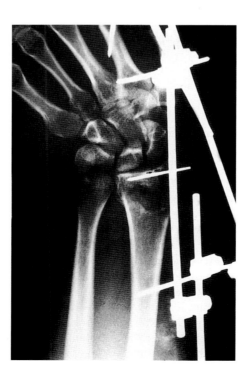

**FIGURE 3.** A similar construct utilizing only a single Kirschner wire. Note the perfect reduction of the joint surface. The osseous defect was not bone grafted in this case.

If a large defect (this is subjective) is created with the disimpaction, the reduced fragment has a tendency to collapse back into the defect, if not supported by more than a few Kirschner wires. Bone graft will work extremely well in providing the additional necessary support.

Obtain bone graft from the olecranon or the iliac crest, or use a substitute material. Insert the cancellous material through the small dorsal incision and use the elevator or small punches to place and pack the graft under the reduced fragment. Use the image intensifier to ensure that the fragment has not moved, that the material does not extrude into the joint, and that adequate fill of the defect is obtained.

Then provide internal fixation using percutaneous 1.6-mm Kirschner wire. Ideally the wires come transversely across from the radial styloid directly under the reduced lunate facet fragment. The K-wire should lie just below the dense subchondral bone, serving to buttress the depressed joint segment. It must stop just before the sigmoid notch; otherwise, the point of the wire will enter the distal radioulnar joint and cause damage to the ulnar head in the postoperative period.

Place a second wire to further support the fragment. It usually is brought in from the ulnar side, more dorsal-to-palmar-oriented than the first wire, which is directly transverse. Localize it with the mini-C arm, insert it under power, and follow across to the palmar cortex. This pin just engages the dorsal, ulnar aspect of the reduced die-punch fragment, coming in from over the ulnar head.

An alternative to the ulnar placement of the second Kirschner wire is to use a modification of the Kapandji intrafocal pinning technique (10). Using this technique, the second wire can be placed directly dorsally—just engaging the proximal end of the reduced fracture fragment—then manually angled distally and power driven forward, engaging the palmar cortex of the distal radius. This pin then serves as a dorsal buttress, supporting this fragment and preventing the fragment from slipping back into extension.

Bone graft can be added following internal fixation if the K-wires seem insufficient to support the reduced fragment until union occurs.

If the defect size is relatively small, the bone quality reasonable, and the K-wire fixation good, bone grafting can be avoided reasonably safely. Overall, the vast majority of our limited open reduction procedures are done without the use of cancellous bone graft.

Check the K-wire placement once again to assure that the pins are not extending too far out through the cortex, into either joint, or too far into the soft tissues. Pins are usually left out through the skin, cut, and bent over. Check the skin and release it where tethering by the pins has occurred. Protect the pin ends appropriately and apply gauze dressings over the tips (Fig. 4A–C).

## POSTOPERATIVE MANAGEMENT

Elevate the limb, encourage finger motion, and initiate a physiotherapy program early for patients that show evidence of excessive swelling, reflex sympathetic dystrophy, or shoulder and elbow stiffness.

If the distal radioulnar joint has not been pinned, it is advisable to begin active and passive pronation and supination routines early on, even with the fixator in place. This regimen can be helpful in the early restoration of limb mobility.

Dress the pin sites both from the external fixator and the percutaneous K-wires, as you prefer. Our own routine is to dress the sites with Betadine-soaked gauze or pieces of scrub sponges also soaked in Betadine. After approximately 2 weeks the sites are left dry, without dressings, unless drainage is present.

Leave the external fixator in place for approximately 6 weeks, rarely more than 8 weeks. Keep the supplemental Kirschner wires in for 4 to 6 weeks. Remove them before or at the same time that the external fixation is removed. The decision

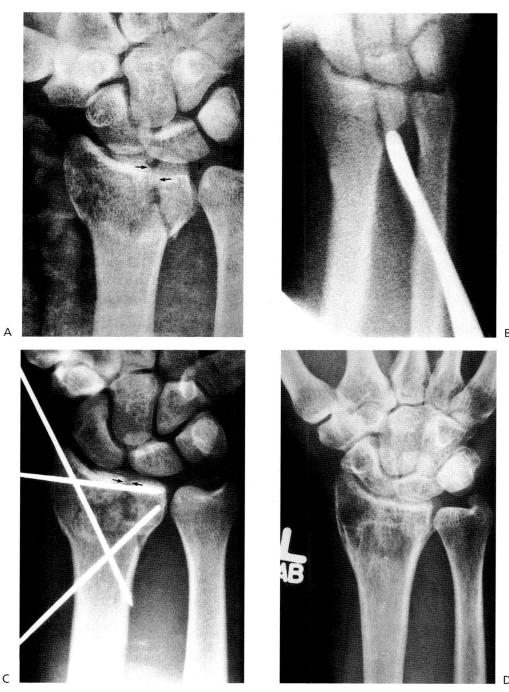

**FIGURE 4.  A:** A joint shearing type of fracture involving the entire lunate facet (*arrows*). Failure of reduction via closed means. **B:** Intraoperative imaging of the elevator in place, teasing the fragment into place. **C:** The Kirschner wire configuration utilized in this particular fracture pattern (*arrows*). The radial sided fracture was minimally displaced; simple pinning was chosen instead of an external fixator. **D:** Two months postoperative, following Kirschner wire removal in the clinic. Note the anatomic position of the healed fracture.

to remove is based on sequential x-rays, showing progressive fracture healing and a lack of migration of the fracture segments.

Generally, it is advisable to repeat x-rays of the wrist at 1 to 2 weeks following the surgical procedure, and then at 4 weeks and immediately before removing any of the fixation devices.

Should x-rays reveal a loss of reduction of the elevated fragments sufficient to result in an unacceptable degree of joint incongruency, it is best to intervene early with a revision of the reduction and internal fixation.

It is probably not advisable to persist with a limited open technique after a few weeks have passed. The fracture will be starting to unite and limited approaches will not predictably be able to manipulate a partially healed fracture. In these rare cases, or in the case of the initial treatment being delayed beyond 2 weeks after the fracture, it is best to move immediately to an open reduction. In this procedure, the fragments can be carefully mobilized, reduced anatomically, and held in place with more rigid, stable internal fixation devices. Ideal devices are the fixed angle blade plates or similar implants that will secure small fragments in somewhat osteopenic bone.

Following pin and external fixator removal, the exercise program concentrates on mobilization of the wrist. Continue it as long as necessary to maximize the range of motion. Emphasize digital motion and function initially, and wrist motion secondarily.

## RESULTS TO BE EXPECTED

We have published a small series of results early on with this technique and have found that the articular surface will remain reduced and reliably heal in a near anatomic position (5) (Fig. 4D). Wrist scores and patient satisfaction remain high (*unpublished data*).

Fernandez has indicated that a matched series of patients, all with unreduced articular surfaces following closed manipulation (even with an external fixator), had equal results in moderate-term follow-up as long as the articular surface was reduced adequately. He found, as we have, that it does not matter which technique—formal open or limited open—is used to achieve the joint reduction. The end result—a level joint—is achieved whichever way will provide the best possible outcome for the patient (6). The limited open technique is associated with less soft tissue morbidity and stiffness and fewer intraoperative difficulties.

## RECOMMENDED READINGS

1. Fernandez, D.L., Jupiter, J.B.: Comparative classification for fractures of the distal end of the radius. *J. Hand Surg.*, 22(4): 563–571, 1997.
2. Knirk, J.L., Jupiter, J.B.: Intra-articular fractures of the distal end of the radius in young adults. *J. Bone Joint Surg.*, 68(5): 647–659, 1986.
3. Axelrod, T.S., McMurtry, R.Y.: Open reduction and internal fixation of comminuted, intraarticular fractures of the distal radius. *J. Hand Surg.*, 15(1): 1–11, 1990.
4. Fernandez, D.L., Geissler, W.B.: Treatment of displaced articular fractures of the distal radius. *J. Hand Surg.*, 16A: 375–384, 1991.
5. Axelrod, T.S., Paley, D., Green, J., McMurtry, R.Y.: Limited open reduction of the lunate facet in comminuted intra-articular fractures of the distal radius. *J. Hand Surg.*, 13(3): 372–377, 1988.
6. Fernandez, D.L., Jupiter, J.B.: Compression Fractures of the Distal Radius. In: *Fractures of the Distal Radius*, Springer-Verlag New York, New York, pp. 189–220, 1996.
7. Kambouroglou, G.K., Axelrod, T.S.: Complications of the AO/ASIF titanium distal radius plate system (pi plate) in internal fixation of the distal radius: a brief report. *J. Hand Surg.*, 23(4): 737–741, 1998.
8. Jupiter, J.B., Lipton, H.: The operative treatment of intraarticular fractures of the distal radius. *Clin. Orthop.*, 292: 48–61, 1993.
9. Ring, D., Jupiter, J.B.: Percutaneous and limited open fixation of fractures of the distal radius. *Clin. Orthop.*, 375: 105–115, 2000.
10. Kapandji, A.: "Reduction-effect" ARUM-type intra-focal pins in the osteosynthesis of fractures of the lower end of the radius. *Ann. Chir. Main Memb. Super.*,10(2): 138–145, 1991.
11. Scheck, M.: Long-term follow-up of treatment of comminuted fractures of the distal end of the radius by transfixation with Kirschner wires and cast. *J. Bone Joint Surg.*, 44A: 337–351, 1962.

# 6

# Intrafocal Pinning with "Arum" Pins in Distal Fractures of the Radius

Adalbert I. Kapandji

Many surgeons use traditional K-wire pinning in fractures of the distal radius, but this method does not prevent postoperative displacement in all cases. For this reason, I have proposed intrafocal pinning (1,2), using "arum" pins (Fig. 1), so named for their resemblance to an arum (lily) flower (3).

Intrafocal arum pinning (IFAP) avoids secondary displacement by introducing the pins directly into the fracture line, where they can act as buttresses. Any subsequent tilt of the distal fragment is avoided, which makes casting unnecessary. Immediate rehabilitation is possible, resulting in better function.

## INDICATIONS/CONTRAINDICATIONS

### Nonarticular Fractures

IFAP can provide superior results in most cases of nonarticular fracture, whatever the type of fracture and degree of displacement, because it allows immediate rehabilitation. Previously, I reserved use of IFAP for fractures with displacement. However, I now advocate it routinely, regardless of the level of displacement, for two reasons. First, nondisplaced fractures often displace later, in spite of a good cast; second, immobilization, even the shortest possible immobilization, may have functional sequelae that impede full recovery.

This procedure also is indicated for fractures with posterior comminution, because the cone penetration of the arum pin compensates in advance for the posterior tilt, and the larger diameter of the cone, compared with a simple pin, provides better support to the border of the distal fragment.

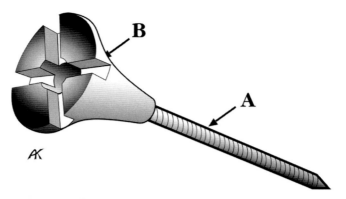

**FIGURE 1.** A: The arum pin has a threaded shaft. B: The concave conical extremity and smoothly convex head prevent damage to tendons. The head has a cruciform groove for the special screwdriver. A small space houses the blunt cut edge of the pin, so it cannot damage the tendons. The nut is named for its shape, which resembles an arum or lily flower.

In fractures with an anterior tilt, one or two anterior pins control displacement without disturbing tendons, nerves, and arteries. This approach is more limited than the one needed for the setting of an anterior plate, and pin fixation is as firm as plate fixation, in my opinion.

### Intraarticular Fractures

Arum pins provide the same benefits for intraarticular as for nonarticular fractures. The most common intraarticular fracture contains a posteromedial fragment (Fig. 2A, B). The presence of this fragment disturbs the congruity of the articular surface of the distal radius and of the sigmoid notch (Fig. 2C). A third pin is used to control the posteromedial fragment (Fig. 2D, E), because the function of the distal radioulnar joint (DRUJ) may be restricted if it is not restored to an anatomic position. The third posteromedial fragment may be combined with a T-shaped fracture in the frontal plane; in this case, the posterior blocking of the distal fragments is better obtained with two posterior pins.

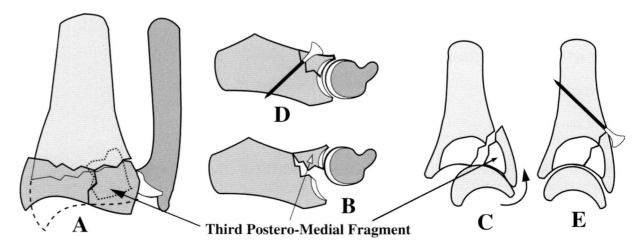

**Third Postero-Medial Fragment**

**FIGURE 2.** The third arum pin in a fracture with a posteromedial fragment. **A:** Front view with a third posteromedial fragment. **B:** Transversal cut: the third posteromedial fragment destroys the radial sigmoid notch. **C:** Side cut: it also destroys the distal radial surface. **D:** The added pin rebuilds the sigmoid notch **(E)** and the distal radial surface.

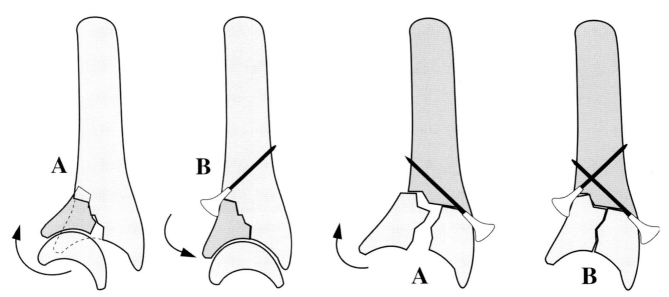

**FIGURE 3.** Anterior border fracture. **A:** This fracture destroys the distal radial surface and allows the anterior subluxation of the carpus. **B:** The anterior arum pin resets the fragment to its site and controls carpal subluxation.

**FIGURE 4.** Fracture of the anterior and posterior borders. **A:** The posterior pin controls the posterior border. **B:** The anterior pin rebuilds the distal radial surface.

Fractures with an anterior fragment may be controlled with an anterior pin (Fig. 3). The combined fracture of the two borders of the distal radial surface (Fig. 4) may be reduced with anterior pins reconstructing the distal radial surface (Fig. 5). Fractures with a sagittal split (Fig. 6) may be controlled with three pins.

In fractures where a posterior tilt is combined with a fracture of the radial styloid process (Fig. 7A, B, C), a lateral pin is used to restore the distal radial articular surface. Associated commonly with this type of fracture is scapholunate dislocation. It is detected with a frontal view, pulling the thumb down to visualize the gap between scaphoid and lunate.

A fracture of the ulnar styloid process is common, causing displacement of the triangular fibrocartilage complex (TFCC). Often this is not visible when the styloid process is intact. As TFCC displacement may compromise DRUJ function, the styloid process is restored to an anatomic position.

Finally, and contrary to what might be expected, multifragment fractures (Fig. 8) may be controlled with three, four, or even five pins. External fixation normally is

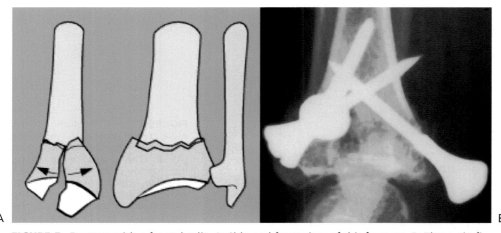

A                                                                                                 B

**FIGURE 5.** Fracture with a frontal split. **A:** Side and front view of this fracture. **B:** Three-pin fixation of the fracture (one pin is set laterally).

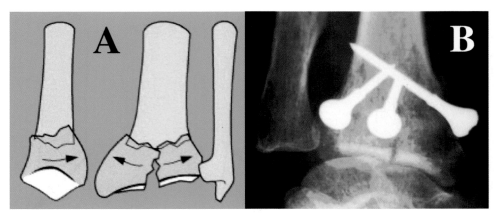

**FIGURE 6.** Fracture with a sagittal split. **A:** Side and front view of this fracture. **B:** Three-pin fixation of the fracture (one pin is set laterally).

indicated in these types of fractures. However, IFAP may be used in these cases. A lateral pin is inserted first, which should provide stable fixation. A second, posterior or anterior pin provides reconstruction of the radial epiphysis, and the remaining pins may be placed. It is also possible to fix a postoperatively displaced fracture (Fig. 9) within a period of fifteen days, as long as consolidation is not yet complete.

If secondary displacement occurs in a multifragment fracture, the functional result still may be good, because of the minimally invasive nature of the surgery and the early rehabilitation.

## SURGERY

### Principles of IFAP

After manual reduction, a threaded K-wire is inserted through a transverse short skin incision, directly into the fracture line. Stable fixation requires three pins

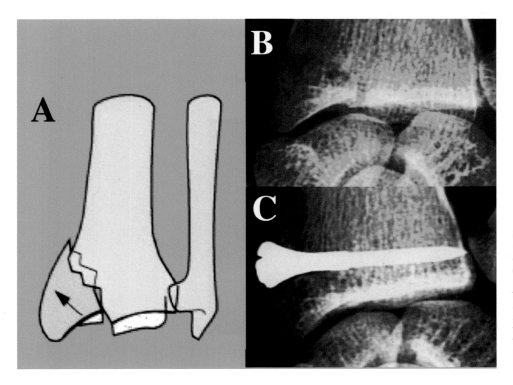

**FIGURE 7.** In a fracture of the radial styloid process, the ascension of the radial styloid process is seen **(A)**. **B:** The frontal x-ray shows interruption of the distal radial surface line, which can pose a risk of arthrosis if it is not corrected. **C:** The arum head of the pin, set in the fracture line, acts in a wedge-like fashion and resets the fragment, rebuilding the distal radial surface line.

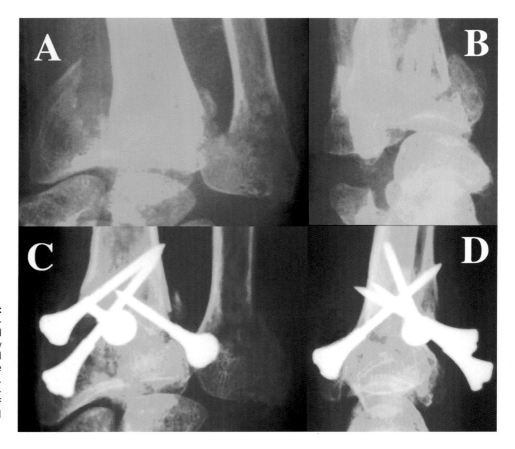

**FIGURE 8.** Complex fracture. **A:** Front view shows significant displacement, with a nondisplaced ulnar head fracture. **B:** Side view shows a posterior margin displaced fracture. **C:** Front view shows the reduced fracture using four pins. The distal radial surface line is normal. **D:** Side view shows that one of the four pins is anterior. The distal radial surface is rebuilt.

inserted in precise points (Fig. 10). The first pin (Fig. 10A) is introduced laterally between the tendons of the extensor carpi radialis and the extensor pollicis brevis. The second pin (Fig. 10B) is inserted posterolaterally, close to Lister's tubercle (care must be taken to avoid damage to the extensor pollicis longus). The third pin (Fig. 10C) is set posteromedially, passing between the extensor digitorum and the extensor carpi ulnaris tendons.

With this approach, the tendons are exposed clearly. To prevent the pins from moving either more deeply or more superficially, I use threaded rather than smooth pins; this ensures that the pins are seated securely in the opposite wall of the radius.

To prevent the blunt, severed edge of the pins from damaging the tendons, I tried "hooding" the pin spike with a metal or plastic cap. This was not a satisfactory solution, because the cap positioning is difficult and the cap often migrated from the pin.

The solution devised subsequently is termed IFAP (3). The pins (Fig. 11A) are 20/10 mm threaded pins of assorted lengths with a special arum nut (Fig. 11B).

Because it is threaded, the pin cannot be expelled. The nut has two advantages: (a) As it penetrates in a wedge-like fashion (Fig. 12A) into the fracture line, it has a "hyper-reduction effect" (Fig. 12B) on the fractured bone that compensates for the posterior compression of the fracture; (b) because the sharp end of the pin (Fig. 13A) could damage the tendons, the rounded shape of the nut and the housing of the pin's sharp edge within the base of the nut protect the tendons from damage (Fig. 13B).

Three pins are necessary (rather than the two-pin technique that I initially proposed), even in treating nonarticular fractures, because posterior blocking of the distal fragment is more effective with two posterior pins rather than with one.

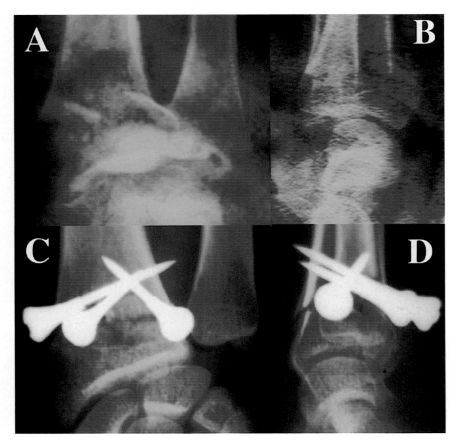

**FIGURE 9.** Displacement after treatment can be repaired using IFAP if the injury is not too old. Front view **(A)** and side view **(B)** show significant tilt and shortening. **C:** Front view shows the fracture perfectly reduced and stabilized with three arum pins. **D:** Side view reveals how the orientation of the distal radial surface becomes normal with two posterior pins.

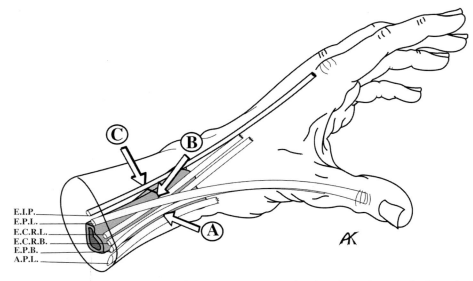

**FIGURE 10.** The three posterolateral pin insertion points for dorsal pinning. A: The lateral pin is set between the extensor carpi radialis brevis and the extensor pollicis brevis. B: The postero-lateral pin is inserted between the extensor pollicis longus and the extensor indicis. C: The posteromedial pin is set close to the medial side of the extensors digitorum and sometimes between the extensors of the fourth and the fifth. A.P.L., abductor pollicis longus; E.C.R.B., extensor carpi radialis brevis; E.C.R.L., extensor carpi radialis longus; E.I.P, extensor indicis proprius; E.P.B., extensor pollicis brevis; E.P.L., extensor pollicis longus.

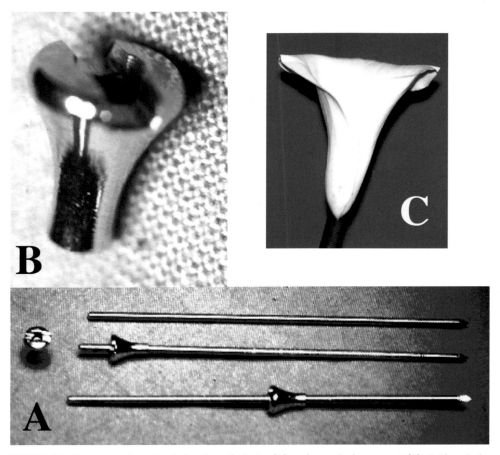

**FIGURE 11.** The arum pin set includes threaded pins **(A)** and a conical arum nut **(B)**. **C:** The pin is shaped like a lily flower ("arum" in French).

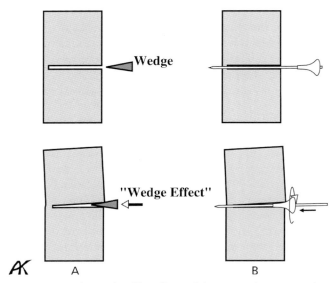

**FIGURE 12.** The wedge-like effect of the arum pin. **A:** A wedge inserted between two pieces widens the space between them. **B:** When the conical nut of the arum is screwed into the fracture line, it widens this space and makes a hypercorrection.

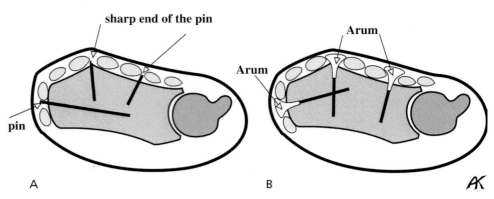

**FIGURE 13.** The risk to tendons. **A:** Traditional techniques of intrafocal pinning, the rough cut end of the pins can damage the tendons. **B:** The smooth shape of the arum nut avoids damage to the tendons.

### Arum Pin Placement

Surgery is performed under general or regional anesthesia and requires the use of a tourniquet. An x-ray amplifier is useful but not necessary. In every case, radiographs are taken after pin placement.

The pin is inserted with a pin-holder, never with a motorized device. Before firmly positioning each threaded pin in the pin-holder, it is prepared with the arum nut in position: at least 1 cm away from the thickness of the bone and in line with the proposed oblique direction of the pin, as visualized on the radiographs. The pin segment caught in the pin-holder becomes unusable, because the pin threads are squeezed by the chuck.

### Fractures with Posterior Tilt

For fractures with posterior tilt, manually reduce the fracture.

- Set each pin through three short, transverse incisions, parallel to the direction of the skin creases. Determine their location on the fracture line by palpation or amplifier; the incisions should be long enough (7–8 mm) to visualize the tendons. The pins should not be set through a simple skin puncture.
- Divide only the skin; dissect the subcutaneous tissues to prevent damage to subcutaneous nerves.
- Separate the tendons from each other by introducing the tips of a fine forceps (Fig. 14) into an intertendinous interval.
- Widen the tips of the first forceps, and insert a second pair of forceps between them.
- Use the second forceps, with closed tips, to "scrape" the bone from top downward (Fig. 14A) to find, by feel, the fracture line. It is easier if the reduction is slightly improved.
- When the fracture line is located, gently introduce the tips of the second forceps into it (Fig. 14B), widen the forceps slightly, and set the pin perpendicularly into the fracture between the forceps. Tilt the pin obliquely (45°) upward (Fig. 14C) until it touches the opposite wall. Screw the pin into the bone with alternative rotatory motion. Any back displacement becomes impossible, and the edges of the two bones' fragments are blocked onto the pin.
- Screw in the arum nut (Fig. 14D) while the fracture reduction is improved slightly (the cone of the arum nut is penetrating safely into the interval of the tendons), then between the two edges of the fracture, creating the "reduction effect," until the narrow part of the cone is completely inside. If the fracture line must be widened further, introduce the beginning of the larger part of the cone.
- Note that the nut must be screwed in a little more than 2 mm (three or four turns), so it may be unscrewed later.

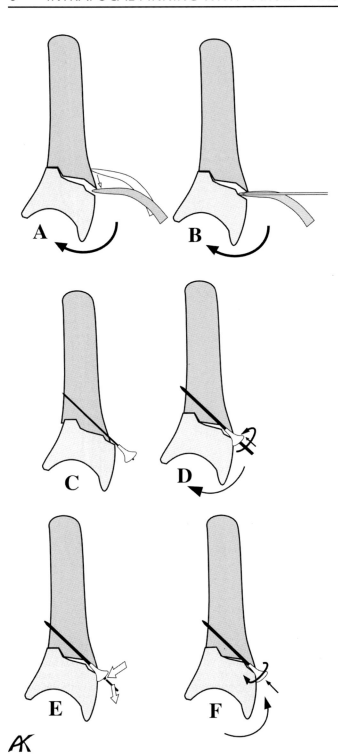

**FIGURE 14.** Introducing the pin into the fracture line. First, reduce the fracture through a small transversal incision. **A:** Use small forceps to "scrape" the dorsal aspect of the radius to locate the fracture line. **B:** Place the pin between the two branches of the forceps and introduce it perpendicularly into the fracture gap. **C:** Tilt the pin obliquely upward until it touches the opposite wall of the radius; with some alternative rotation motions, screw it into the bone. **D:** Screw the arum nut into the fracture line, as the reduction is improved. **E:** Cut the pin as close as possible to the nut; if possible, with the special shears. **F:** Unscrew the arum nut until its cut end is housed in the bottom of the nut.

There is a special pin-holder chuck with a fitting on a screwdriver; when the pin is mounted correctly, it is possible to do the pinning and the screwing without changing the position of the pin-holder. This device provides the advantage of firmly holding the pin as the arum nut is screwed or unscrewed. Also there are special shears, fitted with asymmetrical jaws, to cut the pin (Fig. 14E) close (less than 2 mm) to the nut. With these shears, the depth of the cut may be adjusted. If incompletely cut, the pin may be held during the unscrewing of the nut, while it is bent and broken in the nut.

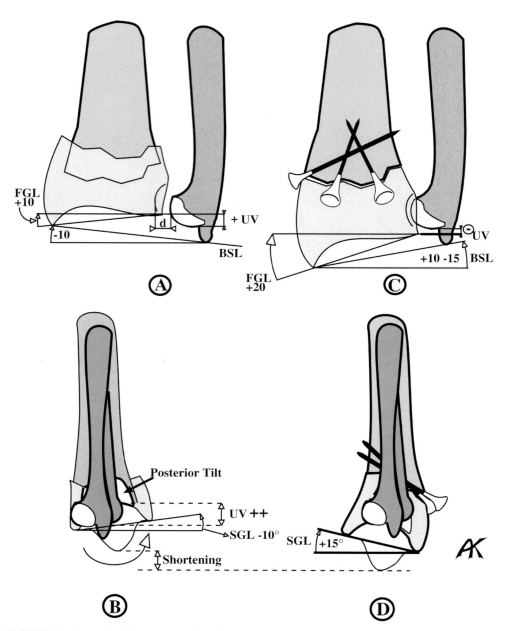

**FIGURE 15.** X-ray criteria. **A:** Front view showing a posterolateral displacement; BSL: the obliquity of this line is inverted, and may become negative; FGL: its value diminishes or becomes negative; UV: it becomes also positive. **B:** Side view showing posterior tilt; SGL: side glenoid line becomes negative; UV: it becomes positive, as a shortening is visible, associated with the posterior tilt; **(C–D)** normal or after reduction. **C:** Front view; BSL: bistyloid line (+10–15°) normal inclination; FGL, or radial inclination angle (+20°); UV, ulnar variance (–2 m/m). **D:** Side view; SGL: side glenoid line (+15°), so the distal radial surface faces downward and slightly forward.

- Gently unscrew the arum nut (Fig. 14F) three or four turns to allow the freshly cut pin end to house itself into the small space located in the base of the arum, so that it cannot harm the tendons. The base of the arum nut should be level with the subcutaneous tissues.
- Use an intradermal suture to close the skin, not only for aesthetic reasons but because this type of suture requires less skin on either side of the incision compared with regular stitches. An intradermal suture keeps the cutaneous wrist perimeter from being diminished and lessens the risk of edema. For this reason, transversal incisions are preferred.

Figure 15 shows the fracture schemas (A, B) before and (C, D) after reduction with proper positioning of the three pins.

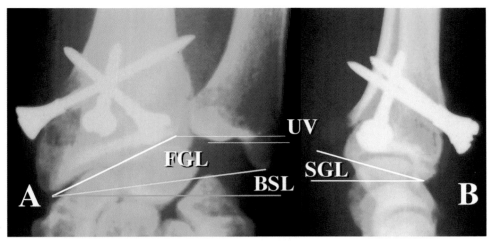

**FIGURE 16.** X-rays results. **A:** Front view after the setting of three pins. **B:** Side view. BSL, bistyloid line; FG, front glenoid line; SGL, side glenoid line; UV, ulnar variance.

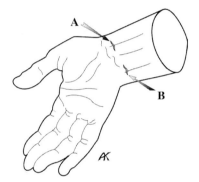

**FIGURE 17.** Two anterior approaches, each using short transversal incisions. **A:** The anterolateral approach (G. Hoël). **B:** The anteromedial approach (A. Kapandji).

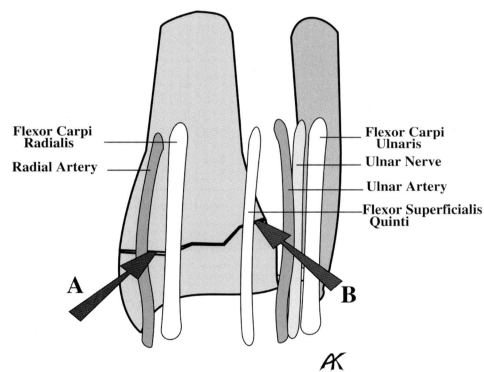

**FIGURE 18.** Two anterior approaches for inserting arum pins. **A:** The anterolateral approach, between the tendon of the flexor carpi radialis and the radial artery. **B:** The anteromedial approach, between the tendons of the flexors digitorum, especially the flexors quinti and the ulnar nerve and artery flanked by the tendon of the flexor carpi ulnaris.

■ Obtain radiographs of the pinned area and compare them with preoperative radiographs to evaluate (Fig. 16) the results of the surgery.

## FRACTURES WITH ANTERIOR TILT

It is possible to insert two anterior pins (Fig. 17) (4). Two methods may be used (Fig. 18).

In the first, insert one anterolateral pin (Fig. 18A), through a short transversal approach on the anterior aspect of the wrist, at the lateral side of the flexor carpi

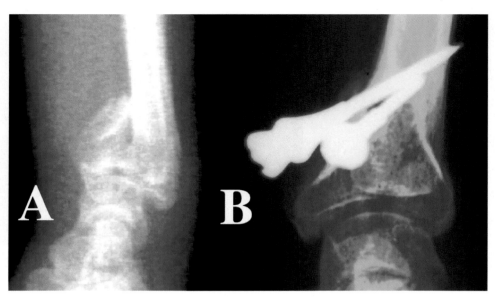

**FIGURE 19.** Side views of arum pins in an anterior tilt fracture. **A:** The fracture with an anterior tilt. **B:** The inserted arum pins. Note that the nut makes an abutment to the distal fragment. One of these pins is set laterally.

radialis. Dissect the subcutaneous tissues as previously described, so that the surface of the radius between the tendon and the radial artery may be visualized and protected. Set the pins as previously described. The arum pin screwed between the two borders is tolerated by both the tendon and the artery.

A second approach is possible for an anteromedial pin (Fig. 18B), at the lateral side of the flexor carpi ulnaris, through the interval between the ulnar artery and nerve and the tendons of the flexor quinti superficialis and profundus. There is no danger to the tendon, nerve, and artery because of the smooth shape of the arum nut.

Thus, this kind of fracture may be reduced and fixed with anterior pins (Fig. 19).

### Number of Pins

A maximum of five pins are inserted around the wrist (Fig. 20), if they are inserted through transverse incisions: two anterior (Fig. 20A, B), one lateral (Fig. 20C), and two posterior (Fig. 20D, E). This configuration allows the fixation of multifragment fractures, particularly in the case of frontal split.

## REHABILITATION

Have the patient begin gentle rehabilitation the day after surgery. I do not advocate casting or splinting, because the advantage of the immediate mobilization and rehabilitation is lost. Even a temporary cast should be avoided, because of the risk of a neuro-algo-dystrophic syndrome. Patients are encouraged to use the hand and wrist.

## POSTOPERATIVE MANAGEMENT

After 5 weeks, remove the pins: Unscrewing the arum nut takes off the pin simultaneously, because the shears squeeze the threading and block the pin in the nut. General or regional anesthesia and tourniquet are necessary during removal, because of the risk of damaging the nerve under local anesthesia.

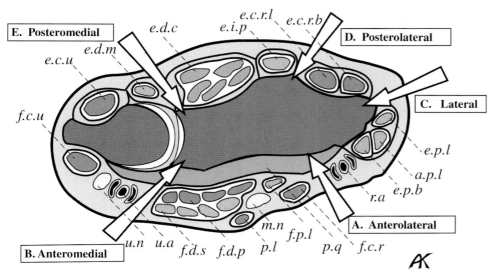

**FIGURE 20.** The five approaches for inserting arum pins around the wrist: Anterolateral (A), anteromedial (B), lateral (C), posterolateral (D), posteromedial (E). a.p.l., abductor pollicis longus; e.c.r.b., extensor carpi radialis brevis; e.c.r.l., extensor carpi radialis longus; e.c.u., extensor carpi ulnaris; e.d.c., extensor digitorum communis; e.d.m., extensor digiti minimi; e.i.p., extensor indicis proprius; e.p.b., extensor pollicis brevis; e.p.l., extensor pollicis longus; f.c.r., flexor carpi radialis; f.c.u., flexor carpi ulnaris; f.d.p., flexor digitorum profundus; f.d.s., flexor digitorum superficialis; f.p.l., flexor pollicis longus; m.n., median nerve; p.l., palmaris longus; p.q., pronator quadratus; r.a., radial artery; u.a., ulnar artery; u.n., ulnar nerve.

## COMPLICATIONS

### Intraoperative Complications

Damage to a nerve branch, which may cause transitory paresthesias (6.75%), can be avoided if the approach is significantly extensive. The skin incision is less than 7 to 8 mm, and the subcutaneous tissues are dissected bluntly not transected.

Damage to tendons is avoided if they are visualized directly and gently detracted.

Some surgeons have reported hyper-reductions, with an undesirable anterior tilt, if pins are set too vertically: Their obliquity must not be greater than 45°. However, the anterior tilt may be counteracted by inserting an anterior pin.

### Postoperative Complications

Most complications with distal radius fractures are caused by early technical mistakes. In one case, sepsis was halted when the pins were removed. IFAP precludes pin expulsion and tendon damage. Damage to the subcutaneous nerves must be avoided due to the risk of neuroma.

### Malunion

Malunion may occur in 4% of cases of posterior or lateral tilt reproduction; for the most part, they do not compromise good function (8). On the whole, the functional results with IFAP are better than with other procedures, except when the DRUJ is involved. Because the distal fragment is compressed upwardly or laterally, dislocation of the DRUJ may jeopardize the pronation-supination motion, as in other types of treatment.

Paradoxically, the main difficulty in cases of malunion is not the flexion-extension restrictions, but rather pronation-supination limitations, which necessitate specific actions on the DRUJ (Kapandji-Sauvé procedure), not on the malunion itself.

Neuro-algo-dystrophic syndrome, the most dangerous complication in all kinds of treatment, is rare (4%) (5–7).

## REFERENCES

1. Kapandji, A.: Ostéosynthèse par double embrochage intra-focal. Traitement fonctionnel des fractures non articulaires de l'extrémité inférieure du radius. *Ann. Chir.*, 30: 903–908, 1976.
2. Kapandji, A.: L'embrochage intra-focal des fractures de l'extrémité inférieure du radius dix ans après. *Ann. Chir. Main.*, 6: 57–63, 1987.
3. Kapandji, A.: Les broches Intra-Focales à "effet de réduction" de type "Arum" dans l'ostéosynthèse des fractures de l'extrémité inférieure du Radius. *Ann. Chir. Main.*, 10: 138–145, 1991.
4. Hoël, G.: La voie antero-externe pour le brochage intra-focal des fracture de l'extrémité inférieure du radius à déplacement antérieur. Communication at The International Symposium on the Wrist - Nagoya March 1991. Monography published under the direction of R. Nakamura, R. Linscheid, and T. Miura. Springer Verlag Editor Tokyo 1992.
5. Dunaud, J. L.: L'embrochage intra-focale "en berceau" des fractures de l'extrémité inférieure du radius. Incidence de ce traitement en matière de réparation des dommages corporels. Memoire pour le CES de réparation juridique du dommage corporel (N° 02100 Saint Quentin), Université R. Descartes Paris V, 1983–1984.
6. Dunaud, J. L., Caron, M., Ben Slama, H., Kharrat, M.: Technique de Kapandji et son évolution dans le traitement des fractures de l'extremité inférieure du radius. Á propos de 159 cas. *Ann. Chir. Main.*, 6: 109–122, 1987.
7. Epinette, J. A., Lehut, J. M., Cavenaille, M., Bouretz, J. C., Decoulx, J.: Fractures de Pouteau-Colles: double embrochage intra-focal "en berceau" selon Kapandji. A propos d'une série homogène de 72 cas. *Ann. Chir. Main.*, 1: 71–83, 1982.
8. McQueen, M., Caspers, J.: Colles' fractures: does the anatomic result affect the final function? *J. Bone Joint Surg.*, 70B: 649–51, 1980.

# 7

# Fixation Using Norian SRS Bone Cement

Colin W. Fennell

## PREOPERATIVE PLANNING

A number of classifications (2) have been proposed to guide the management of distal radius fractures. Use of Norian SRS bone cement may be indicated in those fractures of mid-range complexity. Fractures that are displaced but not highly comminuted, along the articular surfaces in patients who would benefit from an early active rehabilitation program, are appropriate for use of bone cement.

Norian SRS consists of powdered calcium phosphate and calcium carbonate that is mixed in the operating room with calcium phosphate solution to produce an injectable paste. The curing of the paste produces a hardened material at body temperature in approximately 10 minutes. Crystallization continues for 24 seconds; the final product resembles human cancellous bone, both structurally and chemically (3). In fracture fixation, the space-occupying capability of Norian SRS potentially eliminates the need for autogenous or allograft bone graft. In addition to and distinctly different from standard cancellous bone graft, SRS is able to provide structural support in compression (measured by the manufacturer) to be equal to that of human cancellous bone (1,3). However, structure does not provide strength in torsion or shear and cannot be relied on to resist those forces. The SRS material is ultimately removed from the site of implantation by osteoclast activity. The rate of removal as seen radiographically is somewhat location dependent (more peripheral locations are remodeled faster) and volume dependent. Theoretically, rate of removal would be slowed by adjunctive use of bisphosphates, which impair osteoclastic remodeling. Resorption typically is at a rate of 30% to 60% in the first year (4).

The ideal candidate for use of Norian SRS in a distal radius fracture has a displaced fracture with comminution of a degree that is reconstructable by means of manipulation, pin, limited open reduction, or external fixation. The articular surface is reconstructable and reducible (5).

Use of SRS is contraindicated in the case of an unreconstructable joint surface that is not capable of containing the cement within the fracture site. A relative

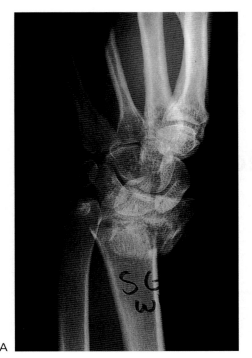
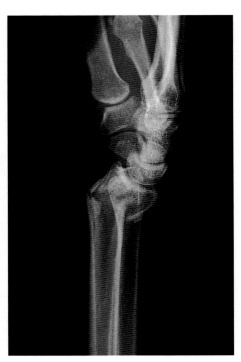

**FIGURE 1.** Anteroposterior view **(A)** and lateral view **(B)** of dorsally displaced distal radius fracture.

contraindication is the fracture that has a shear configuration, such as the radial styloid or volar/dorsal rim fracture. Once the fracture has been stabilized with other techniques, SRS is used to supplement treatment. It is not used alone as a fixation method. Use of SRS in the presence of an open fracture has not been studied to date. At present, an open fracture is a contraindication for cement use.

## PREOPERATIVE PLANNING

The traumatic event is usually a fall on an outstretched hand. On routine examination, the degree of deformity and the presence or absence of open wounds is noted. A neurologic assessment, including both sensory and motor evaluation of the terminal function of the ulnar, median, and posterior interosseous nerve, is carried out. A general history of salient features that preclude operative management is obtained.

Routine radiographic assessment using posteroanterior, lateral, and oblique films is necessary to evaluate the extent of the injury (Fig. 1). If there is to be any delay before surgery, do a closed reduction of the fracture using a hematoma block. Obtain repeat x-rays to evaluate further the status of the fracture. Additional assessment of complex intraarticular fractures may be conducted by computed tomography scan.

Check the radiographs specifically for fracture components that are the result of shear forces, such as the radial styloid, volar, or dorsal lip segments, because SRS will not resist displacement of fragments that are subject to shear forces. Those components must be identified and a plan developed for fixation that would neutralize the stress by pin, plate, or external fixation.

## SURGERY

Equipment required depends on the extent of fixation planned for the fracture. A radiolucent hand table and an image intensifier are necessary. The ability to apply

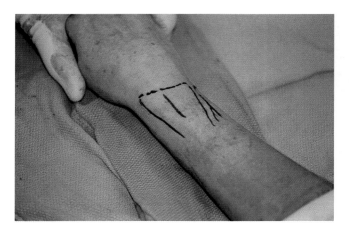

**FIGURE 2.** Closed reduction of fracture performed using fluoroscopic assessment: outline of distal radius and planned incision line.

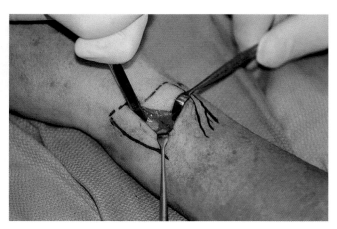

**FIGURE 3.** Make an incision between the second and third dorsal extensor compartments. Dissect down to level of dorsal cortex. Place a flat elevator into the fracture to impact the bone fragments.

longitudinal traction on the hand table or vertically with the traction tower may simplify holding the reduction on occasion. A #15 scalpel, K-wire driver and small retractors, periosteal elevator, irrigation tip, and the Norian SRS injection/mixing set are the instruments required in most cases. The working time of the cement is somewhat temperature sensitive and is reduced by higher temperature; thus, ideally, the operating room should be reduced to 18° to 20°C at the onset of the surgery.

Anesthetic can be general or regional. Bier blocks should not be used, however. As part of the procedure, the tourniquet must be released to permit blood to flow around the cement, allowing it to cure in a hydrated environment at body temperature.

In sterile conditions prepare the hand and forearm, and lay them on the hand table. Use the image intensifier and manipulate the fracture to an acceptable reduction (Fig. 2). Although there is no absolute agreement on what constitutes an acceptable reduction, a fracture with the following parameters is considered well reduced: alignment of the distal lunate facet equidistant with the ulna articular surface, angle of 0° to 10° of volar flexion; radial angle greater than 15°; radial height greater than 1 cm, with radial/ulnar/dorsal/volar translation less than 1 mm; and articular surface congruent to within 1 mm of step and 2 mm of gap.

Make a 2-cm incision over the fracture, typically on the radial side of Lister's tubercle (Fig. 3). Cut the retinaculum longitudinally and expose the dorsum of the distal radius between the second and third dorsal compartments. Introduce a periosteal elevator into the fractured and crushed bone. The extent of damaged bone is typically greater than the radiography suggests.

It is crucial that all damaged bone be compacted to maximize the size of the fracture void, contrary to traditional fracture training to preserve native bone. Micro-fractured bone, however, does not have normal structural strength and will not withstand early functional stress. For the cement implanted to withstand those stresses without shifting, it must be resting on stable compacted bone. Use the periosteal elevator to elevate any articular segment back to an acceptable alignment if this alignment has not already been achieved. Thoroughly irrigate the fracture void to remove any clot and particulate debris. Place the forearm back under the image intensifier and use a probe to map out the extent of the fracture void (Fig. 4).

Use gentle traction to hold the fracture reduced. If no segments of the fracture are likely to be subjected to shear forces, two percutaneous K-wires introduced from the radial styloid across the fracture will provide sufficient interim fixation. Make a small cutaneous cut and reach the styloid with blunt dissection, using a small fine-tip forceps.

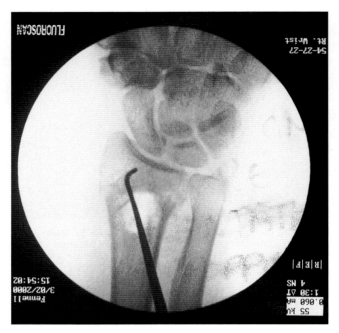

**FIGURE 4.** Use a probe to assess the fracture void to determine the adequacy of the impaction.

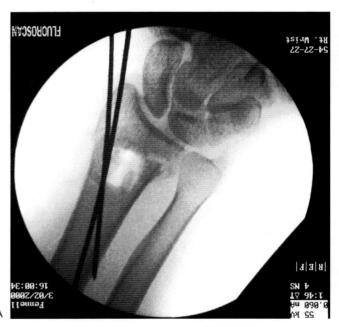
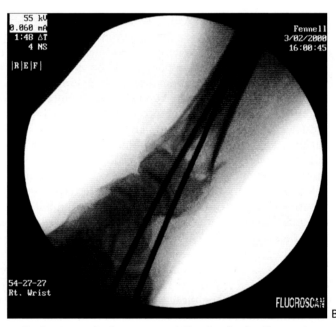

**FIGURE 5.** Introduce percutaneous K-wires across the fracture to stabilize the distal radius segment. Transverse subcortical wires may be used if the fracture also has lunate facet fracturing. Then irrigate the fracture void to remove loose debris. **A:** Anteroposterior view. **B:** Lateral view.

Drive two 0.54 K-wires across the fracture (Fig. 5). If necessary, introduce percutaneous transverse K-wires from the radial side under the subchondral surface to finalize the fixation.

Each recess of the void should be accessible without obstruction. Map out the fracture void. Confirm that the fracture is reduced in an acceptable position, then begin mixing the SRS cement. Mixing of the material is automated and requires approximately 90 seconds.

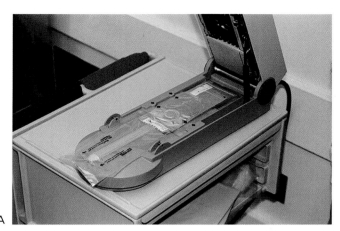

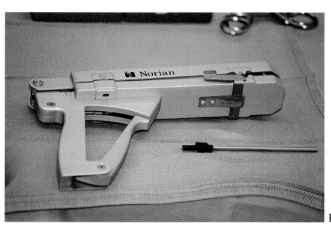

A                                                                                      B

**FIGURE 6. A:** Norian SRS is available with an automated mixer and is mixed in a peel-back pouch. **B:** Once mixed, it is inserted into the injection gun. At room temperature, there is a 5-minute working time with this material.

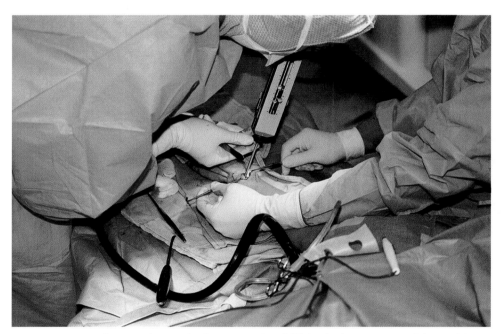

**FIGURE 7.** Insert the cannula into the fracture void and fill the farthest recesses of the void first.

Load the mixed cement tube into the application gun (Fig. 6). Typically, a small-diameter injection needle (#12 or #14 Fr) is used; larger-bore needles are not required, as the SRS cement is thixotropic and will flow easily down a narrow-diameter tube. Large-bore injection needles on occasion will inhibit access to the recesses of the fracture void, thus should not be used routinely.

Injecting the material is similar to using a caulking gun. Use the retrograde filling technique. Fill the furthermost aspect of the fracture first and gradually withdraw the injection needle (Fig. 7). As the void is filled, use the image intensifier at this stage to ensure that the cement is flowing to the full extent of the fracture void and is being contained within the fracture (Fig. 8). Once the fracture void is filled, any excess cement on the dorsal surface can be wiped off with a sponge. Working time during which the cement remains liquid enough to be injected is approxi-

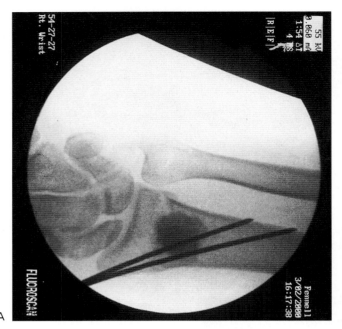
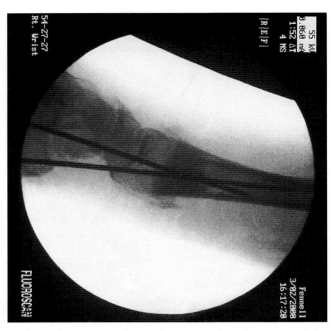

A                                                                                    B

**FIGURE 8.** When the material has filled the hole, use fluoroscopy to confirm the extent of the "fracture fill." **A:** Anteroposterior view. **B:** Lateral view. Deflate the tourniquet and allow the SRS to sit for 10 minutes. Wipe off excess SRS in the soft tissues, using a sponge.

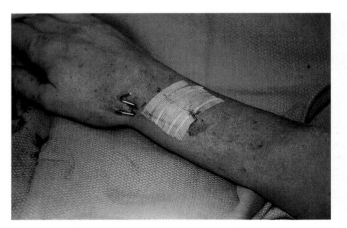

**FIGURE 9.** Close the wound with absorbable sutures.

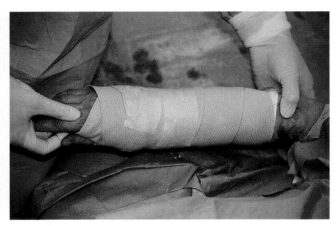

**FIGURE 10.** Use a short-arm volar plaster splint for postoperative protection.

mately 5 minutes—usually far more time than is required to finish the injection. Typically, 2 to 3 cc of material will fill a distal radius fracture void.

Once the injection of cement is complete, deflate the tourniquet to allow blood flow into the limb. The cement requires hydration to crystallize; if kept dry, it will dehydrate and crumble. Allow the cement to set, without being disturbed, for 10 minutes, then examine the fracture under the C-arm; the cement is densely radiopaque and is visualized easily. If cement has been injected into a joint inadvertently, an arthrotomy is recommended to remove the cement. In the few reported cases in which a small amount of cement did enter the joint, no discernible harm occurred.

Cut the K-wires external to the skin and bend them to prevent migration. Close the dorsal retinaculum and skin with absorbable suture (Fig. 9). Dress the pin sites with Betadine ointment, pad them, and apply a volar plaster splint (Fig. 10).

## POSTOPERATIVE MANAGEMENT

The patient can be discharged the same day, usually with nothing more than acetaminophen and codeine for analgesia. Encourage the patient to keep the hand elevated above heart level as much as possible for the next 72 hours. Encourage finger, elbow, and shoulder exercises. Use of the hand for simple assisting activities such as dressing, eating, and grooming, is permitted.

The pins that are not stabilizing shear-sensitive fragments theoretically can be removed in 24 hours. It is often more practical, however, to leave them *in situ* until the splint is removed at 2 weeks. At that time the pins can be taken out, the splint removed, and the hand placed in a removable wrist brace. Have the patient begin wrist range-of-motion and forearm-strengthening exercises at the 2-week stage. In cases in which major shear fragments have been stabilized using pins, pin removal and mobilization should be performed 5 to 6 weeks postoperatively.

## COMPLICATIONS

Pin-track infections are perhaps the most common complication when this technique is used for distal radial fixation. The frequency of infection, however, is no greater with this procedure than with any other technique that uses pins. Because of the structural integrity of the SRS, remove noncritical pins if there is any redness or purulence at the pin site. Preserve pins that were used for maintenance of fragments subjected to shear forces (e.g., radial styloid), however, and treat the patient with oral antibiotics and daily pin care with peroxide. Other complications that have been reported with this technique, such as extensor pollicis rupture or reflex dystrophy, do not appear to occur at a rate any different from what is expected with cast treatment alone.

Intraarticular injection of SRS has been reported. Follow-up x-rays over a 2-year period showed the material to have marginalized in the joint with no evidence of inflammatory or degenerative reaction. Should an intraarticular injection of SRS occur, a miniarthrotomy and evacuation of the material is recommended as soon as such an injection is observed.

## RECOMMENDED READING

1. Constantz, B. R., Ison, I. C., Fulmer, M. T., et al.: Skeletal repair by *in situ* formation of the mineral phase of bone. *Science*, 267: 1796–1799, 1995.
2. Fernandes, D. L., Jupiter, J. B., eds.: *Fractures of the Distal Radius.* Springer-Verlag, New York, 1996.
3. Frankenburg, E. P., Goldstein, S. A., Bauer, T. W., et al.: Biomechanical and histological evaluation of a calcium phosphate cement. *J. Bone Joint Surg.*, 80A: 1112–1123, 1998.
4. Ladd, A. L., Pliam, N. B.: Use of bone-graft substitutes in distal radius fractures. *J. Am. Acad. Orthop. Surg.*, 7(5): 279–290, 1999.
5. Yetkinler, D. N., Ladd, A. L., Poser, R. D., et al.: Biomechanical evaluation of fixation of intra-articular fractures of the distal part of the radius in cadavera: Kirschner wires compared with calcium phosphate bone cement. *J. Bone Joint Surg.*, 81A: 391–399, 1999.

# PART IV

# Nonunions of the Distal Radius

# 8

# Use of the LoCon T Plate with Distal Radius Osteotomy

Gary S. Shapiro and Andrew J. Weiland

Malunion of the distal radius is more common in the wrist than in any other anatomic site. Early and late loss of reduction and consequent malunion occurs in approximately 5% of patients (1).

The malunited distal radius typically is caused by a fall on a pronated outstretched hand, resulting in loss of radial inclination, loss of volar tilt, and radial shortening (2,12). Radial shortening causes a positive ulnar variance, leading to problems with the distal ulna, such as ulnar impaction and disruption of the distal radioulnar joint. Osteotomy can restore or improve the architecture of the distal radius and its relationship with the ulna and carpus (15).

The LoCon T plate is an internal-fixation device that conforms to the dorsal aspect of the distal radius. The low-profile design of the plate allows for reconstruction of the extensor retinaculum and provides rigid internal fixation of the osteotomy site.

## INDICATIONS/CONTRAINDICATIONS

Symptomatic malunion can cause weakness, stiffness, and pain in the wrist. Alterations in the radial inclination, rotation, and tilt create more concentrated forces through the carpus on the contact surfaces of the radius and ulna. Change in volar tilt of 10° to a dorsal tilt of 45° increases the load through the ulna from 21% to 67% (13). Pain and functional impairment correlate with inadequacy of reduction (11). Various prospective studies have focused on the relationship between anatomy and function (5,6). Malunion is defined as (a) loss of volar tilt greater than 20°; (b) radial inclination less than 10°; and (c) radial shortening more than 2 mm.

Malunion may lead to pain, loss of motion, arthritis, weakness, carpal instability, cosmetic deformity, delayed neuropathy, and tendon rupture. Dorsal tilting may produce a carpal collapse pattern similar to that seen in dorsal intercalated segment instability but without interosseous ligament disruption or secondary midcarpal instability (10,14).

Candidates for surgery include manually active patients with pain and loss of function after a malunited fracture. Loss of volar tilt, when associated with shortening of the fracture fragment of the distal end of the radius, may result in dysfunction of the distal radioulnar joint, manifested by limited rotation of the forearm and impingement of the ulna on the radius (9).

In laboratory studies, malalignment of the radius caused reduction of the radioulnar contact area, disruption of the deep portion of the dorsal radioulnar ligament, tightness of the triangular fibrocartilage complex, and limited forearm pronation and supination (8). Further alterations have been found concerning the carpal kinematics, the force transmission through the wrist, and the pressure distribution on the articular surface of the radius and the median nerve.

The aims of radial osteotomy are to restore function and improve the appearance of the wrist by correction of the deformity at the level of the old fracture. The optimal timing of the procedure is controversial. Some surgeons recommend waiting 6 weeks to allow soft tissue swelling to subside and allow for functional range of motion of the fingers (3). We advocate early correction to prevent arthritis, dysfunction of the radioulnar joint, and a longer period of disability, as shown by Jupiter and Ring (7).

Additional procedures on the ulna have been described in addition to radial osteotomy to correct incongruity of the distal radioulnar joint. Fernandez used a Darrach procedure, especially in cases with degenerative changes in the distal radioulnar joint, but expressed concern over loss of grip strength, loss of carpal support by the ulna, and instability of the ulnar stump (2). Functional requirements, patient age, and motivation must also be considered.

Contraindications to corrective osteotomy include significant radiocarpal or intercarpal arthritis, limited functional capacities, extensive osteoporosis, and fixed carpal malalignment.

## PREOPERATIVE PLANNING

Take a detailed history and perform a physical examination to discern the mechanism of injury and previous treatment the patient has received. Ascertain the patient's ability to perform daily activities. Test the wrist and forearm for motion and strength, and compare the limb to the contralateral extremity. Measure flexion/extension, pronation/supination, and radial/ulnar deviation on both wrists, using a goniometer. Test the grip strength of both hands.

The basic radiographic evaluation of a malunited distal radius fracture includes both a posteroanterior and lateral radiograph (Fig. 1). Contralateral wrist films are helpful for comparison of ulnar variance. Three basic radiographic measurements can be obtained from these standard views. In the uninjured wrist, the average sagittal plane volar tilt of the distal radial articular surface is 11° to 12°. The average frontal plane radial inclination measures 22° to 23°. The radial length averages 11 to 12 mm (4) (Figs. 2, 3).

Calculate the size of the opening wedge osteotomy that must be made to restore radial length and reconstruct the deformity in all planes. Posteroanterior views in a neutral forearm rotation and true lateral radiograph serve as guides for the reconstruction. The maximum that can be gained without an accompanying ulnar shortening procedure is 10 to 12 mm of radial length.

A computed tomography scan may be helpful to define further the deformity preoperatively.

## SURGERY

Place the patient in a supine position, with the hand on the arm table. Place a tourniquet on the upper arm set to 250 mm Hg (Figs. 4, 5). Use either regional or

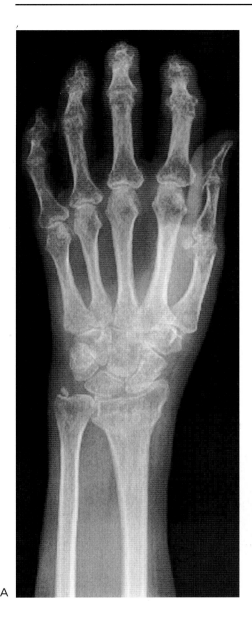

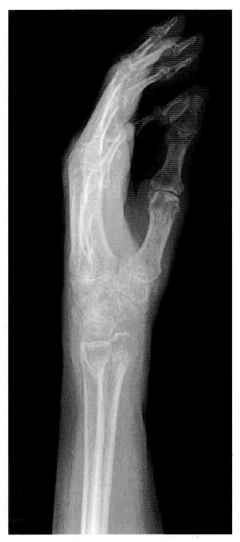

A

B

**FIGURE 1.** Anteroposterior **(A)** and lateral radiographs **(B)** showing radial shortening, dorsal tilt, and loss of radial inclination.

general anesthesia. Administer an intravenous dose of a cephalosporin to nonallergic patients before inflating the tourniquet. If the patient has an allergy, use either clindamycin or vancomycin. Prep and drape the ipsilateral iliac crest. If regional block is used, administer local anesthetic to the iliac crest.

### Dorsal Approach (Freeland and Geisler, Mississippi)

Make a 10-cm longitudinal incision over the dorsal radial side of the distal forearm, just lateral to Lister's tubercle (Figs. 6, 7). Do not incise the dorsal radiocarpal ligament. Incise the extensor retinaculum longitudinally over the third compartment, just ulnar to Lister's tubercle. Identify and resect the terminal branch of the posterior interosseous nerve. Elevate the soft tissue from the distal radius to both sides, reflecting the fourth dorsal compartment ulnarly and the second dorsal compartment radially.

Place small Hohmann retractors on both sides of the radius to enhance exposure (Figs. 8, 9). Take care to protect the first dorsal compartment and the extrinsic fin-

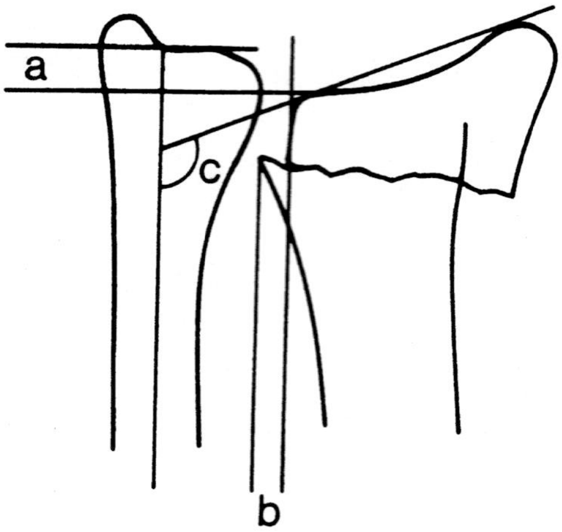

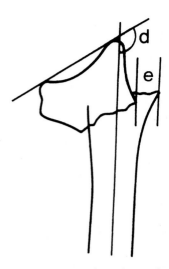

**FIGURE 2.** Anteroposterior radiograph parameters. Radial shortening (a): The difference in level between the distal ulnar surface and ulnar part of the distal radial surface. Radial displacement (b): The displacement of the distal fragment in relation to the radial shaft. Radial angle (c): The angle of the distal surface in relation to the long axis of the radius. (From Abbaszadegam, H., Jonsson, U., Von Sivers, K.: Prediction of instability of Colles' fractures. *Acta Orthop. Scand.,* 60: 646–650, 1989, with permission.)

**FIGURE 3.** Lateral radiographic parameters. Dorsal angle (d): The angle of the distal radial surface in relation to the long axis of the radius. Dorsal displacement (e): The distance of the distal radial fragment in relation to the radial shaft. (From Abbaszadegam, H., Jonsson, U., Von Sivers, K.: Prediction of instability of Colles' fractures *Acta Orthop. Scand.,* 60: 646–650, 1989, with permission.)

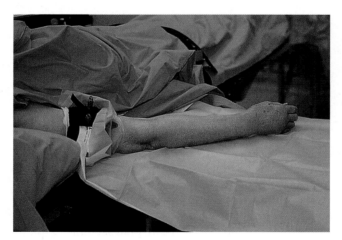

**FIGURE 4.** Right upper extremity positioned on radiolucent table with pneumatic tourniquet in place.

ger extensors. Place a 0.045-mm Kirschner wire into the radiocarpal joint in the plane of the distal radius. Place a second wire ½ cm proximal to the joint, perpendicular to the dorsal cortex. The first and second wires need to be parallel. Place a third wire perpendicular to the proximal fragment. The angle between wires two and three is the correction to be achieved (Fig. 10).

Perform an osteotomy with an oscillating saw through the previous fracture site, 2 to 3 cm proximal and parallel to the articular surface. Do not disrupt the volar cortex. Place a laminar spreader to open the osteotomy. The second and third wires must be parallel to ensure correction of the deformity.

Take a trapezoidal unicortical bone graft from the iliac crest. Place the corticocancellous graft and hold it with K-wires. Check the correction radiographically.

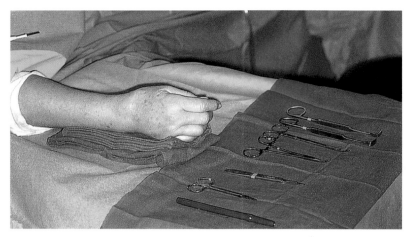

**FIGURE 5.** Arm is prepped and draped in standard sterile fashion.

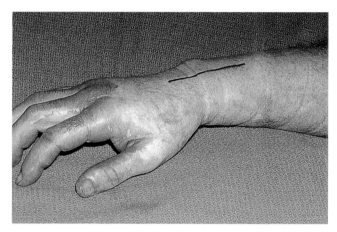

**FIGURE 6.** The dorsal incision is centered over the distal radius, immediately ulnar to Lister's tubercle, extending to the wrist crease.

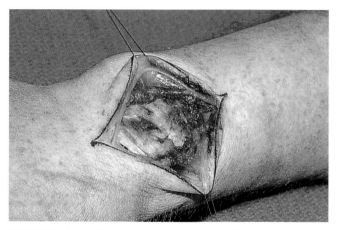

**FIGURE 7.** The subcutaneous tissue is spread bluntly, exposing the dorsal aspect of the extensor retinaculum.

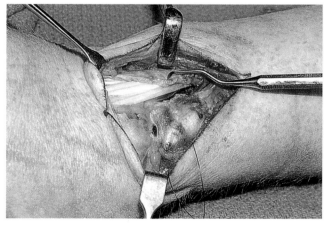

**FIGURE 8.** The extensor retinaculum is incised longitudinally over the fourth dorsal compartment, exposing the tendons of the extensor digitorum communis and extensor indicis proprius. The probe is pointing to the dorsal aspect of the extensor retinaculum.

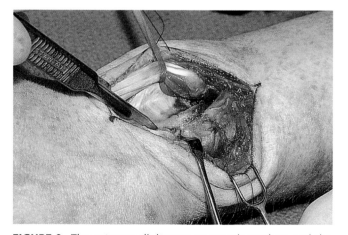

**FIGURE 9.** The extensor digitorum communis tendons and the extensor indicis proprius tendon are retracted ulnarly with a moistened umbilical tape, exposing the infratendinous retinaculum. The distal radial metaphysis is exposed, subperiosteally dissecting the infratendinous retinaculum and periosteum as one continuous layer.

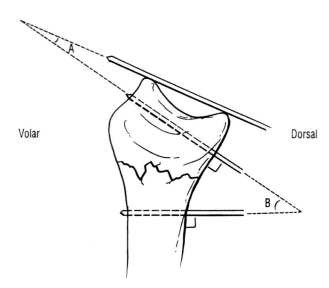

A, 11 degree dorsal of the articular tilt platform;
B, sagittal plane deformity to be corrected.

A

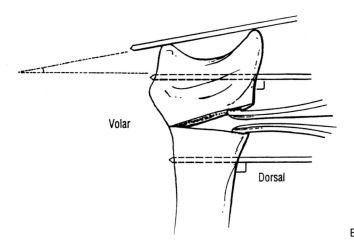

**FIGURE 10. A** and **B:** Preoperative planning of the osteotomy: For correction in the sagittal plane, K-wires are introduced using the angle of dorsal tilt from the lateral radiograph. (From Hunt and Osterman: Surgical Reconstruction of the Upper Extremity, Chapter 33, Figure 33-4 C and F, pp. 659–660, 1999, with permission.)

Once the volar tilt, radial length, and inclination are assessed, put an oblique LoCon T plate in place. Position at least two 2.7- or 3.5-mm cortical screws proximally and distally (Fig. 11).

Transpose the extensor pollicis longus tendon subcutaneously and repair the extensor retinaculum using 3–0 ethibond suture. The low-profile design of the plate allows for easy closure of the retinaculum (Fig. 12). Close using 3–0 vicryl suture in the subcutaneous tissue and 4–0 monocril on the skin. Immobilize the wrist in a sugar-tong plaster splint with the wrist in neutral rotation.

### Volar Approach

Make the incision directly over the flexor carpi radialis (Fig. 13). Carry it through the subcutaneous tissue (Fig. 14). Incise the palmar sheath of the flexor carpi radialis longitudinally and retract the tendon (Fig. 15). Identify the radial artery lying on the soft tissue directly to the radial side of the tendon sheath. Incise the dorsal sheath of the flexor carpi radialis longitudinally, exposing the flexor pollicis longus (Fig. 16). Retract the flexor pollicis longus and flexor carpi radialis ulnarly to expose the pronator quadratus. Retract the radial artery and accompanying veins radially. Incise the insertion of the pronator quadratus longitudinally along the palmar radial border of the distal radius at its insertion, leaving a small cuff of tissue that can be sutured during closure (Fig. 17).

The technique for osteotomy has been outlined. Close the pronator quadratus with 3–0 ethibond suture. Close the subcutaneous tissue using 3–0 vicryl suture and 4–0 monocril on the skin. Immobilize the wrist in a sugar-tong plaster splint with the wrist in neutral rotation.

## POSTOPERATIVE MANAGEMENT

Remove the sutures 10 to 14 days after surgery, and apply a short-arm cast. Immobilize the arm for 4 to 6 weeks. Obtain radiographs postoperatively at 1, 2, and 4 weeks to assess bony alignment. When the short-arm cast is removed, place a removable wrist splint for an additional 2 to 4 weeks.

Expect postoperative stiffness to resolve over a 3- to 6-month period.

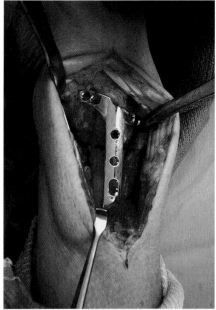
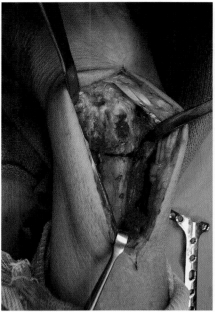
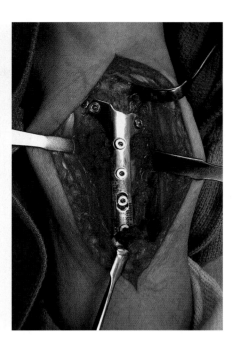

A–C

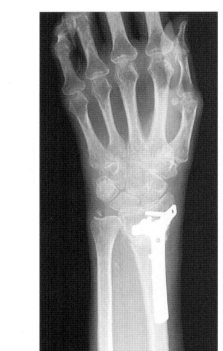
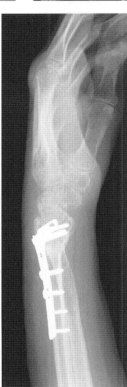

D,E

**FIGURE 11.** The appropriate plate is placed for inspection **(A)**, followed by osteotomy **(B)**, and plate fixation **(C)**. Postoperative anteroposterior radiograph **(D)**; postoperative lateral radiograph **(E)**.

## REHABILITATION

For optimal results after surgery, it is imperative to initiate aggressive therapy by a certified hand therapist. Begin active and passive finger motion immediately. Once the bone has healed, initiate wrist motion. The surgeon must be in close communication with the therapist to maximize results.

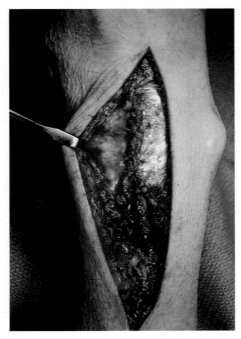

**FIGURE 12.** Close the extensor retinaculum with 3–0 ethibond suture. The low-profile plate allows for facilitated closure.

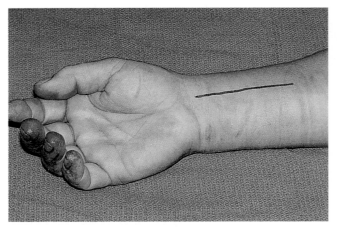

**FIGURE 13.** A longitudinal palmar approach provides excellent exposure of the distal radius for fixation of distal radius fractures, radial osteotomy, and harvesting distal radial bone graft. The incision begins at the juncture of the distal transverse wrist crease and flexor carpi radialis tendon and extends proximally along the radial shaft.

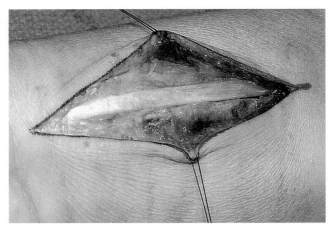

**FIGURE 14.** The subcutaneous tissue is spread bluntly directly over the flexor carpi radialis tendon. The tendon sheath is incised longitudinally.

## COMPLICATIONS

Complications after distal radial osteotomy include failure to achieve the desired alignment, nerve damage, nonunion at the osteotomy site, and limitation of pronosupination due to distal radioulnar joint capsule contracture.

### Illustrative Case

A 61-year-old woman sustained a fracture of her right dominant wrist in November 1999. She was treated with closed pinning and postoperative therapy to

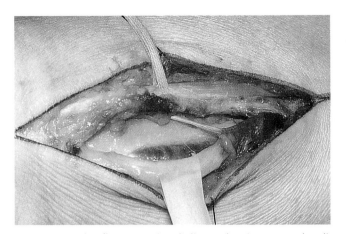

**FIGURE 15.** The flexor carpi radialis tendon is retracted radially with a moistened umbilical tape, and the median nerve and palmar cutaneous branch are identified in the ulnar portion of the incision. A soft rubber drain is placed around the median nerve to protect it from injury during the procedure.

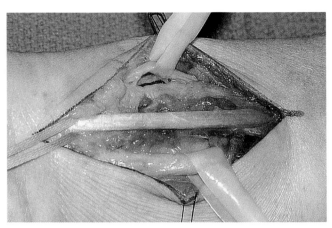

**FIGURE 16.** The radial artery is identified in the deep subcutaneous tissue on the radial side of the flexor carpi radialis tendon. It should be retracted with a soft rubber drain. A longitudinal incision in the dorsal aspect of the flexor carpi radialis tendon sheath exposes the flexor pollicis longus tendon.

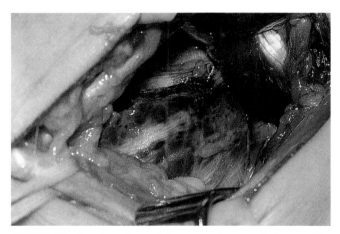

**FIGURE 17.** The insertion of the pronator quadratus on the distal radius is identified and incised longitudinally 5 mm from its insertion on the lateral edge of the distal radial metaphysis. The pronator quadratus then is dissected from the distal radius subperiosteally, reflecting it ulnarly.

regain motion. She presented to the office 6 months later with complaints of cosmetic deformity and weakened grip.

On physical examination, she had range of motion of 45° of flexion and extension with full forearm rotation. Clinically, she had significant deformity.

X-rays revealed the distal radius to have collapsed with respect to radial inclination and increasing positive ulnar variance (Fig. 18). Radial inclination was less than 10°, with a positive ulnar variance of 5 mm. Lateral projection revealed neutral volar tilt.

Due to her high level of activity and poor functional result secondary to the malunion, a corrective osteotomy with ICBG was performed. Her osteotomy site healed at 10 weeks (Fig. 19). She regained full motion of the wrist and has equal grip strength of the contralateral hand.

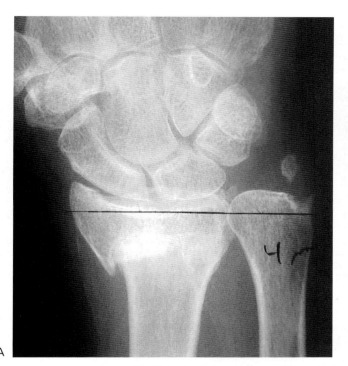
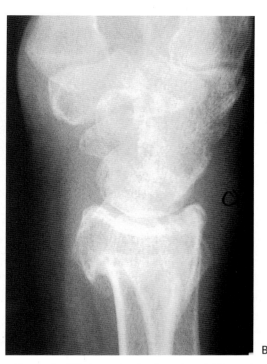

**FIGURE 18.** Anteroposterior **(A)** and lateral radiographs **(B)** show shortening, dorsal tilt, and loss of radial inclination.

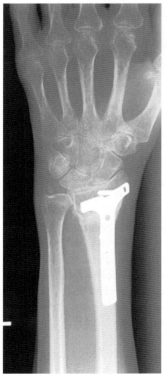
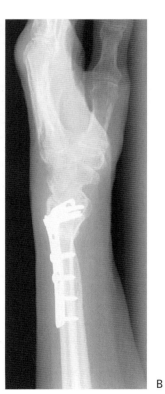

**FIGURE 19.** Anteroposterior **(A)** and lateral radiographs **(B)** after correction of deformity.

## RECOMMENDED READING

1. Cooney, W. P. III, Dobyns, J. H., Linscheid, R. L.: Complications of Colles' fracture. *J. Bone Joint Surg.*, 62: 613–619, 1980.
2. Fernandez, D. L.: Correction of post-traumatic wrist deformity in adults by osteotomy, bone grafting, and internal fixation. *J. Bone Joint Surg.*, 70A: 1164–1178, 1982.
3. Flinkkila, T., Raatikainen, T.: Corrective osteotomy for malunion of the distal radius. *Arch. Orthop. Trauma Surg.*, 120: 23–26, 2000.
4. Friberg, S., Lundstrom, B.: Radiographic measurements of the radio-carpal joint in normal adults. *Acta Radiol.*, 17: 249–256, 1976.
5. Howard, P. W., Stewart, H. D., Hind, R. E., Burke, F. D.: External fixation or plaster for severely displaced comminuted Colles' fractures? A prospective study of anatomical and functional results. *J. Bone Joint Surg.*, 71B: 68–73, 1989.
6. Jenkins, N. H., Jones, D. G., Johnson, S. R., Mintowt-Czyz, W. T.: External fixation of Colles' fractures: an anatomical study. *J. Bone Joint Surg.*, 69B: 207–211, 1987.
7. Jupiter, J. B., Ring, D.: A comparison of early and late reconstruction of malunited fractures of the distal end of the radius. *J. Bone Joint Surg.*, 78A: 739–748, 1996.
8. Kihara, H., Palmer, A. K., Werner, F. W., Short, W. H., Fortino, M. D.: The effect of dorsally angulated distal radius fractures on distal radioulnar joint congruency and forearm rotation. *J. Hand Surg.*, 21: 40–47, 1996.
9. Lidstrom, A.: Fractures of the distal end of the radius. A clinical and statistical study of end results. *Acta Orthop. Scand.*, Suppl. 41, 1959.
10. Linscheid, R. L., Dobyns, J. H., Beaubout, J. W., Bryan, R. S.: Traumatic instability of the wrist: diagnosis, classification, and pathomechanics. *J. Bone Joint Surg.*, 54A: 1612–1632, 1972.
11. McQueen, M., Caspers, J.: Does the anatomical result affect the final function? *J. Bone Joint Surg.*, 70B: 649–651, 1988.
12. Milch, H.: Treatment of disabilities following fractures of the lower end of the radius. *Clin. Orthop.*, 29: 157–163, 1963.
13. Short, W. H., Palmer, A. K., Werner, F. W., Murphy, D. J.: A biomechanical study of distal radius fractures. *J. Hand Surg.*, 12A: 529–534, 1987.
14. Taleisnik, J., Watson, H. K.: Midcarpal instability caused by malunited fractures of the distal radius. *J. Hand Surg.*, 9: 350–357, 1984.
15. Watson, H. K., Castle, T. H.: Trapezoidal osteotomy of the distal radius for unacceptable articular angulation after Colles' fracture. *J. Hand Surg.*, 13A: 837–843, 1988.

# PART V

## Scaphoid Fractures

# 9

# Scaphoid Fractures: Internal Fixation

Timothy J. Herbert and Hermann Krimmer

## INDICATIONS/CONTRAINDICATIONS

Scaphoid fractures (3) are common injuries in young males and normally occur as a result of a fall on the outstretched hand. It has been standard practice to treat the majority of scaphoid fractures with immobilization in plaster; this continues to be the most common method of treatment. Although there has been considerable disagreement over the type and duration of immobilization, currently it is recommended that a long-arm thumb spica cast be used for the first 6 weeks, followed by a short-arm thumb spica cast until clinical and radiologic signs of union are seen (2). In the past, surgery was reserved for the treatment of displaced fractures or for nonunion following conservative treatment.

The problem with this approach is that treatment is often prolonged for many months, particularly if primary healing is not achieved. Few patients can afford such a period of disability, and, as with other fractures, there is increasing demand for immediate and definitive treatment that enables a rapid return of normal function. Although this has led to an increased acceptance of internal fixation as an alternative to conservative treatment (7), many surgeons are reluctant to embrace this philosophy, presumably because of the perceived difficulty of the procedure. However, now that the advantages of internal fixation have been demonstrated (1), it is incumbent on those who treat a significant number of these injuries to master the techniques involved. Fortunately, these techniques have become simplified and refined (4) so that anyone with access to the necessary equipment should consider internal fixation as a viable alternative to immobilization in plaster.

The size, shape, and intraarticular position of the scaphoid bone, together with its precarious vascularity, dictates the use of small, accurately positioned implants capable of providing sufficiently secure fixation to allow for early joint mobilization. In this respect, headless bone screws are particularly suitable, because they

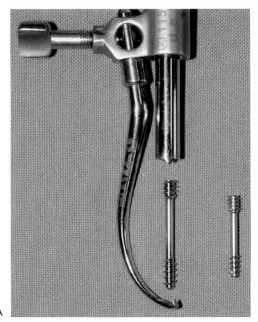
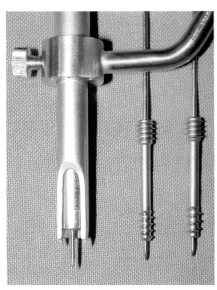

A                                                                                    B

**FIGURE 1.** Different headless bone screws used for scaphoid fixation. **A:** Standard Herbert Screw (normally used with guiding jig) and Mini-Herbert Screw, used for fixation of proximal pole fractures. **B:** Cannulated Herbert Bone Screw (HBS) system, showing drill guide, guide wire, and standard and high-compression screws.

can be buried beneath the articular surface and do not need to be removed later. The smaller the implant, the easier it is to insert and less likely to cause damage (Fig. 1). We believe that there is no longer need for standard bone screws in the treatment of scaphoid fractures.

Recent improvements in the quality and availability of intraoperative x-rays have led to the popularization of percutaneous methods of scaphoid fixation. There are obvious advantages that these methods have over the more traditional open approach (5,6,9,11). At the same time, a new generation of cannulated headless screws has been developed (Fig. 1B), since accurate positioning of the screw within the scaphoid is facilitated significantly by the use of a guide wire, inserted under x-ray control.

*Unstable* scaphoid fractures (*type B*) are an indication for internal fixation, since they are known to have a poor prognosis with conservative treatment. *Stable* scaphoid fractures (*type A2*) should be considered for internal fixation as well whenever treatment in a cast is not appropriate, for example, in the case of professional athletes (10) or patients with financial pressures that dictate an early return to work, which would not be possible in a plaster cast. Similarly, the management of patients with coexisting or multiple injuries is simplified significantly if the scaphoid fracture is internally fixed and plaster can be avoided.

Fractures of the tubercle of the scaphoid (*type A1*) have a good prognosis and rarely need immobilizing. Similarly, internal fixation is not indicated in the skeletally immature unless there is significant displacement, in which case open reduction and K-wire fixation are required.

Internal fixation is contraindicated in the presence of osteoporosis and/or stiffness of the wrist following immobilization in plaster. Under such circumstances, surgery should be delayed for a few weeks and therapy started immediately to overcome the adverse effects of immobilization.

Other contraindications include sepsis, systemic disease, algodystrophy, an uncooperative patient, or lack of the necessary equipment or surgical skills to perform this type of surgery.

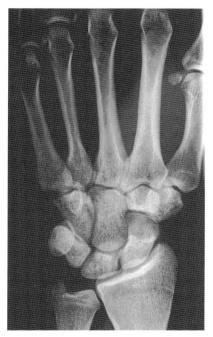
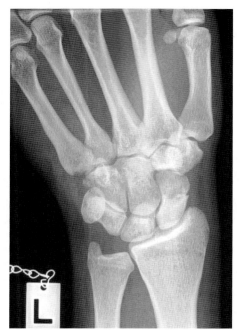
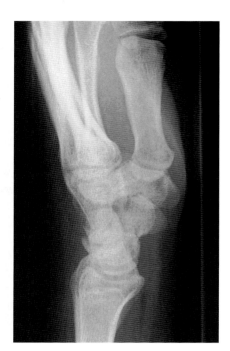

A–C

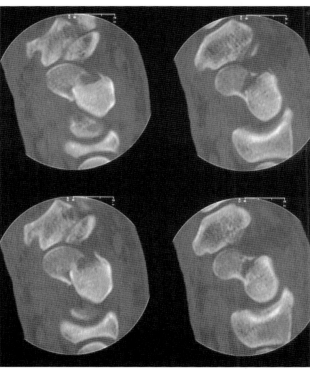

D

**FIGURE 2.** Views used to demonstrate an acute scaphoid fracture, type B2. Posteroanterior in radial deviation **(A)**, posteroanterior in ulnar deviation **(B)**, true lateral **(C)**, computed tomography scan **(D)** in the sagittal plane.

## PREOPERATIVE PLANNING

The diagnosis of an acute scaphoid fracture requires a high index of suspicion and awareness that there is no such thing as a "sprained wrist." High-quality x-rays of both wrists should include, at minimum, posteroanterior views with the wrist in full radial and ulnar deviation, together with true laterals, with the wrist in neutral position. If a fracture is suspected but cannot be demonstrated on the initial x-ray, a computed tomography (CT) bone scan should be ordered (8). A sagittal cut, parallel to the long axis of the scaphoid, is the best way to demonstrate the fracture and any associated deformity (Fig. 2). If the diag-

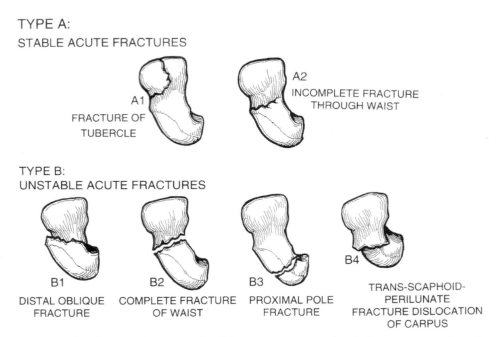

**FIGURE 3.** Classification of acute scaphoid fractures: type A1, tubercle fracture; type A2, undisplaced waist fracture; type B1, distal oblique fracture; type B2, displaced waist fracture; type B3, proximal pole fracture; type B4, comminuted fracture.

nosis is still unclear, arthroscopy is indicated, since acute scapholunate ligament injuries closely mimic scaphoid fracture. Even with high-quality x-rays and CT scans, it can be difficult to determine whether the fracture is stable: Although there may be no obvious displacement, the fracture may have the potential to displace in plaster, as is often the case with proximal pole fractures. For this reason, we prefer to plan management on the basis of fracture pattern, since retrospective studies have shown a close relationship between fracture type and the ultimate prognosis (1,3).

## Classification of Scaphoid Fractures

Figure 3 illustrates the classification of acute scaphoid fractures. Scaphoid fractures are classified as follows:

*Type A2*: Simple, undisplaced fractures of the wrist should be treated by *percutaneous fixation,* using the cannulated screw system.

*Type B1*: Distal oblique fractures are often highly unstable and have the potential to displace or collapse under load. For this reason, *open reduction (volar approach)* and supplementary K-wire fixation normally are required, although it is reasonable to attempt a closed reduction initially. If this is satisfactory, then closed screw fixation is appropriate, although a supplementary, parallel K-wire may be necessary for stability.

*Type B2*: Displaced wrist fractures may be suitable for *percutaneous fixation*, but only if an accurate closed reduction can be achieved. If not, they will require *open (volar)* reduction and fixation.

*Type B3*: Proximal pole fractures require *open (dorsal)* reduction, and should be fixed with a mini-screw, inserted freehand in an antegrade direction.

*Type B4*: Comminuted fractures require *open* reduction, bone grafting, and internal fixation, often via an *extended volar* approach or a *combined volar and dorsal* approach, depending on the extent of the associated carpal injuries. Please see Chapters 7, 8, and 10 for further details.

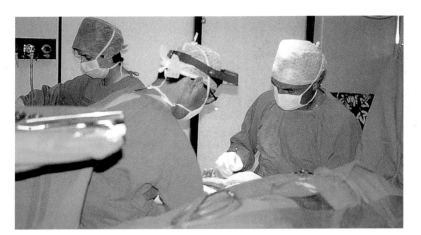

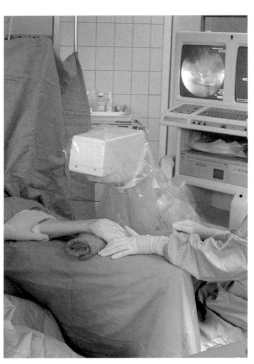

**FIGURE 4.** Setup for volar approach to the scaphoid. Note that the right-handed surgeon is seated to the head of the patient; this position is reversed for a left-handed surgeon or when operating on the opposite limb.

**FIGURE 5.** Position of the hand with the incision marked on the skin.

The appropriate approach and procedure are planned according to the fracture type. However, the surgeon must be prepared to change the approach and technique depending on the findings at the time of surgery. All patients should consent for the harvesting of an iliac crest bone graft.

## SURGERY

Either general or local anesthesia is used. A tourniquet is applied and the limb is placed on an arm extension table. The opposite iliac crest is prepared and draped in the event that a bone graft is required. The operating table is placed in such a way that the C-arm is readily accessible, and the screen clearly visible.

For a volar approach, whether open or closed, the surgeon should be seated with dominant hand at the outer end of the table (Fig. 4). For a dorsal approach, this position is reversed. A radiolucent, hinged handholding device is extremely useful, but if not available, a large, rolled-up towel can be used to aid extension of the wrist.

### Technique One: Percutaneous Fixation

Screen the scaphoid with the image intensifier to confirm that the fracture is suitable for closed treatment, and carefully carry out a closed reduction if required. Identify and mark out the prominence of the scaphoid tubercle, which is more prominent with the wrist in radial deviation. Make a 1-cm longitudinal incision over the tubercle, and carefully dissect off the overlying soft tissues to expose the bone (Fig. 5). Take care to protect the palmar branch of the radial artery as it crosses towards the palm, just proximal to the tubercle.

Position the drill guide firmly on the tubercle, towards its radial side, and insert a 1-mm guide wire through the sleeve. Use the C-arm to check that the entry point

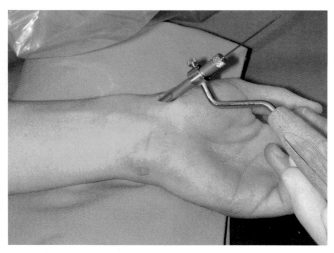

**FIGURE 6.** Guide wire being inserted; note that the drill guide has been carefully positioned on the tubercle and is being used to direct the guide wire toward the proximal pole of the scaphoid at approximately 45° dorsal and 45° ulnar.

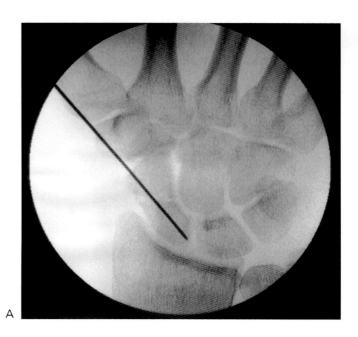

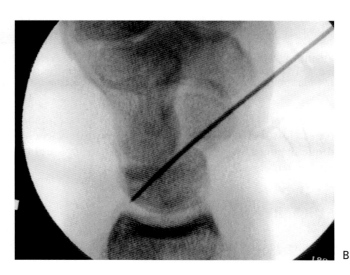

A

B

**FIGURE 7.** Intraoperative screening of guide wire: Note correct line on both posteroanterior **(A)** and lateral **(B)** projections.

is correct. Then, aiming the guide towards the proximal pole of the scaphoid at approximately 45° dorsally and 45° ulnarly in relation to the neutral plane, slowly insert the guide wire under x-ray control (Fig. 6). The optimum position should be along the mid-axis of the scaphoid in both plains and as closely perpendicular to the fracture as possible. The guide wire should enter, but not penetrate, the firm subchondral bone at the apex of the proximal pole (Fig. 7).

Once the guide wire is in the correct position, measure the length using the depth gauge, making sure that the tip of the guide remains firmly on the tubercle (Fig. 8). Set the stop on the cannulated drill to the appropriate length, and, after removing the wire sleeve, pass the drill over the wire and slowly insert it (Fig. 9). Drilling may be carried out by hand, using the handle provided, or by power, provided the driver has a sufficiently fine speed control.

Take care to ensure that the drill follows the same line as the guide wire, to avoid jamming or bending. Once it is fully inserted, check the position again on

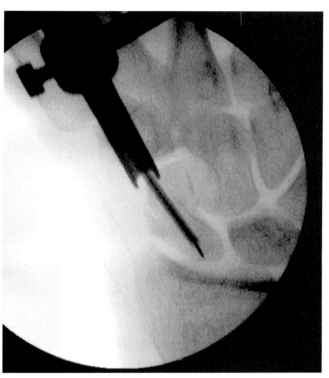

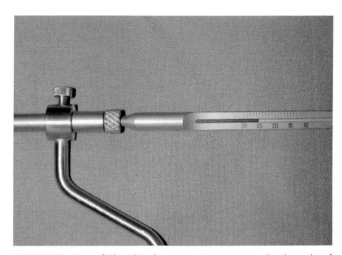

**FIGURE 8.** Use of the depth gauge to measure the length of the scaphoid.

**FIGURE 9.** The cannulated drill is inserted to the predetermined depth under x-ray control.

the image intensifier. Carefully withdraw the drill, making sure that the guide wire remains in position.

Depending on the appearance of the fracture, determine whether a *normal* or *high compression cannulated screw* (Fig. 1) is required, and insert this over the guide wire. Once the trailing threads start to engage in the bone, remove the guide and the guide wire before fully tightening the screw. Ensure that the trailing threads are well buried beneath the surface of the tubercle, and check the final position and stability of fixation again by screening the wrist on the image intensifier (Fig. 10). Release the tourniquet, suture the skin wound, and apply a firm, padded bandage without plaster.

### Technique Two: Open Fixation—Volar Approach

Center the incision over the tubercle of the scaphoid, which is easily palpable with the wrist in full radial deviation. The distal limb of the incision is gently curved toward the base of the thumb. The proximal limb extends for approximately 2 cm along the radial border of the flexor carpi radialis tendon (Fig. 11). The palmar branch of the radial artery (variable) is normally ligated and divided as it crosses into the palm just proximal to the tubercle of the scaphoid (Fig. 12). The sheath of the flexor carpi radialis tendon is incised and the tendon is retracted ulnarward to expose the anterior capsule of the wrist over the scaphoid bone. The incision is deepened distally, dividing the origin of the thenar muscles in line with their fibers, over the palmar surface of the trapezium (Fig. 13).

The capsule is incised longitudinally from the tubercle distally to the tip of the radius proximally. By cutting upward, damage to the underlying articular cartilage of the scaphoid is avoided. At the proximal end of the incision, a condensation of the capsule—the radiolunate ligament—appears as a labrum to the radiocarpal joint. Divide this to provide adequate exposure of the proximal pole of

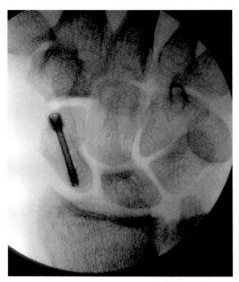
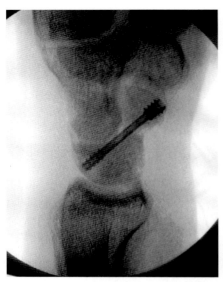

A

B

**FIGURE 10.** X-ray to show correct positioning of the screw on both anterior **(A)** and lateral **(B)** projections; note that the fracture line is now barely visible.

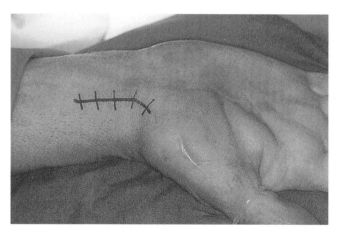

**FIGURE 11.** Palmar skin incision.

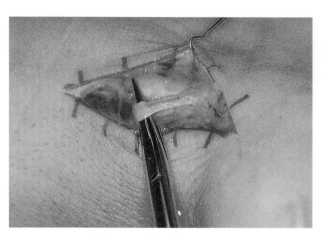

**FIGURE 12.** Superficial palmar branch of radial artery exposed.

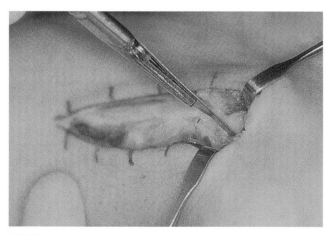

**FIGURE 13.** The thenar muscles are split at their origin over the trapezium to expose the scaphotrapezial joint.

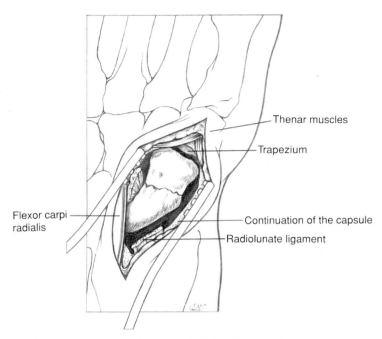

FIGURE 14. Exposure of the scaphoid following capsular incision.

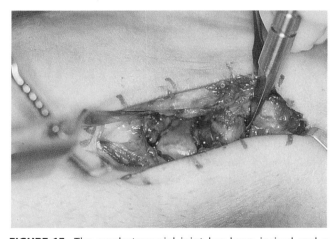

**FIGURE 15.** The scaphotrapezial joint has been incised and a dissector has been inserted to check that there is adequate access to the distal pole of the scaphoid.

the scaphoid. Insert a small self-retaining retractor for excellent visualization of the entire palmar surface of the scaphoid (Fig. 14).

The joint between the scaphoid and trapezium is identified, and the joint capsule is incised by sweeping the knife blade radially around the tubercle of the scaphoid (Fig. 15). This dissection is not carried too proximally or deeply (maximum, 1 cm) to avoid damage to the blood vessels entering the scaphoid along the spiral groove.

Use the fine suction device to aspirate the hemarthrosis. Clear any soft tissue attachment to the fracture site and remove any synovium that may have become trapped between the bone fragments. Carefully examine the fracture and remove or reposition any loose bone fragments. Manipulate the wrist to assess the degree of instability and/or displacement at the fracture site. Examine the scapholunate ligament for possible associated tears.

Accurate reduction of the fracture is carried out at this point, taking care to correct any angular, rotary, or translocation deformity. A K-wire may be used to hold

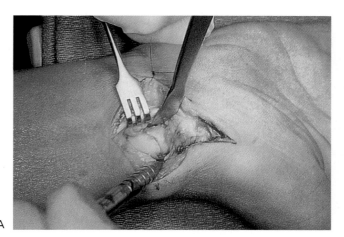

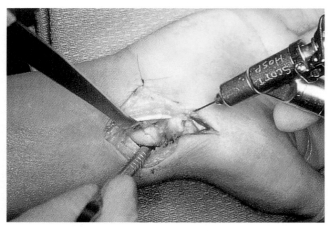

A                                                                                          B

**FIGURE 16. A:** An unstable oblique fracture of the scaphoid (palmar approach, right wrist); the fracture has been reduced using two small bone levers. **B:** A K-wire is passed along the ulnar border of the scaphoid to hold the reduction prior to application of the jig.

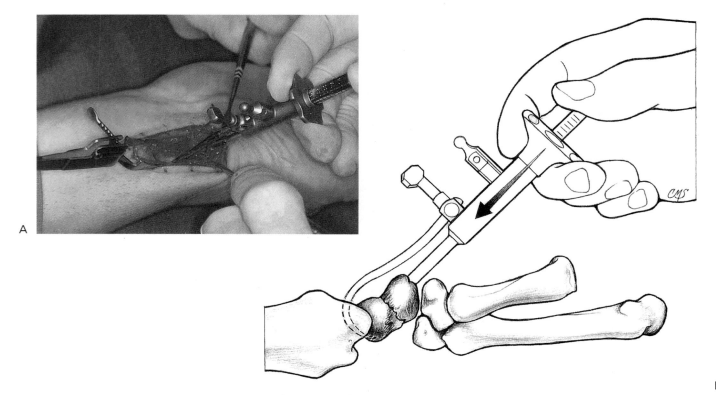

A                                                                                          B

**FIGURE 17. A:** With the elevator in the scaphotrapezial joint, the barrel of the jig is firmly clamped onto the distal pole of the scaphoid. **B:** The fracture is compressed by applying firm thumb pressure on the barrel.

the reduction. This wire is inserted into the tip of the tubercle at its ulnar border, directed proximally and dorsally toward the apex of the proximal pole (Fig. 16). If there is a defect at the fracture site or any tendency for the fragments to collapse under compression, all loose fragments of bone are removed and an adequate corticocancellous bone graft (harvested from the iliac crest) is inserted.

Fixation of the fracture is now performed. It is preferable to use the *guiding jig*, if familiar with the use (Fig. 17), as it holds the fracture firmly reduced and ensures accurate positioning of the screw. X-ray control is not necessary, although

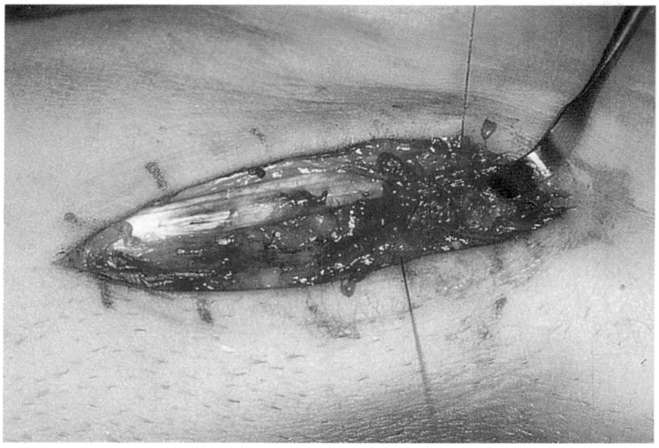

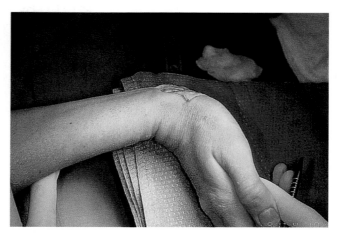

**FIGURE 18.** Capsular repair is carried out using 4–0 nonabsorbable mattress sutures. The capsule over the scaphotrapezial joint is approximated with a single stitch.

**FIGURE 19.** Following capsular repair, the range of motion and integrity of fixation are checked.

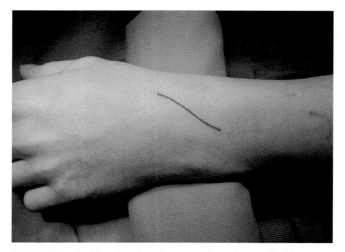

**FIGURE 20.** Incision for dorsal approach to the scaphoid.

if there is any doubt about the alignment of the jig, it is useful to check this by inserting a guide wire through the sleeve provided with the jig.

The *cannulated screw system* may be used as an alternative, as described in the previous section on closed fixation. The palmar wrist capsule is repaired using interrupted mattress sutures. Starting proximally at the radius, the cut ends of the radiolunate ligament are reapposed. Proceeding distally, the capsule is closed over the scaphoid and a single suture is used to approximate the soft tissues over the scaphotrapezial joint (Fig. 18).

The integrity of the soft tissue repair is checked by carrying the wrist through a full range of motion (Fig. 19). The skin is sutured and a firm 4-in. wool and crepe bandage is applied. This normally provides adequate support for the wrist during the period of wound healing while simultaneously allowing sufficient movement to prevent adhesions and joint stiffness.

### Technique Three: Open Fixation—Dorsal Approach

A 3- to 4-cm straight incision, centered on Lister's tubercle, is carried out and deepened; care is taken to protect the dorsal cutaneous branches of the radial nerve (Fig. 20). The second and third extensor compartments are divided carefully (for later repair) and the extensor pollicis longus, extensor carpi radialis longus, and

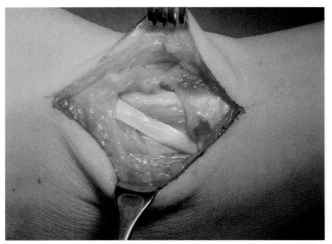

**FIGURE 21.** Extensor tendons are retracted to allow access to the dorsal capsule overlying the proximal pole of the scaphoid.

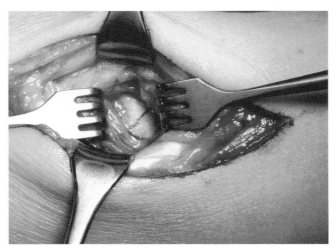

**FIGURE 22.** The fracture is exposed and, where necessary, reduced and held with a temporary K-wire.

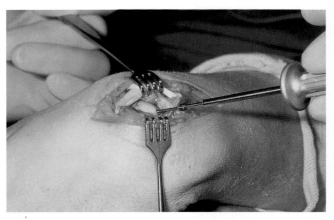

**FIGURE 23.** Fixation carried out by freehand insertion of a Mini-Herbert screw. Note that the screw is being aimed in a volar and radial direction toward the tubercle.

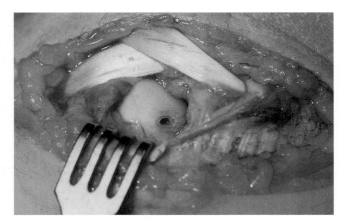

**FIGURE 24.** Note that the implant following insertion of the screw is buried well beneath the articular cartilage of the proximal pole, and that the fracture is well compressed.

extensor carpi radialis brevis tendons are mobilized and retracted radially (Fig. 21). The wrist capsule then is incised longitudinally over the scapholunate joint, taking care not to injure the underlying S-L ligament. The soft tissue attachments along the dorsal ridge carrying the blood supply to the scaphoid are left undisturbed.

The hemarthrosis is aspirated, followed by a careful assessment of the fracture and the integrity of the S-L ligament (Fig. 22). Any loose fragments of articular cartilage are removed and the fracture is carefully reduced, taking care to ensure that there is no malrotation. The fragments normally interdigitate closely, and bone grafting is rarely required. If necessary, a temporary K-wire (1.0 mm) may be used to hold the reduction during insertion of the screw. Insert it along the extreme ulnar border of the scaphoid, using x-ray control and taking care not to enter the midcarpal joint.

Flex the wrist fully to expose the entire proximal pole of the scaphoid. The drill guide for the mini-screw is carefully positioned on the apex of the proximal pole. Freehand drilling is carried out at this point, by hand or power, aiming along the mid-axis of the bone (in other words, in a volar and radial direction, roughly along the line of the abducted thumb) (Fig. 23). Depending on the size of the proximal fragment, a screw of 16- to 20-mm length is usually sufficient, so that drilling only needs to be carried out to this depth. The appropriate mini-screw is then inserted through the drill guide and tightened so that its trailing threads lie well beneath the articular cartilage (Fig. 24). The final position is checked on x-ray control (Fig. 25). The capsule is

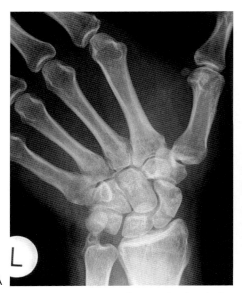 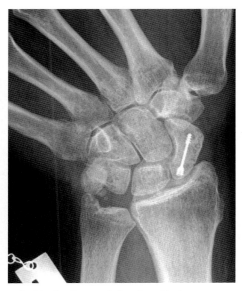

A B

**FIGURE 25.** **A:** X-ray of a proximal pole fracture suitable for internal fixation. **B:** Appearance following fixation with a Mini-Herbert bone screw.

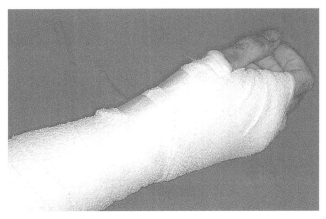

**FIGURE 26.** A firm padded bandage provides adequate protection during the healing period.

repaired with great care using 4–0 Ticron sutures. Reposition the extensor tendons and repair the retinacular compartments.

## POSTOPERATIVE MANAGEMENT

Following wound closure, apply a firm, well-padded bandage (Fig. 26). Do not use plaster, unless fixation is judged inadequate to allow for early wrist motion. Encourage active use of the hand and wrist. Allow the patient to return to clerical or light manual work. Heavy manual work and contact sports should be avoided during the first 6 weeks. Fit a removable splint only if the patient is likely to subject the wrist to excessive strain.

Radiographs are taken again at 6 and 12 weeks. It may be difficult to determine exactly when union has occurred. Provided that there is no increasing lucency at the fracture line or any sign of screw loosening, it is safe to assume that union is complete by 3 months. If there is any doubt, a control CT scan will show the healing process clearly. Upon complete union, allow the patient to resume full normal

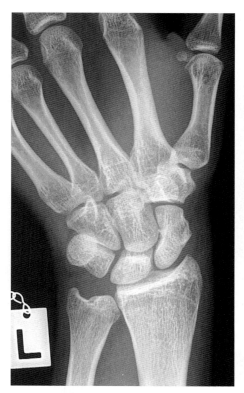

**FIGURE 27.** Initial x-ray of the left scaphoid (posteroanterior in ulnar deviation); note slight deformity of the ulnar cortex, consistent with recent trauma, although the fracture itself cannot be seen.

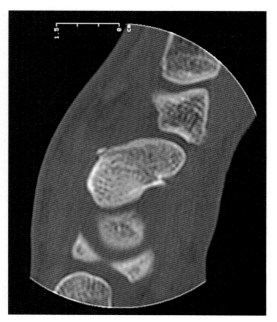

**FIGURE 28.** A computed tomography scan is used to confirm the diagnosis; note that the fracture line is now clear and can be seen to involve both cortices, with the potential for displacement.

activities, including contact sports. If a K-wire has been left in the scaphoid, remove it at this stage.

## ILLUSTRATIVE CASE

A 20-year-old male injured his left wrist during a fall while inline skating. Initial x-ray showed only slight deformity on the ulnar border of the scaphoid (Fig. 27). A CT scan revealed a complete fracture through the waist involving both cortices (Fig. 28). Because there was no significant displacement, the fracture was treated by percutaneous screw fixation, using the cannulated HBS system (Fig. 29). The patient returned to light manual activities without a splint following removal of his sutures at 2 weeks after injury. There was minimal scarring 2 months later (Fig. 30), with symptom-free, normal function of his wrist (Fig. 31). X-rays and CT scan showed sound healing of the fracture (Fig. 32).

## COMPLICATIONS

Complications are rare following internal fixation of the scaphoid, provided that satisfactory fixation has been achieved at the time of surgery and that an early exercise program has been initiated.

Following open surgery, some patients may develop volar scar tenderness; others may have a keloid reaction, requiring revision. A zigzag incision or use of a percutaneous approach may lessen the risk for these complications.

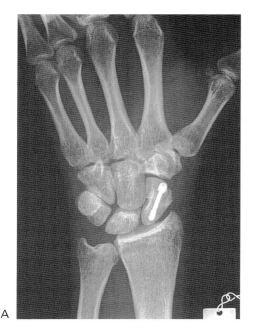
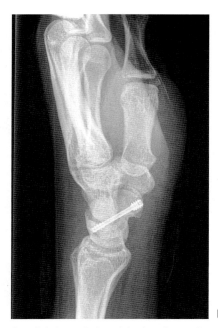

A                                                                                                B

**FIGURE 29.** Postoperative x-rays: Anteroposterior view **(A)** lateral view **(B)** showing satisfactory fixation with a cannulated screw inserted percutaneously.

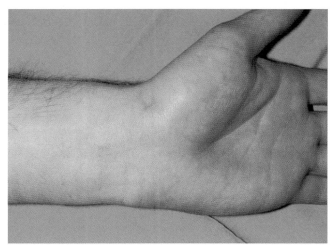

**FIGURE 30.** At 8 weeks, the patient is asymptomatic, and the scar is soundly healed.

When using the open volar approach, faulty positioning of the guiding jig may result in poor screw placement or penetration. This should always be checked radiographically during the procedure; if the jig cannot be applied satisfactorily, the freehand cannulated system should be used instead. With particularly small scaphoids, use of the smaller mini-screw is preferred.

The use of the cannulated screw system carries a risk of the guide wire becoming bent or broken, thus this part of the procedure demands extra caution. In particular, if the guide wire penetrates the bone (unless it is removed immediately), the joint must not be moved, as this likely would cause the wire to bend or break.

As with any surgery around the wrist, take extreme care not to damage the palmar cutaneous or the dorsal radial sensory nerves, since neuromas at these sites can be extremely disabling.

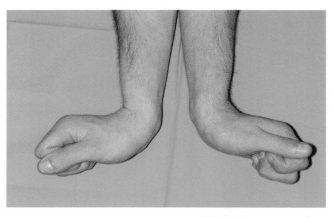
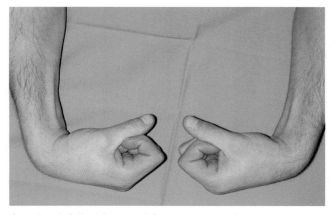

**FIGURE 31.** At 8 weeks, range of motion is full with normal function restored.

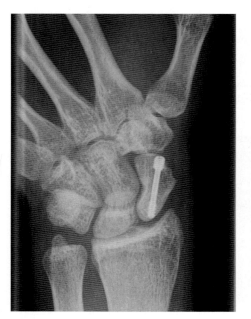
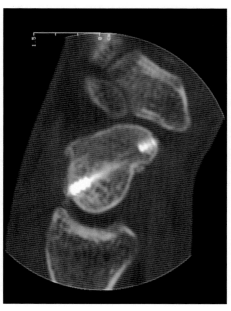

A                                                                                                      B

**FIGURE 32.** At 8 weeks, x-ray **(A)** and computed tomography scan **(B)** confirm sound healing of the fracture.

## RECOMMENDED READING

1. Filan, S. L., Herbert, T. J.: Herbert screw fixation of scaphoid fractures. *J. Bone Joint Surg.*, 78B: 519–529, 1996.
2. Gelberman, R. H., Wollock, B. S., Siegel, D. B.: Current concepts review: fractures and nonunions of the carpal scaphoid. *J. Bone Joint Surg.*, 71A: 1560–1565, 1989.
3. Herbert, T. J.: *The Fractured Scaphoid*, Quality Medical Publishing, St. Louis, 1990.
4. Herbert, T. J., Carter, P.: *Surgical Techniques for Fixation of Scaphoid and Other Small Bones*, Zimmer Inc., Warsaw, Indiana, 1993.
5. Hung, L-K., Pang, K-W.: Percutaneous screw fixation of acute scaphoid fractures. *J. Hand Surg.*, 19B(Suppl. 1): 26, 1994.
6. Inoue, G., Shionoya, K.: Herbert screw fixation by limited access for acute fractures of the scaphoid. *J. Bone Joint Surg.*, 79B: 418–421, 1997.
7. Kozin, S. H.: Internal fixation of scaphoid fractures. *Hand Clin* 13(4): 573–586, 1997.
8. Krimmer, H., Schmitt, R., Herbert, T.: Diagnosis, classification, and treatment of scaphoid fractures. *Der Unfallchirug.*, 103: 812–819, 2000.
9. Ledoux, P., Chahidi, N., Moermans, J. P., Kinnen, L.: Osteosynthese percutanee du scaphoide par vis de Herbert. *Acta Orthop. Belg.*, 61(1): 43–46, 1995.
10. Rettig, A. C., Kollias, S. C.: Internal fixation of acute stable scaphoid fractures in the athlete. *Am. J. Sports Med.*, 24(2): 182–186, 1996.
11. Werber, K. D., Hirgstetter, C.: The early treatment of scaphoid fracture with a scaphoid screw. *J. Hand Surg.*, 19B(Suppl. 1): 26, 1994.

# PART VI

## Scaphoid Nonunions

# 10

# Open Reduction and Internal Fixation—A Dorsal Approach for Small Pole Fragments

H. Kirk Watson and Jeffrey Weinzweig

## INDICATIONS/CONTRAINDICATIONS

If scaphoid fractures are undisplaced and stable, 95% should heal when treated with immobilization (3). However, delayed diagnosis, inadequate treatment, and complicated fracture patterns with displacement contribute to the prevalence of scaphoid nonunion (2,4,6). Chronic symptomatic nonunion of the scaphoid that lasts longer than 3 to 6 months requires surgical intervention to achieve bony healing (1,5,8–11,15). Optimal management of symptomatic scaphoid nonunion usually includes bone grafting.

One of the contraindications to bone grafting is radioscaphoid arthritis, the result of rotary subluxation of the distal pole of the scaphoid, which causes incongruity and destruction between this fragment and the corresponding articular surface of the distal radius (12). Other contraindications include arthritis between capitate and proximal scaphoid pole, and avascular necrosis of the proximal pole (7). Bone grafting will not address sufficiently these additional underlying carpal pathologies. Such cases may require formal scapholunate advanced collapse wrist reconstruction (see Chapters 16–18).

The biconcave technique described for the management of scaphoid nonunion is reliable for addressing problematic or long-standing nonunions without the need for permanent fixation or the use of compression screws (14). The principles employed in this approach to scaphoid nonunion reflect those utilized in performing intercarpal arthrodeses. They include maintenance of the external dimensions and relationships of the carpal bones (in this case, the proximal and distal poles of the scaphoid) and creation of broad cancellous surfaces for grafting (in this case, sufficient biconcave surfaces). Also included are utilization of cancellous bone graft and the use of K-wires that cross only the joints to be fused (in this case, the nonunion site).

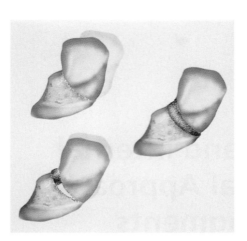

**FIGURE 1.** It is no longer sufficient simply to obtain union. Volar grafting will correct the angulation but not reestablish adequate scaphoid length. Long-standing nonunion usually consists of collapse between the two fragments of bone. Bringing the bone out to length, correcting its angulation, and filling the defect with cancellous bone will achieve the desired result. The dorsal approach allows use of the capitate as a template.

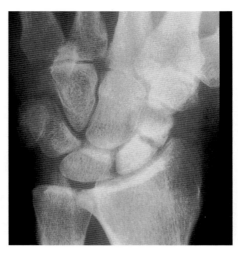

**FIGURE 2.** Long-standing scaphoid nonunion with some sclerosis of the proximal pole will require biconcave bone grafting to achieve union.

The dorsal approach permits correction of the bony angulation and realignment of the scaphoid fragments (Fig. 1). This approach results in an excellent union rate with few complications, yielding functional wrists with minimal loss of wrist motion.

## PREOPERATIVE PLANNING

Preoperative evaluation of patients with persistent symptoms following a scaphoid fracture requires a focused physical examination and radiographic assessment. Symptoms usually include pain, loss of strength, and considerable restriction of motion. Scaphoid nonunion may follow a fracture known to the patient or may be discovered upon initial evaluation.

Physical examination generally reveals periscaphoid swelling and synovitis as well as restricted flexion and extension. Clinical suspicion of scaphoid nonunion usually is confirmed radiographically (Fig. 2). In some cases, tomograms or a computed tomography scan may be useful in identifying the nonunion that is difficult to confirm on plain radiographs. During radiographic evaluation, special attention should be directed toward the radiocarpal joint. Patients who have advanced scapholunate advanced collapse wrist changes, as a result of long-standing scaphoid nonunion, will not benefit from grafting of the scaphoid; in most cases, they will require a capitate-hamate-lunate-triquetrum limited wrist arthrodesis.

## SURGERY

Management of the scaphoid nonunion by bone grafting is done through a dorsal approach. Position the patient supine. Prepare and drape in standard fashion. Use an upper arm tourniquet. We generally do not administer perioperative antibiotics. Perform the procedure under general anesthesia, although regional block can be used. With the arm fully abducted and pronated on the hand table, the surgeon can perform the procedure most comfortably seated on the axillary side of the wrist.

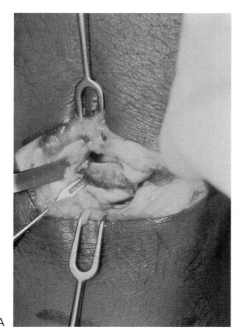
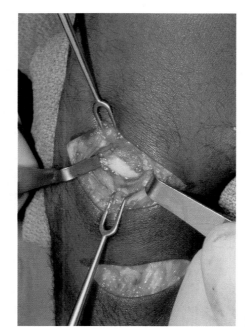

A                                                                                  B

**FIGURE 3. A:** Drilling, rongeuring, and curetting are the methods of choice for removing the bone from the proximal and distal portions of the scaphoid, forming a cancellous concavity. **B:** Note the broad cancellous surface filling the defect between the proximal and distal poles. There is no cortical bone contact between the proximal and distal poles in this patient. Note the proximal incision utilized for distal radius bone graft harvest.

## Technique

Make a transverse incision dorsally over the wrist at the tip of the styloid of the radius. Use blunt spreading technique to protect the branches of the superficial radial nerve, which in most instances are retracted radially. Open the dorsal wrist capsule over the scaphoid between the extensor carpi radialis longus and brevis. Both tendons should be free of their surrounding fascias so that they may be retracted in opposite directions. The extensor pollicis longus usually is retracted ulnarward with the extensor carpi radialis brevis. Cut back the synovial and capsular attachments at the nonunion site from the dorsal ridge of the scaphoid, and open the nonunion.

Dental rongeurs are usually sufficient to form a cancellous concavity in each section of the scaphoid (Fig. 3A). Occasionally, the use of a drill or burr will facilitate the forming of the cavities. Use the drill or burr in a slow mechanical drill (a few hundred revolutions per minute), not a high-speed air drill. Maintain cortical edges on each of the segments.

The average depth of the cavity should be approximately 5 to 8 mm from the surface of the nonunion. If the cancellous bone appears healthy, the cavity can be more shallow. If the proximal pole is small, the depth of the cavity obviously will be considerably less. Concentrate on the radius where, through a transverse incision 2.5 to 3.0 cm proximal to the first wrist incision, bone graft is harvested from the distal radius between the first and second dorsal compartments. Take only cancellous bone.

Run a retrograde 0.045 Kirschner pin out from the concavity of the scaphoid through the distal pole of the scaphoid and out through the volar radial aspect of the wrist. Run a second present pin through the skin across the dorsal surface of the radial edge of the lunate and into the proximal pole, aimed so that it will pass through the proximal pole and out through the distal scaphoid. With these two pins in place and drawn back, densely pack cancellous bone graft into both concavities.

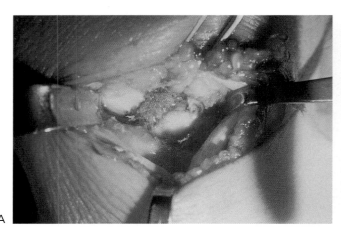
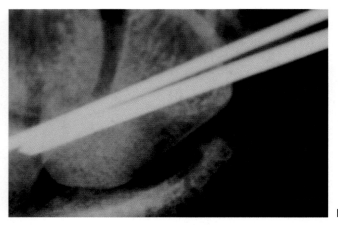

**FIGURE 4. A:** The cancellous concavities have been filled, and the proximal and distal segment cortices are separated with cancellous bone, filling the defect. **B:** Solid scaphoid healing occurred 6 weeks following biconcave bone grafting despite the gap seen between the cortical edges.

The advantage of the dorsal approach is evident in that the alignment of the scaphoid can be easily seen and adjusted. The capitate may be used as a template. The scaphoid is often angled, but there is also a loss of bone stock and shortening. A significant cancellous cap can be left between the two halves of the scaphoid, as is done with a limited wrist arthrodesis (Fig. 3B). The cancellous bone may occupy space on the articular surface between the two halves of the scaphoid; there is no need for concern for the articular surface of the radius. With the scaphoid properly realigned, its typical flexion and length corrected, drive the pins across the nonunion site, securing both poles. Then pack the rest of the cancellous bone between the two halves; it is not uncommon to see 1 or 2 mm of cancellous bone all the way around the nonunion site (Fig. 4A). Cut off pins below skin level. They pass only through the scaphoid. Do not suture the capsule and other soft tissue structures; close the two dorsal skin incisions with 4.0 subcuticular wires. Apply a long-arm bulky dressing incorporating plaster splints.

## POSTOPERATIVE MANAGEMENT

Replace the long-arm splint approximately 48 hours after surgery and apply a long-arm Groucho Marx cast. This cast includes the proximal phalanges of the index and middle fingers, with slight flexion at the metacarpophalangeal and interphalangeal joints, and the thumb to its tip in opposition. If significant sclerosis and cyst formation is observed by x-ray in a long-standing nonunion, maintain the long-arm cast for 4 weeks. If the nonunion is relatively recent with good bone stock on both sides, 3 weeks in the long-arm cast is sufficient.

Apply a short-arm gauntlet cast for an additional 3 weeks. Obtain x-rays out of plaster, and decide whether to remove pins and begin mobilization or continue in the short-arm gauntlet for an additional week or two (Fig. 4B).

## COMPLICATIONS

Potential complications in the management of scaphoid nonunion include persistent nonunion following bone grafting, avascular necrosis, graft extrusion, pin-track infection, and progressive degenerative changes.

The results of 36 patients who underwent biconcave bone grafting for scaphoid nonunion were reviewed (13). Eleven of the 36 fractures were diagnosed at the time of injury. The interval between initial fracture and biconcave bone grafting ranged from 3 months to 20 years (mean, 3 years).

During this interval, 61% of the patients underwent some form of treatment. Nineteen fractures were treated with casts, four surgically, three with palmar bone grafting, and one with an associated styloidectomy. Physical examination demonstrated decreased range of motion, localized synovitis, and a change in the mobility of the scaphoid compared with the opposite wrist. Radiographic examination confirmed the clinical diagnosis of scaphoid nonunion in each case. The distribution of fractures included 50% waist fractures, 28% proximal pole fractures, and 22% distal pole fractures. All 36 patients underwent biconcave bone grafting of the scaphoid nonunion as described.

Thirty-two of the 36 scaphoid nonunions (89%) healed; four patients demonstrated a persistent nonunion. All proximal- and distal-pole nonunions healed. Follow-up ranged from 3 months to 11 years (mean, 5 years). The four failures occurred in the waist fracture group. Two of these patients demonstrated fibrous stability requiring no further treatment. The other two patients underwent an additional procedure—a scaphocapitate fusion in one, and a scaphoid replacement in the other (not acceptable treatment at this time).

The patients with healed scaphoids had flexion/extension averaging 76% that of the opposite wrist; grip strength averaged 88% that of the opposite wrist. One patient with a healed scaphoid nonunion complained of pain with light use of the surgically treated wrist. Postoperative radiographs demonstrated marked static rotary subluxation of the scaphoid, a dorsal intercalated segment instability deformity of the lunate, and a scapholunate angle of 95° (the preoperative films could not be found to determine whether this problem existed prior to surgery). In this group of patients, the scapholunate angle averaged 60° (range, 40° to 95°). No other complications occurred in this series of patients.

## RECOMMENDED READING

1. Andrews, J., Miller, G., Haddad, R.: Treatment of scaphoid nonunion by volar inlay distal radius bone graft. *J. Hand Surg.*, 10B: 214–216, 1985.
2. Cooney, W. P., Dobyns, J. H., Linscheid, R. L.: Nonunion of the scaphoid: analysis of the results from bone grafting. *J. Hand Surg.*, 5: 343–354, 1980.
3. Cooney, W. P., Linscheid, R. L., Dobyns, J. H.: Fractures and dislocations of the wrist. In: *Fractures in Adults, 3e,* vol. 1, edited by C. A. Rockwood, D. P. Green, J. B. Lippincott, Philadelphia, pp. 638–647, 1991.
4. Cooney, W. P., Linscheid, R. L., Dobyns, J. H., Wood, M. B.: Scaphoid nonunion: role of anterior interpositional bone grafts. *J. Hand Surg.*, 13A: 635–650, 1988.
5. Dooley, B. J.: Inlay bone grafting for nonunion of the scaphoid bone by the anterior approach. *J. Bone Joint Surg.*, 50B: 102–109, 1968.
6. Fisk, G.: Carpal instability and the fractured scaphoid. *Ann. R. Coll. Surg. Engl.*, 46: 63–76, 1970.
7. Green, D. P.: Russe technique. In: *Master Techniques in Orthopaedic Surgery, The Wrist,* edited by R. H. Gelberman, Raven Press, New York, pp. 107–118, 1994.
8. Herbert, T. J., Fisher, W. E.: Management of the fractures scaphoid using a new bone screw. *J. Bone Joint Surg.*, 66B: 114–123, 1984.
9. Mack, G. R., Bosset, M. J., Gelberman, R. H.: The natural history of scaphoid nonunion. *J. Bone Joint Surg.*, 66A: 504–509, 1984.
10. Schneider, L. H., Aulicino, P.: Nonunion of the carpal scaphoid: the Russe procedure. *J. Trauma*, 22: 315–319, 1982.
11. Stark, H. H., Rickard, T. A., Zemel, N. P., Ashworth, C. R.: Treatment of ununited fractures of the scaphoid by iliac bone grafts and Kirschner wire fixation. *J. Bone Joint Surg.*, 70A: 982–991, 1988.
12. Vender, M. I., Watson, H. K., Wiener, B. D., Black, D. M.: Degenerative change in symptomatic scaphoid nonunion. *J. Hand Surg.*, 12A: 514–519, 1987.
13. Watson, H. K., Pitts, E. C., Ashmead, D., Makhlouf, M. V., Kauer, J.: Dorsal approach to scaphoid nonunion. *J. Hand Surg.*, 18A: 359–365, 1993.
14. Watson, H. K., Weinzweig, J. Scaphoid nonunion: biconcave bone grafting. In: *The Wrist*, edited by H. K. Watson, J. Weinzweig, Lippincott Williams & Wilkins, Philadelphia, pp. 901–905, 2001.
15. Zaidemberg, C., Siebert, J. W., Angrigiani, C.: A new vascularized bone graft for scaphoid nonunion. *J. Hand Surg.*, 16A: 474–478, 1991.

# 11

# Russe Bone Graft Technique

David P. Green

The Russe bone graft technique has been called the *Matti-Russe procedure*, as the concept of excavating the bone by removing all the necrotic bone, cartilage, and fibrous tissue at the fracture site was described by Hermann Matti (4) in 1937 (Fig. 1). Matti used a dorsal approach and filled the cavity with a plug of cancellous bone. In 1960, Russe (5) modified the operation by suggesting a palmar approach as less likely to cause damage to the blood supply of the scaphoid. He also used an oblong piece of cancellous bone that he packed into the scaphoid like "a dentist filling a cavity in a tooth." He later substituted a single corticocancellous graft for the oblong piece of cancellous bone. Eventually the operation evolved into using two corticocancellous grafts (Fig. 2), which he described in the German literature in 1980 (6), but never in English. I learned of the two-graft technique when Russe visited San Antonio in 1976; he later sent me a detailed description of the operation as he currently was performing it.

## INDICATIONS

The prime indication for Russe bone grafting is an established nonunited scaphoid, regardless of whether there has been a prior period of cast immobilization. The length of time since the original injury is inconsequential provided none of the contraindications listed below is present.

A relative indication for the operation, in my opinion, is the untreated patient who presents 3 to 6 months following the initial injury and in whom there is a nonunited scaphoid. This patient's fracture might heal without surgical intervention, but in some selected patients I recommend a Russe bone graft to enhance the chances of union, since the wrist will have to be immobilized for 4 to 6 months in any case.

## SURGICAL ALTERNATIVES

The main surgical alternatives to Russe bone grafting at the present time are screw fixation (with or without bone graft) and vascularized bone grafts. Choices

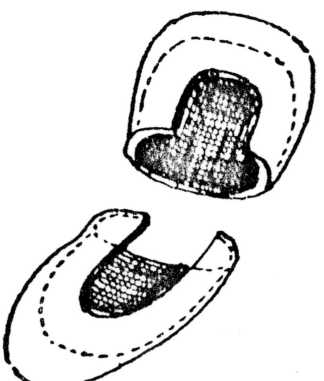

**FIGURE 1.** Matti's original illustration, which demonstrates his "excavation concept" of removing all dead bone, cartilage, and fibrous tissue from within the cavity of the scaphoid. (From Matti, H.: Uber die behandlung der navicularefraktur und der refractura patellae durch plombierung mit spongiosa. *Zentralbl. Chir.*, 41: 2353–2359, 1937, with permission.)

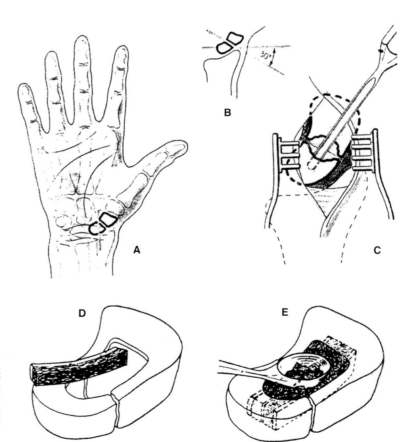

**FIGURE 2.** **A–E.** Russe demonstrated his two-graft technique in the German language literature in 1980, but he never published this in English. [From Russe, O.: Die kahnbeinpseudarthrose, behandlung und ergebnisse (mit film). *Hefte. Unfallheikd.*, 148: 129–134, 1980, with permission.]

for screw fixation include the Herbert (3), Whipple, and Acutrak, but are not limited to those. The rate of successful healing appears to be about the same for Russe bone grafting and screw fixation, but the latter has the advantage of requiring minimal postoperative immobilization.

More recently, vascularized bone grafts have become increasingly popular. Easy access to ideal sources of vascularized bone grafts makes them a logical choice for the treatment of all scaphoid nonunions, not just those with avascular necrosis. It is the opinion of this author that the Russe bone graft, which was for several decades the gold standard of scaphoid nonunion treatment, will soon be obsolete.

## CONTRAINDICATIONS

There are four contraindications to Russe bone grafting of the scaphoid, as outlined in the following sections.

### Small Proximal Pole

If the proximal pole is less than one-third, there is insufficient bone stock to provide adequate purchase on the two corticocancellous grafts. Taleisnik (8) has suggested that the original Matti-Russe operation using a plug of cancellous bone is applicable to such fractures, but my preference is for insertion of a Herbert screw from the proximal approach as described by Herbert and reported by DeMaagd and Engber (1).

### Severe Carpal Instability

If there is a significant "humpback" deformity of the scaphoid (angulation secondary to palmar collapse at the fracture site) with resulting dorsiflexion intercalated segment instability (DISI), the Russe bone graft will not correct the deformity satisfactorily, and a palmar wedge graft is required.

### Totally Avascular Proximal Pole

Russe stated that if the proximal pole is completely avascular, his operation will not achieve desired results. There is no completely reliable and consistently predictable method of determining avascular necrosis preoperatively as there is a lack of a precise definition of avascular necrosis. Total avascular necrosis is defined as the complete absence of any viable osteocytes microscopically and the absolute absence of any visible evidence of bleeding within the bone on direct observation at operation (see the Technique section for further discussion). The orthopaedic and radiology literature is replete with references that equate increased density on radiographs with avascular necrosis, but it is my conviction that this assumption can be misleading. Increased radiographic density of the proximal pole does not mean that the fragment is totally avascular, only that there is relative ischemia of the bone. A distinction between relative ischemia and complete avascular necrosis must be made, but cannot be done with plain radiographs.

Magnetic resonance imaging (MRI) is the best way to assess vascularity preoperatively, but it is still difficult to determine complete avascular necrosis positively.

Intraoperative biopsy of bone can be misleading as well because of the patchy pattern of avascular necrosis (9). Biopsy specimens are likely to contain both viable and dead osteocytes, therefore it would be necessary to make serial sections of the entire proximal pole to prove the existence of complete avascular necrosis conclusively.

### Arthritis

The presence of radioscaphoid arthritis is another contraindication to Russe bone grafting. Achieving union of the fracture in the presence of significant post-traumatic arthritis is not likely to relieve the patient's symptoms, although minimal changes between the tip of the radial styloid and distal pole of scaphoid might be acceptable.

## PREOPERATIVE PLANNING

Most patients with a scaphoid nonunion will have pain with use, especially with heavy gripping and extension of the wrist. Consistent physical findings are tenderness in the anatomic snuffbox, some limitation of wrist motion, diminished grip strength, and pain on resisted pronation of the forearm. Accurate preoperative measurements of range of motion and grip strength should be recorded for later comparisons.

It is important to take enough radiographs to evaluate the fracture adequately and to have a consistent method that provides comparable views for later comparison. The scaphoid series that I use includes: (a) posteroanterior view with the wrist in ulnar deviation, which best shows the scaphoid in profile; (b) anteroposterior view with fist compression, which is most likely to reveal scapholunate dissociation, if present; (c) lateral view with the wrist in neutral for measuring the carpal bone angles and the amount of midcarpal instability; and (d) oblique view, which provides a slightly different rotation of the scaphoid and shows the dorsoulnar side of the carpus in profile.

The following elements should be examined in the radiographs: location and direction of the fracture site; size of the proximal pole; presence of resorption or sclerosis along the edges of the fracture line; arthritic changes (seen first between the tip of the radial styloid and distal pole of scaphoid); presence and severity of midcarpal instability; increased gap between the scaphoid and lunate; and relative density of the proximal and distal poles of scaphoid.

Based on what is seen in the routine scaphoid series, additional studies may be indicated. If there appears to be significant DISI, the Sanders-type computed tomography (CT) scan (7) provides the best picture of the humpback deformity.

As noted, MRI provides more accurate assessment of vascularity of the proximal pole than plain radiographs, and if the MRI suggests that the proximal pole is totally avascular, a vascularized bone graft should be considered rather than a Russe bone graft. The MRI can be done in the configuration of the Sanders-type CT scan (i.e., along the true axis of the scaphoid), which allows identification of a humpback deformity as well as avascularity, and precludes the need for obtaining a CT scan in addition to the MRI.

## SURGERY

### Technique

With a tourniquet in place on the upper arm and inflated to standard pressure, the palmar-radial aspect of the wrist is exposed through a 4-cm straight longitudi-

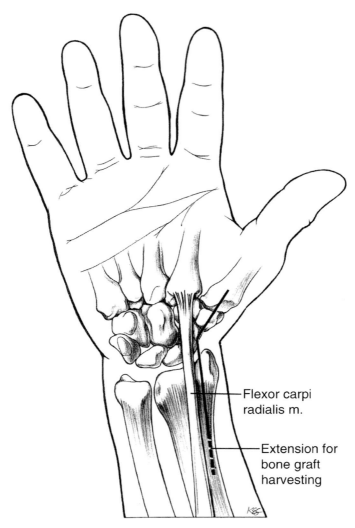

**FIGURE 3.** A longitudinal skin incision is made just to the radial side of the flexor carpal radialis tendon, with an oblique extension over the thenar eminence. The palmar cutaneous branch of median nerve, which runs along the ulnar side of the flexor carpal radialis tendon over the tubercle of scaphoid, must be avoided.

nal incision that parallels the flexor carpi radialis (FCR) tendon, with a 2-cm extension directed radially over the thenar eminence (Fig. 3).

The incision should be radial to the FCR tendon and the tubercle of scaphoid to avoid damage to the palmar cutaneous branch of median nerve. If the distal radius is to be used as the donor site for bone graft, the longitudinal incision is extended an additional 2 to 3 cm proximally. (Although longitudinal incisions in the wrist frequently develop into unattractive scars, this is rarely, if ever, the case following Russe bone grafting because of the 4 to 6 months postoperative immobilization required.) Open the sheath of the FCR tendon and retract the tendon to the ulnar side. Expose the wrist joint capsule by cutting directly through the posterior (dorsal) aspect of the sheath. This exposure through the sheath of FCR obviates the need to expose the radial artery, although it is usually necessary to divide the small volar branch of the artery that crosses the wound transversely at the level of the palmar wrist crease. Incise the wrist capsule in line with the wound, preserving the cut ends of the palmar ligaments for later repair. The nonunion site imme-

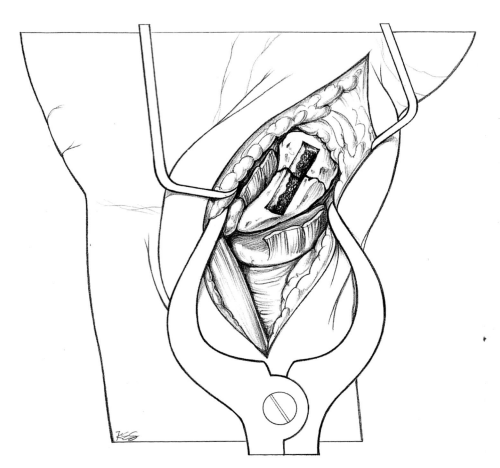

**FIGURE 4.** A 4 mm × 12 mm cortical window is made on the palmar surface of the scaphoid, centered over the nonunion site.

diately comes into view (keep in mind that the waist of the scaphoid is at the level of the palmar wrist crease).

Insert a Gelpi retractor beneath the capsular flaps; longitudinal traction on the thumb by an assistant provides additional exposure by bringing the scaphoid out from beneath the palmar lip of the radius. If there is a fibrous union present, the fracture may appear on the surface to be healed, but the soft nonunion site can be identified easily by gentle probing with a Keith needle or scalpel blade. Using small, sharp osteotomes, a 4-mm × 12-mm window is cut into the palmar cortex of the scaphoid, centered over the nonunion site (Fig. 4). The proximal and distal poles are thoroughly excavated, using no power tools. Although it is certainly easier to do this part of the operation with a power burr, it was Russe's admonition that this not be done because power instruments burn the bone. Therefore, small osteotomes, gouges (3 to 5 mm), and curettes are used to create the cavities. Excavation of the distal pole is usually easy because the bone is generally soft, but in the proximal pole the bone is often very sclerotic and dense. This is the tedious part of the operation, and extreme care must be taken to avoid penetration of the proximal pole; it is imperative to leave the articular cartilage and cortical shell of the proximal pole undamaged. I have found it useful to insert a Freer elevator beneath the proximal pole to provide a counterforce while using the gouges and curettes to scoop out the interior of the bone (Fig. 5). Excavation of the proximal pole must be sufficiently deep to accommodate the two corticocancellous bone grafts but not so deep as to penetrate the cortical shell. Patience and very careful use of hand tools during this part of the operation will be rewarded with an intact cortical shell and undamaged articular cartilage.

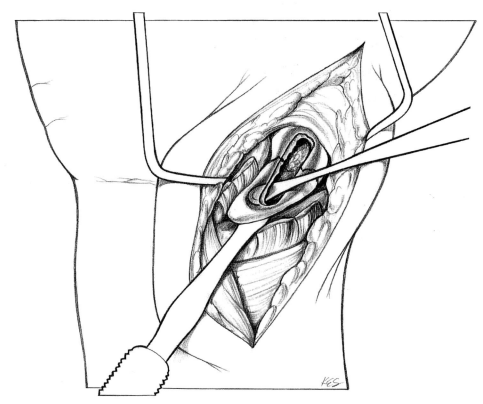

**FIGURE 5.** Excavation of the proximal pole is the most difficult part of the operation because the bone is frequently quite dense, and the cortical shell must not be damaged. Russe discouraged the use of power tools, therefore I use small curettes and gouges to loosen up and remove the bone. It is helpful to insert a Freer elevator behind the proximal pole to provide a gentle counterforce that serves to minimize the chance of inadvertently penetrating the cortical shell.

As the proximal pole is excavated, the surgeon carefully scrutinizes the cancellous interior, assessing the vascularity of the bone. Bone appearance ranges from lush red cancellous bone that looks like freshly harvested iliac bone graft (normal) to chalk-white brittle bone without a trace of red color (totally avascular bone). In my experience, totally avascular bone is uncommon (approximately 10%), but diminished vascularity is usually found. Often the palmar one-third to one-half of the proximal pole may have reasonably good vascularity and the remaining dorsal portion very poor blood supply. The surgeon should note observations of the vascularity and record it in the dictated operation note, for in my opinion this is the single most important factor in predicting the success or failure of the graft (2). Because there is no way to quantify the degree of vascularity scientifically, I assign arbitrary designations: *Normal* or *good* (Fig. 6A) denotes lush red cancellous bone; *fair* (Fig. 6B) is characterized by a diffuse pale red or pink color; *poor* (Fig. 6C) is manifested as tiny punctate bleeding points widely scattered on a yellow background; and *none* (Fig. 6D) means totally avascular bone, which is chalk-white and brittle. If there is any question regarding vascularity the tourniquet can be deflated, but in my experience this is not necessary, since there is usually no difference in the bleeding from the bone with or without the tourniquet.

If the distal radius is to be the donor site, detach the pronator quadratus muscle from its radial insertion and retract it to expose the palmar cortex. Using osteotomes and no power instruments, two 3 mm × 16 mm grafts are taken from the radius (Fig. 7) and immediately inserted into the prepared scaphoid cavity with their cortical surfaces facing outward (Fig. 8). Russe believed this would provide maximum stability. A thin layer of cancellous bone is left attached to the cortical

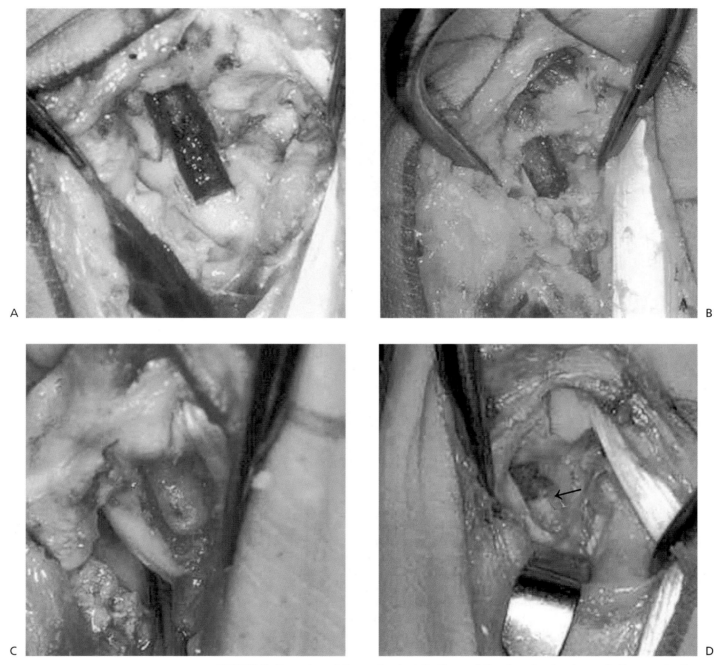

**FIGURE 6.** Examples of the author's definitions of the four levels of vascularity seen in the scaphoid at operation. **A:** *Good or normal*: The bone is lush red throughout, similar to what is seen when harvesting fresh iliac crest bone graft. **B:** *Fair*: The bone has a diffuse, fairly homogenous, pale red or pink color. **C:** *Poor*: Tiny punctate bleeding points are widely scattered on a yellow background. **D:** *None*: The chalk-white appearance of the proximal pole signifies complete or total avascular necrosis. Note the sharp line of demarcation at the fracture site *(arrow)* between the avascular proximal pole and the normal vascularity of the distal pole.

grafts, making the thickness of each graft approximately 2 to 3 mm. It is impossible to insert two grafts into the scaphoid if they are thicker than this. If the ilium is used as the donor site, more trimming of the grafts will be necessary because of the increased thickness of both cortical and cancellous bone (Fig. 9). Regardless of the donor site (radius or ilium), it is imperative to select an area in which the cortical bone is flat. If a curved piece is taken, it is impossible to insert the two

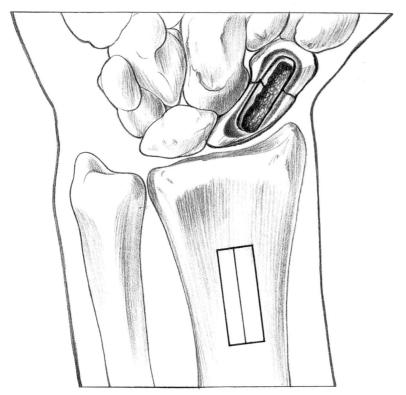

**FIGURE 7.** If bone graft is to be taken from the distal radius, the skin incision is extended proximally to expose a flat surface of the palmar cortex just proximal to the flare of the metaphysis. The grafts (approximately 3 mm × 16 mm) are removed using a sharp osteotome. Cancellous chips are harvested with a small curette from the distal radius after the cortical grafts have been removed.

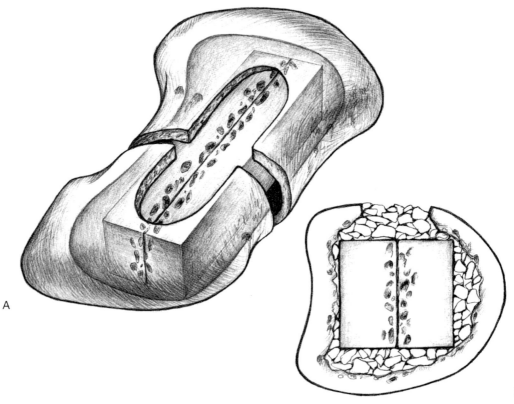

A

**FIGURE 8.** The grafts are wedged tightly into the cavity with the cortical surfaces facing outward **(A)** to provide maximum rotational stability. **B:** The remainder of the cavity is filled with 2-mm cancellous chips.

B

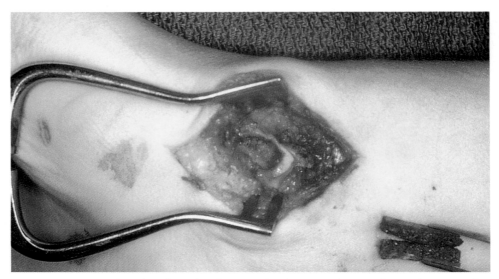

**FIGURE 9.** Bone grafts taken from the iliac crest (as these were) generally require more trimming of cancellous bone to fit into the scaphoid cavity. Grafts taken from the distal radius have a more ideal configuration.

grafts with cortical surfaces facing outward; if the radius is used, the donor site must be proximal to the curved metaphyseal portion of the bone. Having used both ilium and distal radius, my preference is the latter because cortical bone of the distal radius is ideally suited to provide almost the exact configuration required for these small corticocancellous grafts. In addition to this advantage, there is much easier access to the distal radius, and it is less painful as compared to the iliac crest donor site. Although some surgeons still prefer iliac bone graft, in my experience there is no significant difference in healing between the two types of bone graft.

Trim the grafts very carefully to provide the best possible fit. The grafts should be wedged in very tightly, requiring some manual distraction of the thumb to place them in the cavity; a small impactor is used to tamp the grafts firmly into the floor of the cavity. Occasionally, if the excavation is not done completely along the edges of the fracture line, a prominent transverse ridge remains that prevents adequate seating of the grafts. This ridge is removed most efficiently with a small bone rongeur. If the cortical grafts are inserted correctly, good stability of the fracture site is achieved, and there should be no need for supplemental internal fixation. (Supplemental internal fixation has been unnecessary in all of the over 150 Russe bone grafts I have performed.)

Through the cortical window in the distal radius, small (2 mm) cancellous chips are harvested and packed around the corticocancellous grafts. Russe said that he used "cortical bone for stability, cancellous bone for osteogenesis."

Carefully approximate the palmar ligaments and reattach the pronator quadratus. I use interrupted 3–0 chromic sutures, but any type of material is probably satisfactory. I prefer subcuticular closure (4–0 Prolene) of the skin to avoid crosshatches in the scar. If the radius was used for the donor site, suction catheter drainage is used for 24 hours postoperative. A short-arm plaster thumb spica splint is incorporated into the surgical dressing.

## POSTOPERATIVE MANAGEMENT

At 10 days, remove the sutures, take routine scaphoid series radiographs, and apply a fiberglass short-arm thumb spica that leaves the interphalangeal joint of the thumb and the metacarpophalangeal joints of the fingers free. Unless there is a need for a cast change (much less of a problem with fiberglass than plaster) the patient is seen only at 2, 4, and 6 months postoperatively for clinical and radiographic examination. Clinical features to assess healing include lessening tenderness in the snuffbox and less pain on resisted pronation. All radiographs must be taken out of plaster, and each new set of films should be compared with all previous films in sequence to evaluate the progression of healing. Discontinue postoperative immobilization when there is radiographic evidence of union: This is virtually never less than 4 months, usually 6 months. If the fracture is not healed by 6 months, healing is unlikely with further immobilization, and the cast thus is discontinued. A CT scan is useful if there is any question of healing on the plain radiographs.

When the cast is discontinued, the patient is seen by a hand therapist for a home program of range-of-motion and grip-strengthening exercises. If the cast is removed at 4 months, or if the patient is likely to be stressing the wrist in athletic or other activities, the wrist is fitted with an orthoplast thumb spica, which is gradually weaned over the next several weeks, depending on the level of stress. Emphasize the importance of grip-strengthening exercises to the patient, and explain that maximum grip strength may take 12 to 18 months to achieve.

I allow patients to participate in sports postoperatively if they wear either the fiberglass cast or orthoplast splint. Unprotected use of the wrist is not allowed until the fracture is observed radiographically to have healed solidly, good range of motion has been restored, and grip strength is at least 50% to 75% of normal.

## COMPLICATIONS

### Failure to Heal

Failure to achieve union of the fracture is the most common complication of Russe bone grafting. I believe that healing is directly related to the degree of vascularity in the proximal pole (2). In my prospective study of 103 Russe bone grafts done from 1976 to 1991, union rates were as follows, using the definitions of vascularity previously described: (a) good vascularity, 38/42 (90%); (b) fair to poor vascularity, 30/49 (61%); (c) completely avascular, 2/12* (17%) (1).

In the event of failure to heal, I do not attempt to redo the graft. Rather, the patient is given a supervised home therapy program for several months. If the symptoms subside to a tolerable level, no further surgery is done. However, the patient is advised that he will probably need another operation at some time in the future, probably a proximal row carpectomy or wrist arthrodesis. If the symptoms are severe enough to interfere with normal activities, one of these operations is done at that time.

### Penetration of the Bone Grafts

Care must be taken to ensure that the cortical shell is not penetrated either proximally or distally during the excavation process. If this does occur, it is imperative to be certain that the corticocancellous grafts do not extend into the radiocarpal or scaphotrapezial joints.

---

* The two scaphoids with totally avascular proximal poles were treated with external electrical stimulation (EBI) beginning 10 to 14 days postoperatively as an adjunct to standard short-arm thumb spica cast immobilization. Both of these fractures healed. Two similar cases treated with EBI subsequently (not in this series) did not heal.

**Persistent Dorsal Intercalated Segment Instability**

As noted previously, severe dorsiflexion instability of the carpus cannot be corrected with a Russe bone graft; if this operation is done in a patient with significant DISI, that deformity will remain postoperative even if the scaphoid unites. A better choice for such patients is a volar wedge graft.

## ILLUSTRATIVE CASE FOR TECHNIQUE

A 27-year-old right-handed mechanic sustained a Smith's fracture of the left distal radius in December 1987, which was treated with closed reduction under local anesthesia. Following 6 weeks of cast immobilization and physical therapy, the patient continued to have pain in the left wrist; he was referred for evaluation in October 1988. At that time, it was learned that he apparently sustained a nonunion of the scaphoid identified by another orthopaedic surgeon in 1982 (although the date of the original injury was never established) and that he was not treated initially or in 1982.

The patient pointed to the dorsum of the wrist and the snuffbox area as the sites of the pain, which was aggravated by extension and forearm rotation. Physical examination revealed tenderness in both sites. Wrist range of motion was limited to 40° extension, 30° flexion, 10° radial deviation, and 30° ulnar deviation, with nearly normal forearm rotation (60° pronation, 75° supination). There was pain at the limits of all motion, especially extension, and resisted pronation was particularly painful. Grip strength was 40 pounds left, 90 pounds right. Neurologic examination was normal.

Radiographs (Fig. 10A, B) demonstrated a well-established nonunion of the left scaphoid with essentially equal density in both poles. There was mild dorsiflexion instability with a 90° scapholunate angle and a 25° radiolunate angle. Posttraumatic degeneration was present between the radial styloid and the distal pole of scaphoid. There was slight loss of radial length and palmar tilt residual from the previous fracture. There was a nonunion of the ulnar styloid.

This patient presented a difficult management problem because of (a) mild deformity of the distal radius and some radioulnar joint derangement from the previous distal radius fracture, and (b) mild posttraumatic arthritis owing to the long-standing nature of the scaphoid fracture. A wrist arthrodesis was considered, but at operation the radioscaphoid arthritic changes were found to be quite limited. Therefore, a Russe bone graft was done, using the distal radius as the bone graft donor site, combined with a minimal radial styloidectomy (Fig. 10C). Vascularity of the proximal pole was found to be good during excavation of the bone at operation. Postoperative immobilization was achieved by short-arm thumb cast for 4 months, at which time the nonunion was clinically and radiographically healed. He wore an orthoplast thumb spica for the next few weeks as he underwent a supervised home exercise program. He returned to work as a diesel mechanic at 6 months postoperatively, and when last seen at 1 year postoperatively (Fig. 10D), he reported mild discomfort at the base of the thumb but no wrist pain. Range of motion of the wrist was still limited to 30° extension and 35° flexion, with full pronation and supination. Grip strength was 60 pounds left, 100 pounds right.

This case illustrates several points: (a) Successful union was achieved with a Russe bone graft many years after the original injury; (b) posttraumatic arthritis between the radial styloid and scaphoid is a relative contraindication to the Russe operation, but in this case the changes were mild and amenable to a limited radial styloidectomy; and (c) good vascularity in the bone as seen at the time of operation was probably the most important factor in achieving union.

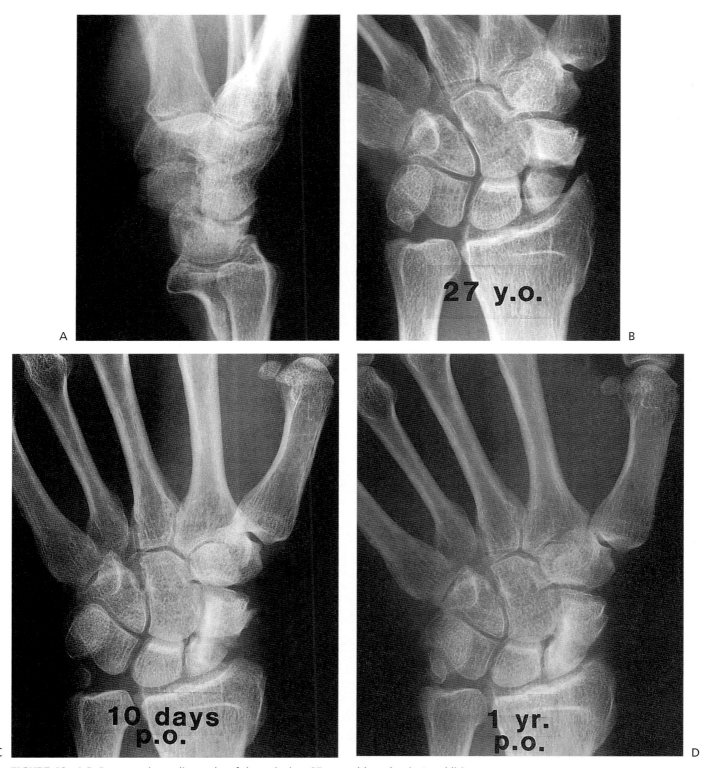

**FIGURE 10. A,B:** Preoperative radiographs of the wrist in a 27-year-old mechanic. In addition to a well-established nonunion of the scaphoid with mild dorsal intercalated segment instability, there are residual changes from the fracture of distal radius sustained 1 year earlier. **C:** Radiographs taken 10 days postoperatively show the cortical grafts in the scaphoid and the minimal radial styloidectomy. **D:** Final follow-up at 1 year shows solid healing of the fracture.

## RECOMMENDED READING

1. DeMaagd, R. L., Engber, W. D.: Retrograde Herbert screw fixation for treatment of proximal pole scaphoid non-unions. *J. Hand Surg.*, 14A: 996–1003, 1989.
2. Green, D. P.: The effect of avascular necrosis on Russe bone grafting for scaphoid non-union. *J. Hand Surg.*, 10A: 597–605, 1985.
3. Herbert, T. J.: Use of the Herbert bone screw in surgery of the wrist. *Clin. Orthop.*, 202: 79–92, 1986.
4. Matti, H.: Uber die behandlung der navicularefraktur und der refractura patellae durch plombierung mit spongiosa. *Zentralbl. Chir.*, 41: 2353–2359, 1937.
5. Russe, O.: Fracture of the carpal navicular. Diagnosis, non-operative treatment, and operative treatment. *J. Bone Joint Surg.*, 42A: 759–768, 1960.
6. Russe, O.: Die kahnbeinpseudarthrose, behandlung und ergebnisse (mit film). *Hefte. Unfallheikd.*, 148: 129–134, 1980.
7. Sanders, W. E.: Evaluation of the humpback scaphoid by computed tomography in the longitudinal axial plane of the scaphoid. *J. Hand Surg.*, 13A: 182–187, 1988.
8. Taleisnik, J.: Bone graft technique (original Russe method). In: *Operative Hand Surgery*, 2nd ed., edited by D. P. Green, Churchill Livingstone, New York, pp. 825–829, 1988.
9. Urban, M. A., Green, D. P., Aufdemorte, T. B.: The patchy configuration of scaphoid avascular necrosis. *J. Hand Surg.*, 18A: 669–674, 1993.

# 12

# Treatment with Reverse Flow Vascularized Pedicle Bone Grafts

Allen Thorpe Bishop and Richard A. Berger

## INDICATIONS/CONTRAINDICATIONS

With prompt appropriate diagnosis and treatment, over 90% of scaphoid fractures unite. Failure to diagnose acute injury, or to treat displaced scaphoid fractures operatively in a timely manner, increases the risk of nonunion (1,2). The development of scaphoid foreshortening and associated carpal instability with elapsed time contributes to the risk of nonunion (1). In addition, fractures of the proximal third heal less readily, in part secondary to operative avascularity in the proximal fragment (3).

Most scaphoid fractures that fail to heal with inlay or wedge conventional grafts probably have impaired vascularity as a contributing factor, as demonstrated by sclerosis of the proximal pole seen in x-ray and MRI imaging, as well as absence of punctate bleeding at the time of surgery (4–8). The use of conventional grafts such as the Matti-Russe volar inlay graft may be contraindicated in the presence of an avascular fragment (9).

Vascularized bone grafts have been proposed as appropriate methods to increase the rate and frequency of healing in fractures with poor prognosis. As early as 1965, Roy-Camille used the palmar tubercle of the scaphoid based on an abductor pollicis brevis muscle pedicle for this problem (9). In recent years, palmar distal radius grafts (10–14), dorsal radius grafts (14,15), and free iliac grafts (16,17) have demonstrated improved results as compared to conventional grafts in difficult circumstances. These include displaced acute fractures with small proximal fragments or bone deficiency requiring grafting, failed conventional grafts, and nonunion of proximal pole fractures, especially when associated with avascular necrosis. Inlay bone grafting coupled with vascular bundle implantation may be considered as an alternative (18,19). A recent experimental study has demonstrated the superiority of vascularized grafts as compared to conventional grafts in healing simulated carpal fracture nonunions with an avascular segment (20).

Vascularized bone grafts are contraindicated in proximal pole fractures whose size and geometry do not allow stable placement of the graft. Fractures with associated degenerative change involving the entire scaphoid fossa or midcarpal joint require a salvage procedure rather than an attempt to achieve union. Pedicled dorsal distal radius grafts are contraindicated in skeletally immature wrists due to the risk of physeal damage. In rare cases, absence of the potential donor vessels described below may require use of alternative pedicles or even a free vascularized graft. Relative contraindications would include acute nondisplaced scaphoid fractures and comminuted distal radius fracture or prior surgery potentially damaging the donor area. Systemic factors (including advanced age, vascular disease, and tobacco use) may indicate the need for an alternative method.

## PREOPERATIVE PLANNING

### Physical Examination

Typical physical findings are tenderness at the level of the fracture. This may be found in the anatomic snuffbox or directly distal to Lister's tubercle, depending on the location of the fracture. Documentation of bilateral wrist range of motion and grip strengths should be made, as well as efforts to rule out concurrent pathology that may affect the outcome of planned surgical procedures.

### X-Ray

The character of the fracture can be assessed adequately with standard x-ray views. These include posteroanterior (PA), lateral and "scaphoid" views, supplemented by comparison views of the contralateral wrist. Inspection of these images should include an assessment of the location and orientation of the fracture, as well as any comminution. PA and lateral intrascaphoid angles are measured and compared to the published standard and the contralateral wrist. The bone is inspected for density changes and the carpus for evidence of degenerative change and instability, including loss of carpal height and altered intercarpal and radiocarpal angles. Trispiral or computed methods provide valuable supplementary information in many cases, frequently demonstrating the deformity and/or arthritis to be more severe than anticipated on plain films alone. Appropriate positioning of the wrist in the CT gantry is necessary to optimize imaging of the scaphoid. The goal of these studies is to quantify the deformity, including angular and translational displacement. This evaluation will provide the best means to achieve an anatomic reconstruction.

### MRI

Although there is controversy regarding its correlation with the presence of punctate bleeding, MRI remains the only preoperative or noninvasive means of evaluating bone viability. In cases in which fracture location or other imaging studies suggest that there is an avascular proximal fragment, an MRI study is desirable prior to surgery.

### Vascular Anatomy of the Distal Radius

A thorough understanding of the vascular anatomy of the distal radius is essential prior to performing this procedure (21). The radial, ulnar, anterior interosseous and

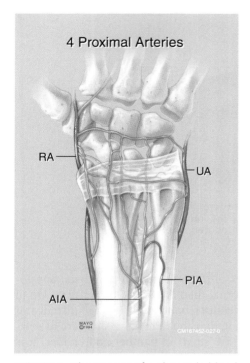

4 Proximal Arteries

RA

UA

PIA

AIA

MAYO
©1994

CM167452-027-0

**FIGURE 1.** The sources of orthograde blood flow to the distal radius include the radial artery (RA), anterior interosseous artery (AIA), and the posterior interosseous artery (PIA). The ulnar artery (UA) does not supply the radius directly. (Reproduced by permission of the Mayo Foundation.)

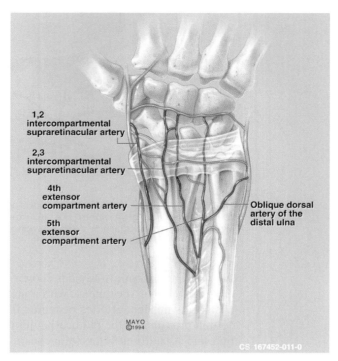

1,2 intercompartmental supraretinacular artery

2,3 intercompartmental supraretinacular artery

4th extensor compartment artery

5th extensor compartment artery

Oblique dorsal artery of the distal ulna

MAYO
©1994

CS 167452-011-0

**FIGURE 2.** Four longitudinal vessels may supply the dorsal distal radius with nutrient vessels. These include two deep vessels, the fourth and fifth extensor compartment arteries. These vessels lie on the surface of the bone on the radial aspect of the fourth or fifth extensor compartment. Two superficial vessels are identified on the surface of the extensor retinaculum: the 1,2- and 2,3-intercompartmental supraretinacular arteries. Each provides nutrient vessels to the radius through a bony tubercle separating the first from the second or second from the third dorsal compartments artery (PIA). The ulnar artery (UA) does not supply the radius directly. (Reproduced by permission of the Mayo Foundation.)

posterior interosseous arteries contribute nutrient vessels supplying the distal radius. The posterior division of the anterior interosseous artery and the radial artery form the primary sources of orthograde blood flow to the distal dorsal radius (Fig. 1).

The vessels directly supplying nutrient branches to the dorsal radius and ulna are described best by their relationship to the extensor compartments of the wrist and extensor retinaculum. They are considered *compartmental* when lying within an extensor compartment and *intercompartmental* when located between compartments.

There are two consistent intercompartmental vessels. They lie superficial to the retinaculum and are described further as *supraretinacular.* These two vessels, the 1,2 and 2,3 intercompartmental supraretinacular arteries (1,2 and 2,3 ICSRA), are located superficial to the retinaculum between their numbered compartments (Fig. 2). The retinaculum under these vessels is adherent to an underlying bony tubercle separating the compartments, allowing nutrient vessels to penetrate bone.

The 1,2 supraretinacular artery (1,2 ICSRA) is the most commonly used vascular pedicle for scaphoid nonunions (Fig. 2). It originates from the radial artery approximately 5 cm proximal to the radiocarpal joint and courses beneath the brachioradialis muscle to lie on the dorsal surface of the extensor retinaculum. Distally, it enters the anatomic snuffbox to anastomose to the radial artery and/or the radiocarpal arch. It is accompanied by venae comitantes and is the smallest of the four vessels. The distal anastomosis is the "ascending irrigating branch" previously described by Zaidemberg et al. (15). Its superficial location makes its dissection straightforward.

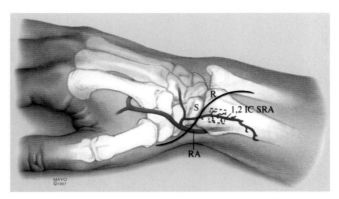

**FIGURE 3.** A curvilinear dorsal radial incision is used to expose the scaphoid and graft donor site. IC, intercarpal; RA, radial artery; SRA, supraretinacular arch; S, scaphoid. (Reproduced by permission of the Mayo Foundation.)

A previous anatomic study has shown the vessel to be present with a distal anastomosis in 94% of specimens, with a mean internal diameter of 0.30 mm (21). Up to 60% of its nutrient arteries penetrate into cancellous bone at an average distance of 15 mm proximal to the radiocarpal joint. Although its pedicle has a short arc of rotation and its nutrient artery branches to bone are small in number and caliber, it is ideally located for grafts to the scaphoid.

## SURGERY

Pedicled bone grafts based on the 1,2 ICSRA are useful for most scaphoid nonunions. A single dorsal approach is used for both graft harvest and exposure of the scaphoid. The extremity is elevated and a tourniquet inflated. Exsanguination with elastic wrap makes vessel identification more difficult and should be avoided. A gentle curvilinear dorsal radial incision is used to expose the scaphoid and bone graft donor site (Fig. 3). Branches of the superficial radial nerve are identified and protected. The subcutaneous tissues are retracted gently, and the 1,2 ICSRA and venae comitantes are visualized on the surface of the retinaculum between the first and second extensor tendon compartments (Fig. 4A, B). The vessels are dissected towards their distal anastomosis with the radial artery (within the anatomic snuffbox). The first and second dorsal extensor compartments are opened to either side of the bone graft site, creating a cuff of retinaculum that includes the 1,2 ICSRA (Fig. 5A, B). The graft is centered approximately 1.5 cm proximal to the radiocarpal joint to include the nutrient vessels. Prior to elevation of the bone graft, a transverse dorsal-radial capsulotomy is made to expose the scaphoid nonunion site (Fig. 6A, B).

### Dorsal Inlay Graft

In proximal pole fracture nonunions, a dorsal inlay graft is most appropriate. Fibrous tissue is removed from the nonunion site with curettes. A high-speed burr prepares a slot that spans the fracture site to receive the bone graft (Fig. 7A, B). If the proximal pole fragment is small, the graft may be placed within the concavity of the proximal pole instead. After preparation of the nonunion site, the graft is elevated. The 1,2 ICSRA and accompanying veins are ligated proximal to the graft. The graft dimensions and location are measured to conform to the prepared scaphoid slot, and centered 1.5 cm proximal to the joint line. The vessels are mobilized carefully distal to the outlined graft. An osteotome is used to elevate the graft, performing the distal osteotomy in two stages, moving the pedicle radial

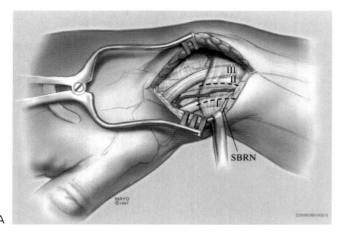
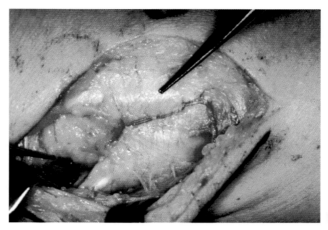

**FIGURE 4.** **A** and **B:** The 1,2 intercompartmental supraretinacular artery (ICSRA) is visualized on the surface of the extensor retinaculum between the first and second dorsal compartments. (Reproduced by permission of the Mayo Foundation.)

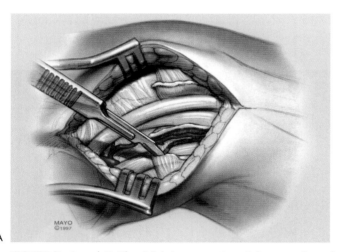
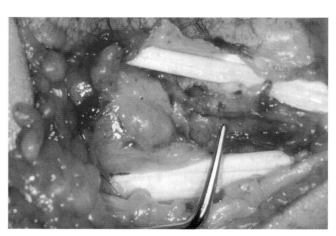

**FIGURE 5.** **A** and **B:** The 1,2 intercompartmental supraretinacular artery (ICSRA) is isolated by opening the extensor retinaculum overlying the first and the second dorsal compartments. The retinaculum is adherent to the radius at this level into which 1,2 ICSRA nutrient vessels pass at a mean 1.5 cm proximal to the radiocarpal joint. (Reproduced by permission of the Mayo Foundation.)

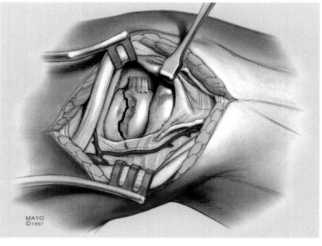
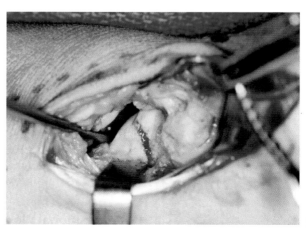

**FIGURE 6.** **A** and **B:** A dorsal radial capsulotomy is made to expose the scaphoid nonunion once the vascular pedicle is identified and protected. (Reproduced by permission of the Mayo Foundation.)

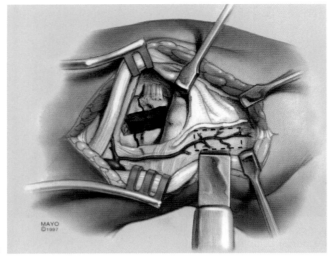
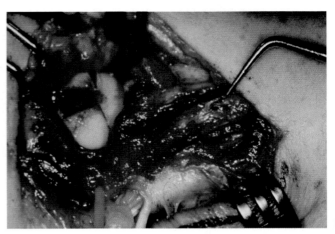

**FIGURE 7. A** and **B:** Dorsal inlay graft. A high-speed burr or sharp osteotome prepares a slot spanning the nonunion site when a dorsal inlay graft is used. (Reproduced by permission of the Mayo Foundation.)

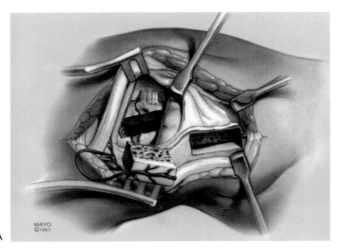
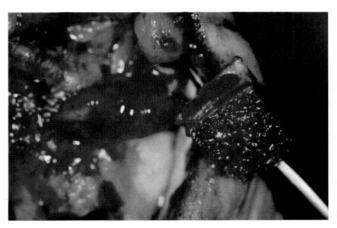

**FIGURE 8. A** and **B:** Dorsal inlay graft. The graft is elevated using harp osteotomes centered 1.5 cm proximal to the joint line. Distally, the pedicle must be carefully elevated from the radial sty-loid to prevent inadvertent injury. (Reproduced by permission of the Mayo Foundation.)

then ulnarward to prevent injury. The graft is gently levered out to create a distally based pedicle. Once elevated, the tourniquet is deflated, and the bone graft vascularity is observed (Fig. 8A, B).

The graft is resized as needed using bone cutters and transposed beneath the radial wrist extensors to the scaphoid. The graft is gently press fit into the prepared scaphoid slot (Fig. 9A, B). Supplemental internal fixation with K-wires or a scaphoid screw is performed next. Method of internal fixation is dictated by size of the proximal fragment and surgeon's preference. Either device may be placed safely antegrade without jeopardy to the pedicle. The wrist capsule and extensor retinaculum are closed, protecting the vascular pedicle. A bulky postoperative dressing incorporating a long-arm plaster thumb spica splint is applied.

### Interpositional Wedge Graft for Scaphoid Nonunion

When scaphoid foreshortening and angular (humpback) deformity is present, an interpositional bone graft is required. A vascularized wedge graft may be placed

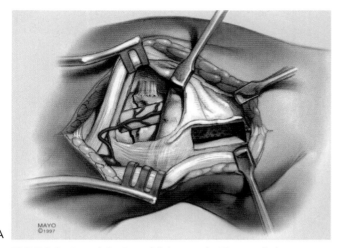

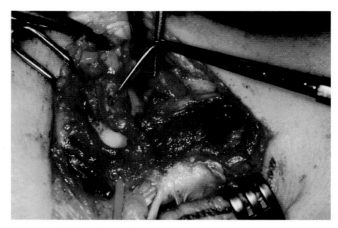

A

B

**FIGURE 9. A** and **B:** Dorsal inlay graft. The graft is transposed to the scaphoid and gently impacted into the prepared slot. (Reproduced by permission of the Mayo Foundation.)

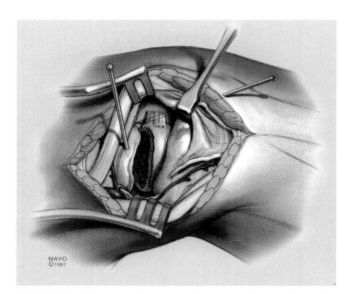

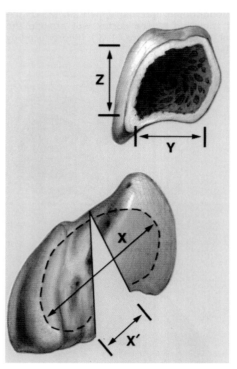

**FIGURE 10.** Wedge graft. A vascularized wedge graft may be placed from the same approach to correct a humpback deformity. Dorsal intercalated segment instability collapse is corrected by flexing the wrist under image intensification to correct lunate extension and is maintained with one or two radiolunate pins. Extension of the wrist then corrects scaphoid shortening. (Reproduced by permission of the Mayo Foundation.)

**FIGURE 11.** Wedge graft. Fibrous tissue is removed, and the internal and external dimensions of the defect are noted. Both the internal dimension (X) and volar cortical gap (X') are measured. (Reproduced by permission of the Mayo Foundation.)

through a dorsoradial approach as an alternative to conventional iliac crest graft. The incision is placed as before and the scaphoid prepared prior to graft elevation. Any DISI carpal collapse is corrected by flexing the wrist until the lunate is in neutral flexion/extension. Its position is fixed with a radiolunate pin. Extension of the wrist then corrects the scaphoid shortening (Fig. 10). Fibrous tissue is removed and the dimensions of the defect noted (Fig. 11). When used as a wedge, the 1,2 ICSRA pedicled graft is oriented to place the vessels and radial cortex pal-

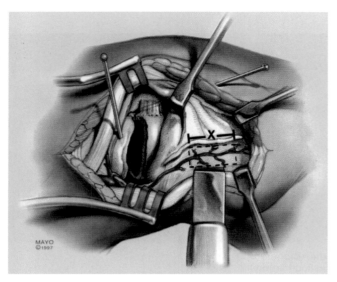

**FIGURE 12.** Wedge graft. A graft is planned sufficiently long enough to fill the longitudinal internal dimension (X) of the defect. Subsequent trimming of the cortex will provide the needed volar cortical length (see Figure 11, X'). (Reproduced by permission of the Mayo Foundation.)

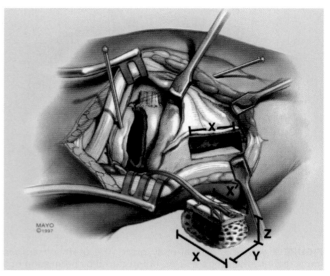

**FIGURE 13.** Wedge graft. A graft sufficiently large enough to correct the scaphoid shortening and fill any internal defect is planned with the 1,2 intercompartmental supraretinacular artery pedicle placed palmarly. (Reproduced by permission of the Mayo Foundation.)

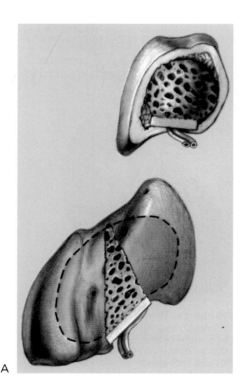

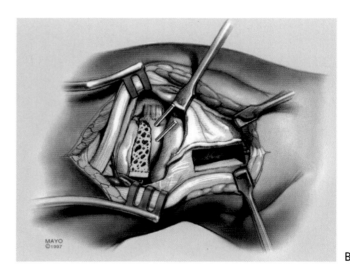

**FIGURE 14. A** and **B:** Wedge graft. The graft is placed and secured carefully with K-wires or a compression screw. (Reproduced by permission of the Mayo Foundation.)

marly for stability. A graft sufficiently large to fill the internal scaphoid defect is harvested as previously described (Fig. 12). The graft is trimmed carefully to match the dimensions of the defect, often requiring a greater length of internal cancellous than palmar cortical bone (Fig. 13). The graft is inserted into the defect and secured with K-wires or compression screw fixation (Fig. 14A, B). The wound is closed and the wrist splinted as previously described.

## POSTOPERATIVE MANAGEMENT

Active and passive range-of-motion (ROM) exercises of the digits and shoulder, as well as anti-edema measures, may begin immediately. The postoperative dressing and sutures are removed 10 to 14 days later, and a long-arm thumb spica cast in neutral forearm rotation is placed for 6 weeks. Radiographs and CT or trispiral tomograms are obtained to evaluate fracture healing. A short-arm thumb spica cast is continued until evidence of healing is seen on tomograms. In our experience, the mean healing time has been 11.1 weeks (range, 8 to 16 weeks) (22). Occasionally, incorporation of the graft to the proximal pole is delayed. Consider electromagnetic field or ultrasound bone stimulation if there is failure to unite by three months. After the fracture has healed, wrist motion and strengthening exercises commence.

## COMPLICATIONS

Complications of vascularized pedicle grafts include persistent pain due to progression of degenerative arthritis, delayed or nonunion of the fracture, malunion, loss of motion, and transient sensory neuropraxia. Our patients have not experienced permanent loss of motion or sensory changes as a result of this procedure. Nonunion is relatively uncommon after vascularized bone grafting (9–11,14,15). In our experience, it typically occurs at the proximal pole-graft interface, particularly when the proximal pole is exceedingly small. Further attempts at gaining union are recommended as described above provided that fixation is stable. A symptomatic nonunion or degenerative change may require a standard salvage procedure such as scaphoid excision with midcarpal arthrodesis, proximal row carpectomy, or total wrist arthrodesis.

## ILLUSTRATIVE CASE FOR TECHNIQUE

A 29-year-old male truck driver was seen 1 year following a fall onto his right wrist from an all-terrain vehicle. He initially treated himself with a brace, and sought medical treatment only after his pain persisted. Tomograms at initial consultation 12 months following injury demonstrated a displaced proximal pole fracture nonunion (Figs. 15, 16). He underwent open reduction and internal fixation with a 1,2 ICSRA pedicle inlay graft at approximately 1 year post-injury (Figs. 4B–9B). At 8 weeks, tomograms demonstrated a healed fracture with bridging bony trabeculae (Figs. 17, 18). At 27 months' final follow-up, he returned to work without restrictions and had achieved a scaphoid score of 8.

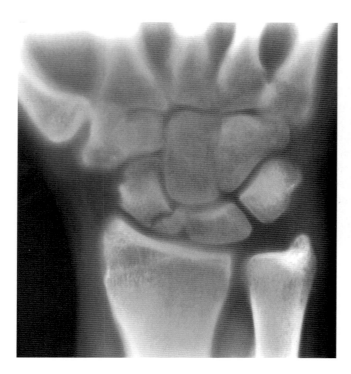

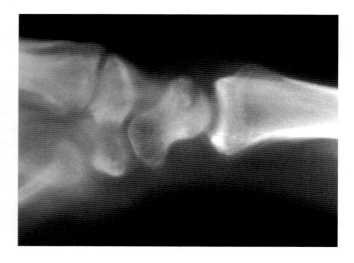

**FIGURES 15** and **16.** AP and lateral trispiral tomographs demonstrate a displaced proximal pole fracture nonunion.

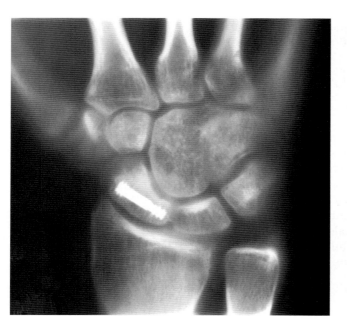

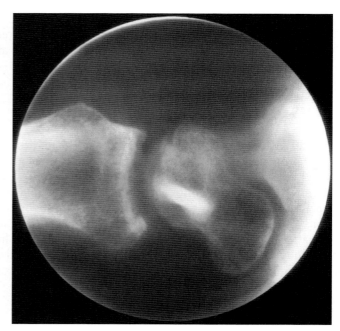

**FIGURES 17** and **18.** AP and lateral trispiral tomographs taken 8 weeks after surgery demonstrate a healed fracture with bridging bony trabeculae.

# REFERENCES

1. Szabo, R. M., Manske D.: Displaced fractures of the scaphoid. *Clin Orthop.*, 280: 30, 1988.
2. Cooney, W. P. III, Dobyns, J. H., Linscheid, R. L.: Nonunion of the scaphoid: analysis of the results from bone grafting. *J. Hand Surg [AM].*, 5 (4): 343, 1980.
3. Hull, W. J., House, J. H., Gustillo, R. B., et al.: The surgical approach and source of bone graft for symptomatic nonunion of the scaphoid. *Clin Orthop.*, 115: 241, 1976.
4. Green, D. P.: The effect of avascular necrosis on Russe bone grafting for scaphoid nonunion. *J. Hand Surg [AM].*, 10 (5): 597, 1985.
5. Stark, A., Brostrom L. A., Svartengren G.: Scaphoid nonunion treated with the Matti-Russe technique. Long-term results. *Clin Orthop.*, 214: 175, 1987.
6. Mazet, R. J., Hohl, M.: Radial styloidectomy and styloidectomy plus bone graft in the treatment of old ununited carpal scaphoid fractures. *Ann Surg.*, 152: 296, 1960.
7. Carter, P. R., Malinin, T. I., Abbey, P. A., et al.: The scaphoid allograft: a new operation for treatment of the very proximal scaphoid nonunion or for the necrotic, fragmented scaphoid proximal pole. *J. Hand Surg [AM].*, 14 (1): 1, 1989.
8. Mulder, J. D.: The results of 100 cases of pseudarthrosis in the scaphoid bone treated by the Matti-Russe operation. *J. Bone Joint Surg Br.*, 50 (1): 110, 1968.
9. Roy-Camille, R.: Fractures et pseudarthroses du scaphoide moyen utilisation d'un gretion pedicule. *Actualites de Chirugie Orthopedique Raymond Poincare*, 4: 197–214, 1965.
10. Braun, R. M.: Proximal pedicle bone grafting in the forearm and proximal carpal row. *Orthop Trans.*, 7 (1): 35, 1983.
11. Kawai, H., Yamamoto K.: Pronator quadratus pedicled bone graft for old scaphoid fractures. *J. Bone Joint Surg Br.*, 70 (5): 829, 1988.
12. Kuhlmann, J. N., Mimoun, M., Boabighi, A., et al.: Vascularized bone graft pedicled on the volar carpal artery for non-union of the scaphoid. *J. Bone Joint Surg Br.*, 12 (2): 203, 1987.
13. Leung, P. C., Hung, L. K.: Use of pronator quadratus bone flap in bony reconstruction around the wrist. *J. Hand Surg [AM].*, 15 (4): 637, 1990.
14. Steinman, S. A, Bishop, A. T., Berger, R. A.: Vascularized bone grafting for scaphoid non-union. American Society for Surgery of the Hand 51st Annual Meeting. Nashville, TN, 1996.
15. Zaidemberg, C., Siebert, J. W., Angrigiani, C.: A new vascularized bone graft for scaphoid non-union. *J. Hand Surg [AM].*, 16 (3): 474, 1991.
16. Pechlaner, S., Hussl, H., Kunzel, KH. [Alternative surgical method in pseudarthroses of the scaphoid bone. Prospective study]. *Handchir Mikrochir Plas Chir.*, 19 (6): 302, 1987.
17. Beck, E.: [Russe surgical procedures in treatment of scaphoid pseudarthrosis (Russe I, Russe II)]. *Handchir Mikrochir Plas Chir.*, 24 (2): 59, 1992.
18. Hori, Y., Tamai, S., Okuda, H., et al.: Blood vessel transplantation to bone. *J. Hand Surg [AM].*, 4 (1): 23, 1979.
19. Fernandez, D. L., Eggli S.: Non-union of the scaphoid. Revascularization of the proximal pole with implantation of a vascular bundle and bone-grafting [see comments]. *J. Hand Surg [AM].*, 77 (6): 883, 1995.
20. Sunagawa, T., Bishop, A. T., Muramatsu K.: Role of conventional and vascularized bone grafts in scaphoid nonunion with avascular necrosis: A canine experimental study. *J. Hand Surg [Am].*, 25 (5): 849, 2000.
21. Sheetz, K. K., Bishop, A. T., Berger, R. A.: The arterial blood supply of the distal radius and ulna and its potential use in vascularized pedicled bone grafts. *J. Hand Surg [AM].*, 20 (6): 902, 1995.
22. Steinmann, S. P., Bishop, A. T., Berger, R. A.: Vascularized bone graft for scaphoid nonunion. *(Submitted)* 2000.

# PART VII

# Carpal Instability

# 13

# Acute Scapholunate Dissociation: Ligamentous Repair

Steven F. Viegas

## INDICATIONS/CONTRAINDICATIONS

The most frequently recognized carpal instability is acute scapholunate dissociation. The prime indication for workup and treatment of acute scapholunate dissociation is a history of a traumatic injury to the wrist that has occurred within 3 weeks of presentation in which the injury, physical findings, and radiographic studies are consistent with this condition.

A relative indication is a wrist initially evaluated at a later interval—3 weeks to 3 months after the injury. Trauma that occurred 3 months or longer prior to presentation is not categorized as acute but is not a contraindication for treatment.

Radiographic or arthroscopic findings of arthritis in the radioscaphoid or capitolunate joint contraindicate treatment of the injury with the method described here.

A relative contraindication to the technique described here is acute scapholunate dissociation that has other associated ligamentous disruptions or carpal fractures. There should be a high index of suspicion for ligamentous injury and possible carpal instabilities with any significant wrist injury, including distal radius fractures. The associated injuries do not preclude treating scapholunate dissociation in the same way, but it is necessary to assess scapholunate dissociation in light of other associated injuries and to modify the treatment plan appropriately.

## PREOPERATIVE PLANNING

### History and Physical Examination

The history reveals whether or not the magnitude of trauma was sufficient to result in injury to the ligaments of the wrist. Typically, the mechanism of injury

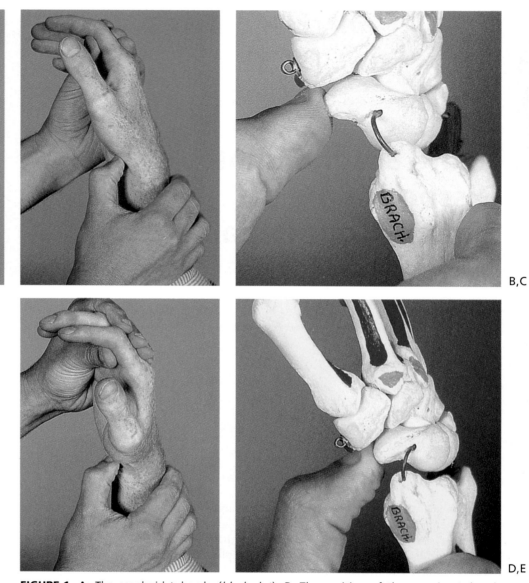

A

B,C

D,E

**FIGURE 1. A:** The scaphoid tubercle (*black dot*). **B:** The position of the examiner's hands when beginning to perform a scaphoid stress test on a patient; the patient's hand is in ulnar deviation. **C:** The examiner's hand placement in relation to the skeletal anatomy. **D:** The patient's hand passively moved to radial deviation. **E:** With counterforce opposing the palmar flexion and more prominence of the scaphoid tubercle, the scaphoid rides out of the scaphoid fossa.

that results in scapholunate dissociation is a hyperextension force to the wrist with concomitant forearm pronation and intracarpal supination.

The physical examination focuses on both the injured and the uninjured extremities. The contralateral side provides an excellent normal baseline for the patient's range of motion and level of constitutional ligamentous laxity. When attempting to assess whether acute scapholunate dissociation exists, one elicits tenderness at the level of the scapholunate joint, particularly at the dorsal aspect of the scapholunate joint, 1 cm distal to Lister's tubercle. The Watson test or scaphoid stress test is useful as well to detect abnormal mobility of the scaphoid (4) (Fig. 1). Occasionally during this test a painful, audible snap is elicited, which is diagnostic of this condition.

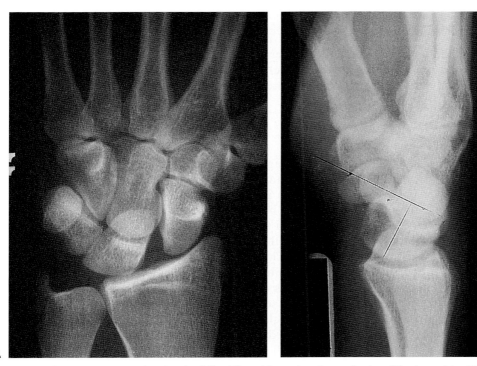

**FIGURE 2.** A posteroanterior clenched-fist **(A)** and lateral radiograph view **(B)** of a wrist with a dorsal intercalated segment instability of the wrist.

## Radiographic Diagnosis

Obtain radiographs including standard posteroanterior, lateral, radial deviation, ulnar deviation, oblique, and anteroposterior (AP) supinated clenched-fist radiographs of the wrist and hand. Obtain radiographs of the contralateral wrist for comparison. Significant scapholunate dissociation results in a carpal instability dissociative type of lesion that typically appears as a dorsal intercalated segment instability (DISI) pattern of carpal malalignment. This carpal instability pattern includes the following radiologic features:

1. *Scapholunate gap*: The intercarpal distance between the scaphoid and lunate on the AP radiograph is increased compared with the other intercarpal spacing. A scapholunate gap greater than 3 mm is considered diagnostic of scapholunate dissociation. The scaphoid gap has been called the *Terry Thomas sign* after the English film comedian's dental diastema. In both biomechanical and clinical studies, the increase in scapholunate intercarpal distance has been most noticeable in the AP supinated clenched-fist radiographic view (Fig. 2A).
2. *Shortened scaphoid*: The scaphoid assumes a flexed posture due to its dissociation from the surrounding carpus. It appears foreshortened on posteroanterior and AP radiographic views.
3. *Cortical ring sign*: The flexed posture of the scaphoid results in an end-on view of the scaphoid tubercle/distal scaphoid and, therefore, a more prominently visualized, circular cortex of the scaphoid. A cortical ring to proximal pole distance of less than 7 mm is considered abnormal.
4. *DISI pattern of the carpus*: The scaphoid assumes a flexed and dorsally subluxed posture; the lunate assumes an extended and palmarly subluxed posture; and the capitate lies in a flexed posture (Fig. 2B).
5. *Taleisnik's V sign*: When the scaphoid is flexed, the palmar edge of the scaphoid outline intersects with the palmar margin of the radius at a more acute

angle than that observed in the normal wrist, in which there is a more gentle, wider C-shaped pattern of intersection.

Scapholunate dissociation is observed alone or in combination with fractures. Carpal alignment is assessed routinely during the evaluation of distal radius fractures, including radial styloid fractures.

### Arthrography

Arthrograms of the wrist, although helpful in identifying ligamentous injuries, do not reveal completely the magnitude of such disruption. Dissections of the wrist in cadavers demonstrate a 28% incidence of scapholunate interosseous disruption. In dissections in which both left and right wrists could be evaluated, it was noted that the presence of a scapholunate interosseous ligament disruption on one side was associated with a 66% incidence of disruption of this ligament on the contralateral side (2). These disruptions, however, were not typically associated with a significant instability of the carpal bones.

Therefore, although reasonable as part of the workup, a positive arthrogram is not considered pathognomonic for scapholunate dissociation, particularly in the older population. A secondary or relative dorsal intercalated segment instability deformity resulting from a displaced distal radius fracture can occur solely as a result of a distal radius fracture. The DISI pattern of deformity can result, even following a distal radius fracture, from radius malalignment or ligamentous disruption or a combination of the two.

### Arthroscopy

If a patient has a history, has physical findings, and has a diagnostic workup consistent with acute scapholunate dissociation, a manual examination under anesthesia and an arthroscopic examination (including proximal wrist and midcarpal joint examinations) may be helpful (see Chapter 2). Wrist arthroscopy helps to confirm whether the ligamentous disruption is acute in nature and to identify concomitant chondral or osteochondral lesions.

Arthroscopic examination of the wrist is a critical step in the workup of a patient when normal clinical and radiographic assessment of a patient's ligament disruption is limited or impaired, as in a wrist with a concomitant distal radius fracture (see Chapter 2). An arthroscopic examination can exclude the presence of a ligament tear as well, as in the case of a wide scapholunate joint space, which can be a normal anatomic finding in a patient with a lunotriquetral coalition (1).

Arthroscopically assisted closed reduction with percutaneous pinning of the scapholunate dissociation is offered as an alternative treatment. My treatment of choice, however, is to confirm the diagnosis and the acute status of the lesion by a combination of history, physical findings, and radiographs and proceed to open reduction and repair of the soft tissues.

## SURGERY

Position the patient supine with the hand on an arm table. Place a tourniquet on the upper arm. Use regional or general anesthesia. Examine the involved wrist manually and, if indicated, examine arthroscopically the proximal wrist joint and midcarpal wrist joint.

Perform arthroscopic examination with the hand in the upright position and with the assistance of traction. Once the diagnosis of acute scapholunate dissocia-

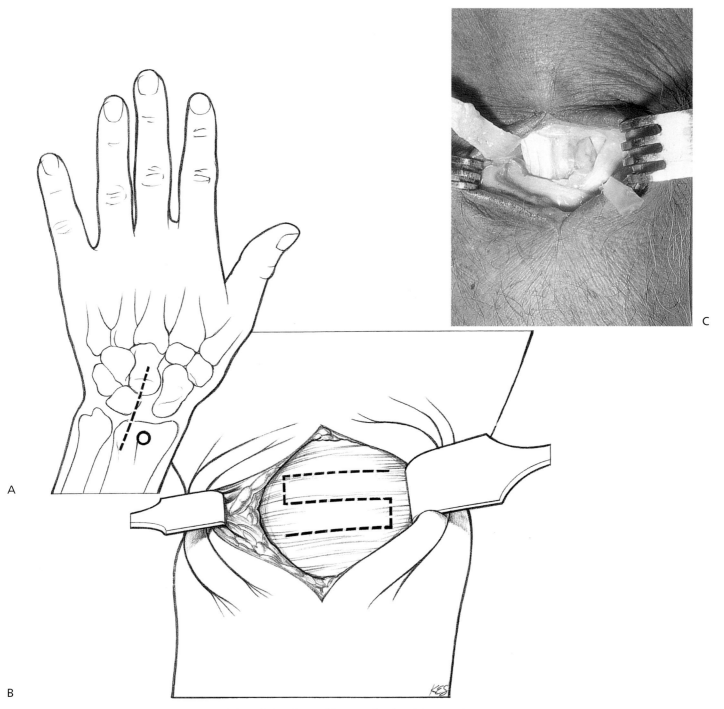

**FIGURE 3. A:** Palpable Lister's tubercle (O) and the planned longitudinal incision. **B:** The step-cut incision in the extensor retinaculum with the arms of the retinaculum retracted. **C:** Intraoperative photo showing the reflected radial and ulnar flaps of the extensor retinaculum, revealing some of the extensor tendons.

tion has been made and the absence of degenerative changes is confirmed, take the extremity out of traction and place it in pronation on the hand table.

## Technique

Make a dorsal longitudinal incision over the dorsum of the wrist just ulnar to Lister's tubercle (Fig. 3A). Carry the skin incision down to the extensor retinacu-

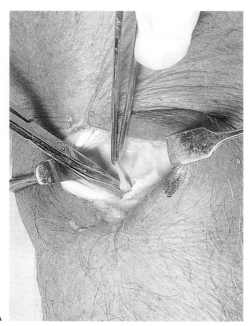
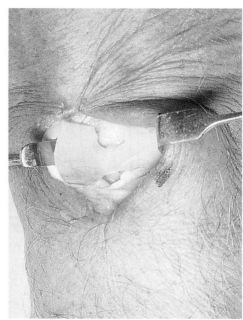

A                                                                                          B

**FIGURE 4.  A:** Terminal branch of the posterior interosseous nerve being dissected off the radius where it lies just to the radial side of the fourth dorsal compartment. **B:** A piece of colored background is placed behind the dissected nerve to allow better visualization of the nerve.

lum. Save the dorsal venous complex of the wrist whenever possible, and extend the dissection plane radially and ulnarly over the extensor retinaculum.

Make a step-cut incision in the extensor retinaculum over the fourth dorsal compartment, leaving a radial- and an ulnar-based flap (Fig. 3B). Identify the terminal branch of the posterior interosseous nerve at the floor of the fourth dorsal compartment lying immediately to the ulnar side of the septum that separates the third and fourth compartments (Fig. 4). Take a segment of the terminal branch of the posterior interosseous nerve, resecting the nerve proximal to the distal end of the radius.

Retract the extensor tendons and make a transverse incision through the wrist capsule just proximal and parallel to the dorsal intercarpal (DIC) ligament. Often, the DIC is not identified easily from the dorsal approach; running a probe or closed forceps from distal to proximal over the dorsal capsule helps isolate the thickened band of tissue that is the DIC ligament (Fig. 5). If necessary, extend the capsular incision proximally and radially, running parallel to the radial aspect of the dorsal radiocarpal ligament. The DIC ligament can be reflected distally if it is an acute injury. If it is a chronic injury, the DIC ligament likely has contracted and already lies distal to its normal level of attachment to the lunate and the dorsal groove of the scaphoid.

Typically, the central, more membranous portion of the scapholunate interosseous ligament is avulsed from the scaphoid within the scapholunate articulation. The more substantial dorsal distal portion of the scapholunate interosseous ligament complex and the DIC ligament also are avulsed from the dorsal proximal pole of the scaphoid (Fig. 6). Often, the DIC also is avulsed from the dorsal aspect of the lunate (3).

Examine the proximal wrist and midcarpal joints through the capsular incisions for any osteochondral or chondral lesions. Excise free fragments. Perform a trial reduction of the scapholunate joint manually.

If it is difficult to obtain the reduction, 0.062-in. K-wires can be used as joysticks in the scaphoid and lunate or a Richard's scaphoid staple reduction clamp can be used to assist in the reduction. Make a single hole using a 0.062-in. K-wire in the dorsal aspect of the proximal pole of the scaphoid and a second hole in the dorsal-radial aspect of the lunate, taking into account the palmar-flexed position of the scaphoid and the extended position of the lunate.

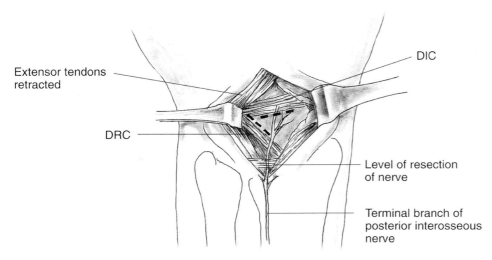

**FIGURE 5.** The lateral V-shaped incision in the dorsal capsule of the wrist, which parallels the dorsal radiocarpal (DRC) and the dorsal intercarpal (DIC) ligaments.

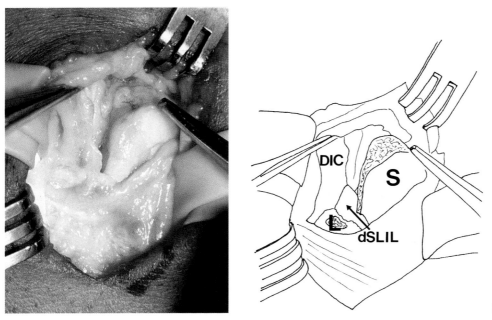

**FIGURE 6.** Intraoperative photograph **(A)** and illustration **(B)** demonstrating the flexed posture of the scaphoid (S) with its prominent proximal pole and the extended position of the lunate (L). The dorsal segment of the scapholunate interosseous ligament and the dorsal intercarpal ligament (DIC) have been avulsed off the proximal dorsal aspect of the scaphoid, and the DIC has also been avulsed off the dorsal aspect of the lunate. dSLIL, dorsal component of the scapholunate interosseous ligament.

Once the scaphoid and lunate have been derotated properly, place the arms of the scaphoid fracture reduction clamp into the holes and use the reduction clamp to reduce the scapholunate joint anatomically. While maintaining the scapholunate reduction, insert 0.045-in. K-wires percutaneously to stabilize the scapholunate joint, maintaining the reduction (Fig. 7). Once the scapholunate joint has been pinned, remove the joysticks or the reduction clamp. Examine the scapholunate alignment in the proximal and midcarpal joints; obtain radiographs confirming the reduction anatomically and radiographically in both AP and lateral projections (Fig. 8).

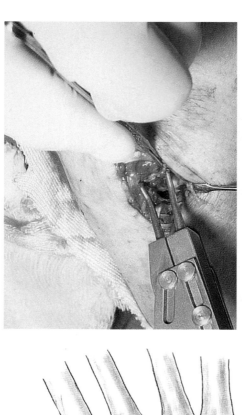
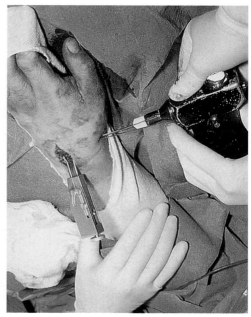

A

B

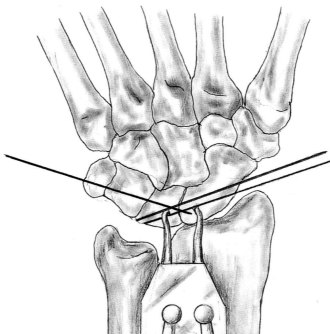

K-wires placed
percutaneously across
scapholunate and
triquetrolunate joints

Reduction clamp holds
scapholunate joint in
reduction

C

**FIGURE 7.** Reduction clamp **(A)** inserted into the prepared holes in the scaphoid and the lunate to facilitate **(B)** the reduction of the scapholunate diastasis, and percutaneously placed K-wires maintaining the anatomic alignment of the reduced scapholunate joint. **C:** Pin placement with reduction clamp still in place.

Once the reduction has been confirmed radiographically, place one or more 2.0- or 2.5-mm suture anchors in the dorsal aspect of the proximal pole of the scaphoid, from which point the dorsal segment of the scapholunate interosseous ligament and the DIC have been avulsed (Figs. 9, 10). Place additional small holes in the dorsal rim of the proximal half of the scaphoid in the area where the dorsal segment of the scapholunate interosseous ligament has been avulsed, to promote ligament reattachment and ingrowth

z

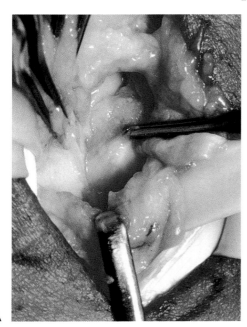
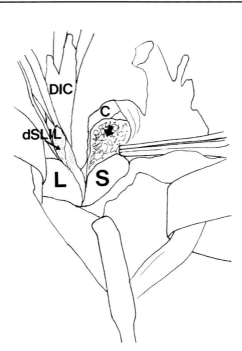

A                                                                              B

**FIGURE 8.** Intraoperative photograph **(A)** and **(B)** illustration demonstrating the reduced scaphoid (S) and lunate (L). The area (*large arrow*) where the dorsal component of the scapholunate interosseous ligament (dSLIL) (*small arrow*) was avulsed from the scaphoid is evident. C, capitate; DIC, dorsal intercarpal ligament.

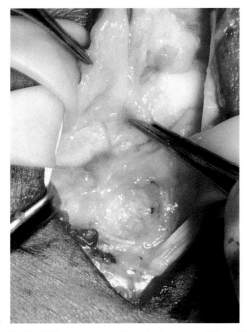
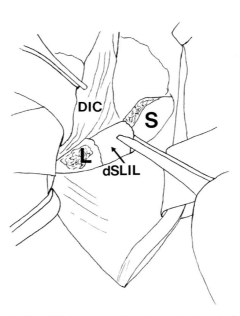

A                                                                              B

**FIGURE 9.** Intraoperative photograph **(A)** and illustration **(B)** demonstrating the avulsed end of the dorsal component of the scapholunate interosseous ligament (dSLIL). The dSLIL is placed back easily onto its attachment site on the scaphoid (S) once the scaphoid and lunate (L) have been reduced and pinned. DIC, dorsal intercarpal ligament.

into bone. Then pass the sutures to anchor both the dorsal portion of the scapholunate interosseous ligament and the DIC ligament to their origins on the scaphoid.

If the DIC is avulsed from the lunate, use a similar technique to reattach the DIC ligament to the dorsal aspect of the lunate (Figs. 11, 12). Finally, repair the capsular incision

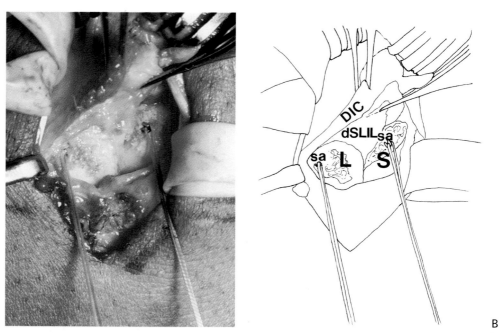

A                                                                                                    B

**FIGURE 10.** Intraoperative photograph **(A)** and illustration **(B)** demonstrating the suture anchors (sa). Suture anchor placed into the scaphoid (S) where the dorsal component of the scapholunate interosseous ligament (dSLIL) and the dorsal intercarpal ligament (DIC) was avulsed. Another suture anchor is shown placed into the dorsal aspect of the lunate (L) where the DIC was avulsed.

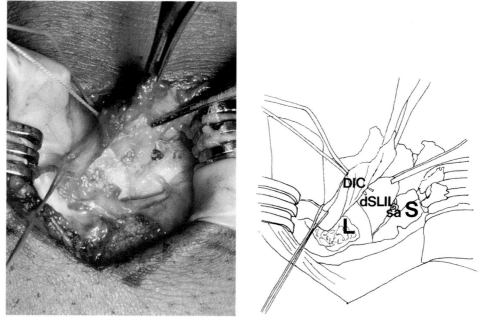

A                                                                                                    B

**FIGURE 11.** Intraoperative photograph **(A)** and illustration **(B)** demonstrating the suture, anchored into the scaphoid (S), passing first through the dorsal component of the scapholunate interosseous ligament (dSLIL) and then the dorsal intercarpal ligament (DIC). The suture, which is anchored to the lunate (L), is seen passing through the DIC ligament.

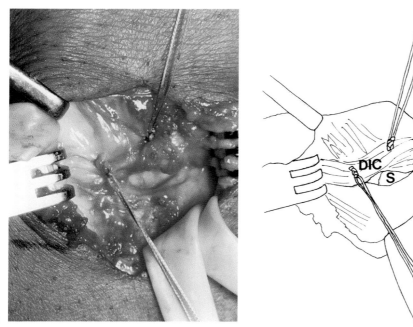
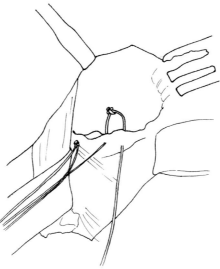

A                                                                                                    B

**FIGURE 12.** Intraoperative photograph **(A)** and illustration **(B)** demonstrating the avulsed dorsal component of the scapholunate interosseous ligament and the dorsal intercarpal ligaments (DIC) sutured back to the scaphoid (S), as well as the avulsed DIC sutured back to the dorsal aspect of the lunate.

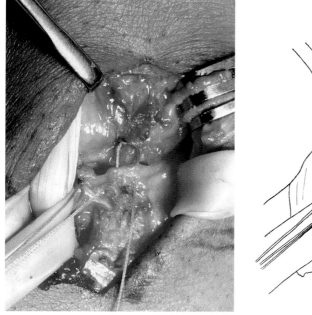

A                                                                                                    B

**FIGURE 13.** Intraoperative photograph **(A)** and illustration **(B)** demonstrating use of the same sutures to repair and slightly advance, in a vest-over-pants fashion, the capsule over the dorsal intercarpal ligament.

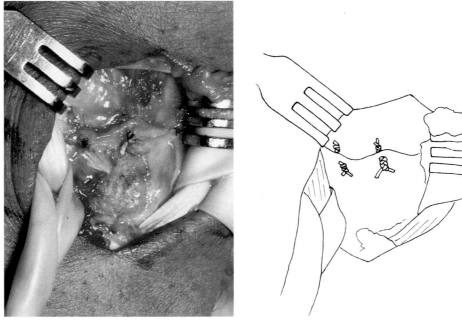

A                                                         B

**FIGURE 14.** Intraoperative photograph **(A)** and illustration **(B)** demonstrating the sutured capsular repair.

using the same sutures (Figs. 13, 14). Close the extensor retinaculum and the skin using simple interrupted sutures.

## POSTOPERATIVE MANAGEMENT

Immobilize the wrist and forearm in a long-arm splint with the forearm in pronation for 4 to 6 weeks. Immobilize the wrist in a short-arm splint for an additional 6 to 8 weeks. Obtain radiographs postoperatively at 1, 2, and 4 weeks to assess carpal alignment and pin position.

Remove sutures at 2 weeks. Treat signs of pin-track inflammation and drainage with antibiotics until pin removal. Remove pins at 12 weeks, place the wrist in a removable short-arm palmar splint, and initiate gentle active range-of-motion exercises.

The postimmobilization period of stiffness resolves over a 3- to 6-month period with activities of daily living or the addition of formal therapy. The small degree of flexion loss of the wrist that is usually present is due to dorsal scarring and capsular and ligamentous reefing.

## COMPLICATIONS

An increase in the intercarpal scapholunate distance in the postoperative period indicates a loss of fixation and disruption of the ligamentous repair. If this situation occurs, consider reexploring the wrist to repair or reconstruct the scapholunate ligaments.

Pin problems include pin-track infections, which should be treated with antibiotics until at least 10 weeks following surgery. Breakage or bending of the pins is a possibility that can be minimized if pins of adequate diameter and sufficient number are used for carpal fixation, along with adequate splinting.

## RECOMMENDED READING

1. Metz, V. M., Schimmerl, S. M., Gilula, L. A., Viegas, S. F., Saffar, P.: Wide scapholunate joint space in lunotriquetral coalition: a normal variant? *Radiology*, 188: 557–559, 1993.
2. Viegas, S. F., Patterson, R. M., Hokanson, J. A., Davis, J.: Wrist anatomy: incidence, distribution and correlation of anatomy, tears and arthritis. *J. Hand Surg.*, 18A: 463–475, 1993.
3. Viegas, S. F., Yamaguchi, S., Boyd, N. L., Patterson, R. M.: The dorsal ligaments of the wrist: anatomy, mechanical properties and function. *J. Hand Surg.*, 24A: 456–468, 1999.
4. Watson, H. K., Ashmead, D. IV, Makhlouf, M. V.: Examination of the scaphoid. *J. Hand Surg.*, 13A: 657–660, 1988.

# 14

# Dynamic Scapholunate Instability: Dorsal Capsulodesis

Charles A. Goldfarb and Richard H. Gelberman

## INDICATIONS/CONTRAINDICATIONS

Scapholunate dissociation, the most common cause of carpal instability, likely results from an injury to the scapholunate interosseous ligament and the long radio-lunate ligament. There is a resultant loss of the normal relationship between the scaphoid and the lunate, and the scaphoid excessively palmar flexes (while the lunate dorsiflexes) with radial deviation of the wrist. This may occur only with wrist motion (dynamic instability) or the scaphoid and lunate may assume an abnormal relationship at rest (static instability). Plain radiographs are normal with dynamic instability and the diagnosis is made on clinical examination with elicitation of tenderness over the scapholunate interosseous ligament and a positive Watson scaphoid shift sign. In static instability, plain radiographs are abnormal and the diagnosis is made with any one of the following criteria: a scapholunate angle of more than 70°, a scapholunate angle more than 15° greater than the contralateral wrist, or a radio-lunate angle greater than 10° on the lateral radiograph (a normal scapholunate angle is 47°, normal radiolunate is 0°); a scapholunate gap of 3 mm or greater on the pos-teroanterior (PA) radiograph; or a decrease in the scaphoid ring to scaphoid proximal pole distance to less than 8 mm on the PA radiograph (Figs. 1, 2).

Dorsal capsulodesis uses a leash of dorsal wrist capsule to tether the distal pole of the scaphoid and prevent excessive scaphoid flexion (Fig. 3). When effective, the painful clunking of the scaphoid against the radius is prevented and the risk of progression of the instability is decreased.

The primary indication for dorsal capsulodesis is dynamic scapholunate disso-ciation after the failure of nonoperative treatment. Our conservative management protocol includes splinting of the wrist in 20° of extension, activity modification, and oral antiinflammatory medications. While we have found that most patients with symptomatic instability ultimately require operative intervention, a 12-week trial of nonoperative management is recommended for all patients.

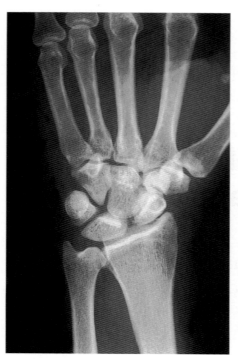

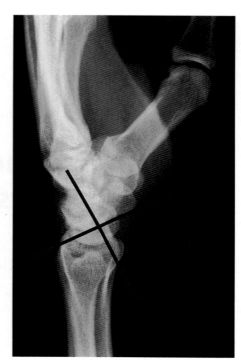

**FIGURE 1.** Posteroanterior radiograph of static scapholunate instability with an abnormal scapholunate gap of 4 mm. The ring to proximal pole distance is decreased to 5 mm.

**FIGURE 2.** In a lateral wrist radiograph of the same patient, the scapholunate angle measures 85°, which is significantly higher than acceptable.

The management of static scapholunate dissociation is controversial. Typically, we treat an acute, static injury with ligamentous repair through a dorsal approach and do not perform a concomitant capsulodesis. Furthermore, while some authors have recommended dorsal capsulodesis and scapholunate repair for chronic, static deformities, we do not recommend capsulodesis in these cases (5).

While the surgical indications for dorsal capsulodesis are controversial, certain absolute contraindications exist: a static scapholunate dissociation in which a bony reduction cannot be easily obtained, an injury to the scapholunate ligament as part of a larger wrist ligamentous injury (perilunate injury), and the presence of arthrosis at any of the carpal articulations. An occult dorsal ganglion may present in a similar fashion to dynamic scapholunate instability, with dorsal wrist pain and often with a positive Watson scaphoid shift test. An ultrasound is used to identify the ganglion and these patients may be treated with ganglion excision alone.

## PREOPERATIVE PLANNING

The most important aspect of preoperative planning for dorsal capsulodesis is an accurate diagnosis of dynamic scapholunate instability based on history, physical examination, and radiographic studies. Patients with dynamic scapholunate instability complain of dorsal wrist pain and clicking or clunking of the wrist with motion. A traumatic incident, usually a fall on an extended wrist, may be recalled. The physical examination includes a global assessment of joint laxity (Fig. 4) and a careful examination of the contralateral wrist for asymptomatic instability. Typically, the affected wrist examination reveals dorsal scapholunate interval tenderness and a positive Watson scaphoid shift test.

The Watson scaphoid shift test (Fig. 5) is performed with the patient sitting with the involved elbow on the examination table and the forearm in neutral rotation and perpendicular to the table. While seated opposite the patient, the examiner's

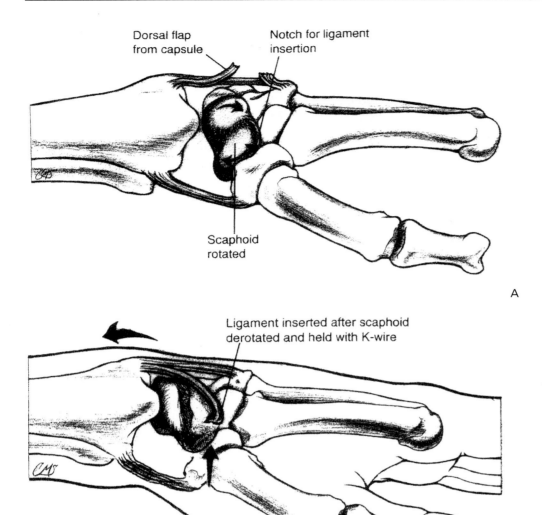

FIGURE 3. A and B: A graphic representation of the concept of dorsal capsulodesis to stabilize the scaphoid from excessive palmar flexion.

thumb is placed over the scaphoid tuberosity with the index and long fingers overlying the dorsal distal radius. While applying an axial load and radially deviating the wrist, the examiner applies a dorsally directed pressure to the scaphoid tuberosity, palpating for a dorsal clunk and attempting to elicit dorsal wrist pain in the area of the scapholunate interosseous ligament (9). The test is considered positive when there is a palpable clunk and associated pain along the dorsum of the wrist in the area of the scapholunate interosseous ligament.

Radiographic assessment includes standard PA and lateral radiographs, which, by definition, should be normal for dynamic instability. A stress series, including true PA radiographs in radial deviation, ulnar deviation, and in neutral with a loaded fist, is also obtained, although these are almost always normal. Cineradiographs, arthroscopy, and arthrogram are all more definitive means of confirming the diagnosis, but in a patient with dorsal wrist pain localized to the scapholunate interosseous space, a history of painful clicking, a positive Watson test, normal plain radiographs, and a failed trial of conservative treatment, operative intervention is recommended without further testing.

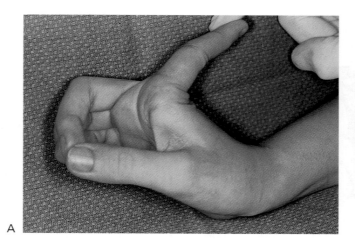

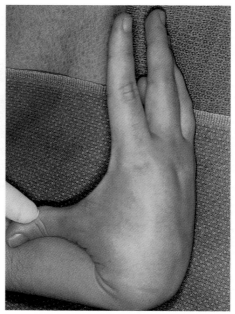

**FIGURE 4. A** and **B:** Globally increased joint laxity is uncommon, but should be recognized preoperatively.

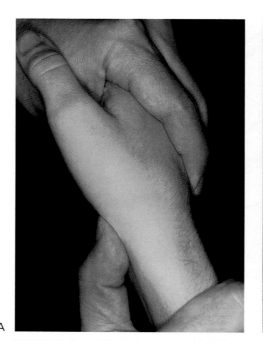

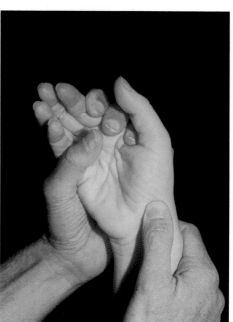

**FIGURE 5. A** and **B:** Watson scaphoid shift test. With axial loading and radial deviation of the wrist, dorsally directed pressure along the volar proximal pole of the scaphoid causes an audible and dorsally painful clunk.

## SURGICAL TECHNIQUE

The patient is seen in the preoperative holding area to confirm the operative side and sign the operative site. The patient is placed supine on the operating room table with the affected extremity on a hand table. A regional anesthetic is administered, a nonsterile tourniquet is placed, and a sterile preparation is performed with Povidone-iodine. After draping the patient, an examination under anesthesia is performed to confirm the diagnosis. The radial styloid and Lister's tubercle are palpated and marked and the scapholunate interval noted 1 cm distal to the tubercle. A 3-cm trans-

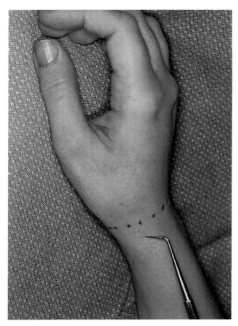

**FIGURE 6.** A transverse incision at the level of the radial styloid in the dorsal wrist crease is outlined. The pointer marks the radial styloid.

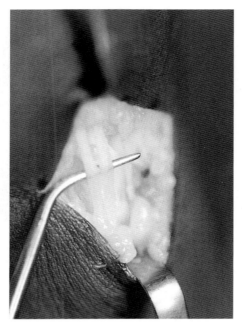

**FIGURE 7.** The identification of the superficial branch of the radial nerve.

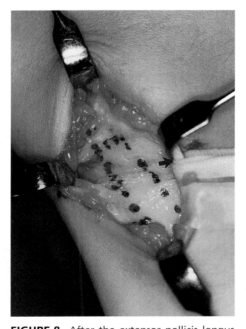

**FIGURE 8.** After the extensor pollicis longus *(arrow)* is translated ulnarward and the extensor carpi radialis brevis translated radially, the capsule is easily exposed. The planned capsular incision is marked and must be at least 1 cm in width.

verse incision is marked (Fig. 6) and incised at the level of the styloid in the dorsal wrist crease. Once the dermis has been incised, blunt dissection with scissors is performed. Divisions of the superficial branch of the radial nerve are identified and tagged with a vessel loop for protective purposes (Fig. 7). Similarly, the radial artery is identified and tagged. The extensor pollicis longus is exposed and retracted ulnar-

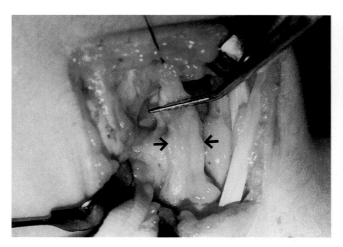

**FIGURE 9.** The length of the flap should be checked as shown. Excess tissue can be trimmed after completion of the capsulodesis. The capsular flap is marked with arrows.

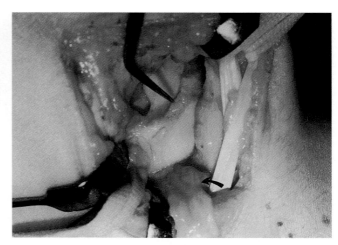

**FIGURE 10.** The dorsal ridge of the scaphoid is identified with the pointer. Note the capsular flap proximally, marked with the arrow.

ward, and the interval between the second and third dorsal compartments is used to expose the distal radius and the dorsal wrist capsule. The scapholunate articulation is identified. A marking pen is used to outline a capsular flap that is at least 1 cm wide and based proximally on the distal radius (Fig. 8). The long axis of the thumb metacarpal is a landmark for distal direction of the planned flap. Care must be taken to avoid narrowing the flap, as this can compromise its strength. The flap extends at least 1.5 cm distally to allow sufficient length for the capsulodesis (Fig. 9). After the flap is created, the dorsal ridge of the scaphoid is identified and the adjacent scaphoid blood supply protected (Fig. 10). A 3-mm round cutting carbide burr or small rongeur is used to roughen the dorsal scaphoid distal to the dorsal ridge to provide an adequate surface for healing of the capsular flap (Fig. 11). A stab incision is then made with a #15 blade on the radial aspect of the scaphoid and a 0.062-in. Kirschner wire is introduced under direct vision to the distal aspect of the scaphoid. The K-wire is then driven through the scaphoid and into the capitate while the wrist is in ulnar deviation and the scaphoid is held extended (Fig. 12). The position of the scaphoid and the K-wire are confirmed with fluoroscopic imaging (Fig. 13). Two 2.5-mm Statak suture anchors (Zimmer,

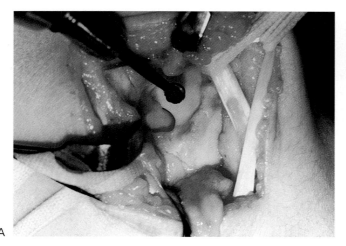

A

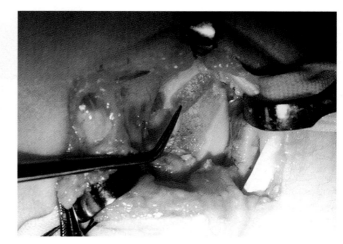

B

**FIGURE 11.  A** and **B:** A burr is used to make a trough distal to the dorsal ridge.

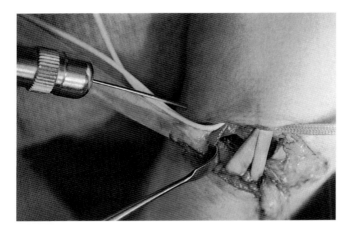

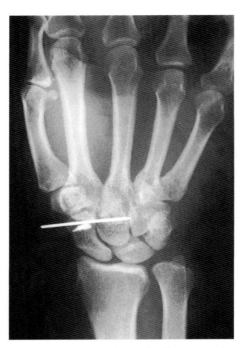

**FIGURE 12.** A 0.065-in. Kirschner wire is placed under direct vision. The wrist is held extended and in ulnar deviation to extend the scaphoid while the K-wire is placed.

**FIGURE 13.** The radiograph illustrates the extended scaphoid with the Kirschner wire holding the scaphoid to the capitate.

Warsaw, IN) with size 0 nonabsorbable suture are placed distal to the dorsal ridge in the previously prepared bed (Fig. 14). The wrist is held in 20° extension for the remaining portion of the case and the Statak suture is then passed through the dorsal capsule and tied securely, thus tethering the scaphoid (Fig. 15). The K-wire is cut and buried subcutaneously.

The tourniquet is released and adequate hemostasis achieved. The subcutaneous layer is closed with 3–0 vicryl and the skin closed with a 4–0 monocryl running

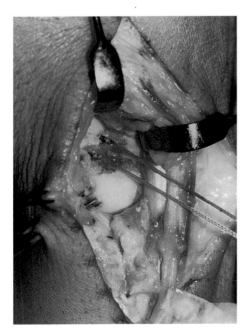

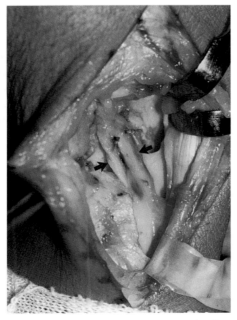

**FIGURE 14.** Suture anchors are then placed in the prepared bed.

**FIGURE 15.** The suture is tied over the flap to secure it into the bed, as marked between the black arrows.

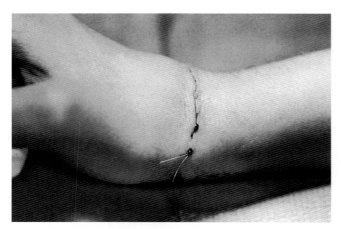

**FIGURE 16.** The wound is closed with a subcuticular stitch. The wrist must be held in 20° extension during closure to prevent injury to the flap.

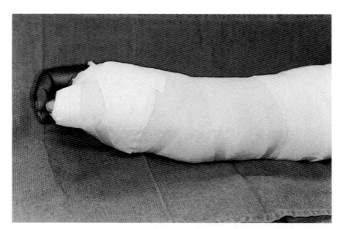

**FIGURE 17.** The wrist is dressed in a bulky dressing while held in 20° extension.

subcuticular stitch (Fig. 16). We do not routinely insert a drainage system if adequate hemostasis is achieved. A sterile dressing and a short-arm spica splint in 20° wrist extension complete the procedure (Fig. 17).

## POSTOPERATIVE MANAGEMENT

A wound check is performed 10 days postoperatively and a short-arm spica cast is placed with the wrist in 20° extension. At 6 weeks the cast is discontinued, the K-wire is removed in the office under local anesthesia, and gentle range-of-motion exercises are begun. Strengthening exercises are instituted at 8 to 10 weeks and resumption of normal activity allowed at 3 months. Rarely is formal occupational therapy required. Range of motion is typically outstanding, although a loss of 10° to 20° of wrist flexion is not unusual. Most patients have a negative Watson scaphoid shift test postoperatively.

## COMPLICATIONS

The most common technical error is to make the capsular flap too narrow, which may provide an inadequate tether for the scaphoid. The flap must be kept at least 1 cm wide. We use a 0.062-in. K-wire to avoid the complication of a broken wire and we bury the K-wire to decrease the possibility of pin-track infection. Care is taken to place the K-wire distal and somewhat volar in the scaphoid to avoid compromising the position of the suture anchors.

Finally, the branches of the superficial branch of the radial nerve are identified and protected with both the exposure and the placement of the K-wire. Care in mobilizing and protecting the branches can help avoid a nerve injury and postoperative neuroma.

## ILLUSTRATIVE CASE FOR TECHNIQUE

A 13-year-old right-hand-dominant female gymnast presented with 8 months of right wrist pain. The patient sustained her initial injury during a gymnastics competition. She was evaluated by a local orthopedic surgeon, was found to have dorsal wrist pain with normal plain radiographs, and was diagnosed with a type I Salter-Harris fracture of her distal radius. Splinting for 6 weeks improved her symptoms and she was cleared to return to gymnastics 3 months later. Two weeks

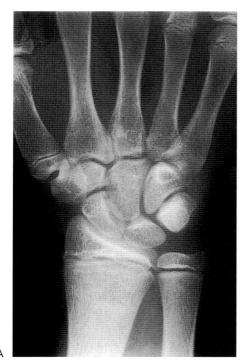
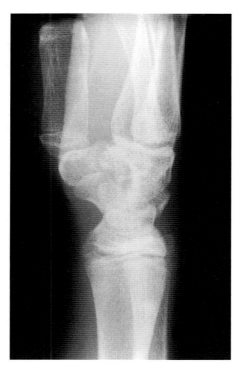

A                                                                              B

**FIGURE 18. A:** Normal preoperative anteroposterior radiograph. **B:** Lateral radiograph.

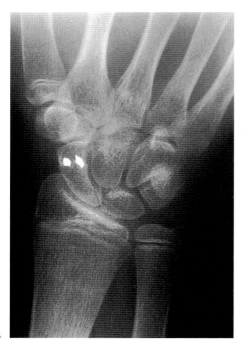
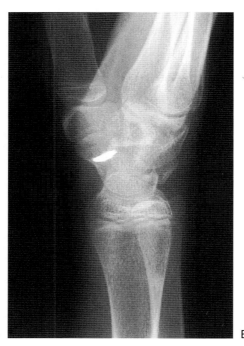

A                                                                              B

**FIGURE 19. A:** Postoperative anteroposterior radiograph revealing the suture anchors. **B:** Post-operative lateral radiograph revealing the suture anchors.

after her return, she reinjured her wrist. She was referred for further evaluation and treatment.

The patient's pain was activity-related and confined to the dorsal wrist. Physical examination revealed dorsal tenderness at the scapholunate interval. There was no tenderness elsewhere in the carpus or at the distal radioulnar joint. A Watson scaphoid shift sign created an audible and dorsally painful clunk. There was no evidence of generalized joint laxity and the left wrist was asymptomatic. The patient's grip strength was markedly diminished at 10 lb for the affected right wrist and 50 lb for the unaffected left wrist. Pinch strength was similarly decreased at 6 lb on the right and 10 lb on the left. Radiographs of the wrist were normal (Fig. 18).

The patient was diagnosed with dynamic scapholunate instability and a trial of splinting was begun. The patient returned to clinic 4 weeks later with no significant improvement. With an 8-month history of pain and a failure of conservative care on two separate occasions, the patient was an excellent candidate for surgical intervention. A dorsal capsulodesis was performed (Fig. 19).

The patient was seen for a wound check at 10 days postoperatively and placed into a short-arm thumb spica cast in 20° of wrist extension. Five weeks postoperatively, the patient's cast was discontinued and the buried K-wire was removed in clinic. Active motion was begun and strengthening exercises instituted at 10 weeks postoperatively. She returned to gymnastics at 3 months and has done well with no further wrist pain.

## RECOMMENDED READING

1. Blatt, G.: Capsulodesis in reconstructive hand surgery: dorsal capsulodesis for the unstable scaphoid and volar capsulodesis following excision of the distal ulna. *Hand Clin.*, 3: 81–102, 1987.
2. Blatt, G.: Dorsal Capsulodesis for Rotary Subluxation of the Scaphoid. In: *Master Techniques in Orthopaedic Surgery: The Wrist*, edited by R. H. Gelberman, Raven Press, New York, pp. 147–165, 1994.
3. Deshmukh, S. C., Givissis, P., Belloso, D., Stanley, J. K., Trail, I. A.: Blatt's capsulodesis for chronic scapholunate dissociation. *J. Hand Surg.*, 24B: 215–220, 1999.
4. Hwang, J., Goldfarb, C., Gelberman, R., Boyer, M.: The effect of dorsal carpal ganglion excision on dynamic scapholunate instability. *J. Hand Surg.*, 24B: 106–108, 1999.
5. Lavernia, C. J., Cohen, M. S., Taleisnik, J.: Treatment of scapholunate dissociation by ligamentous repair and capsulodesis. *J. Hand Surg.*, 17A: 354–359, 1992.
6. Linscheid, R. L., Dobyns, J. H., Beabout, J. W., Bryan, R. S.: Traumatic instability of the wrist: diagnosis, classification, and pathomechanics. *J. Bone Joint Surg.*, 54A: 1612–1632, 1972.
7. Taleisnik, J.: Carpal Instability: current concepts review. *J. Bone Joint Surg.*, 70A: 1262–1267, 1988.
8. Taleisnick, J.: Post-traumatic carpal instability. *Clin. Orthop.*, 149: 73–82, 1980.
9. Wintman, B. I., Gelberman, R. H., Katz, J. N.: Dynamic scapholunate instability: results of operative treatment with dorsal capsulodesis. *J. Hand Surg.*, 20A: 971–979, 1995.
10. Wyrick, J. D., Youse, B. D., Kiefhaber, T. R.: Scapholunate ligament repair and capsulodesis for the treatment of static scapholunate dissociation. *J. Hand Surg.*, 23B: 776–780, 1998.

# 15

# Acute Lunate and Perilunate Dislocations: Open Reduction and Ligamentous Repair

Robert M. Szabo and Craig C. Newland

## INDICATIONS/CONTRAINDICATIONS

The typical presentation of a wrist with an acute perilunate dislocation includes swelling, pain, and deformity following acute trauma. The primary dislocation occurs at the midcarpal joint, where the capitate usually is displaced dorsally to the lunate. When the capitate is displaced, the scaphoid must either fracture or rotate. If a fracture does not occur, the ligaments supporting the proximal pole of the scaphoid rupture, allowing dorsal rotation of the proximal pole; a dorsal perilunate dislocation results. If the scaphoid fractures, the distal fragment moves with the capitate and distal carpal row and the proximal pole remains attached to the lunate, resulting in a dorsal transscaphoid perilunate dislocation.

Radiographs corroborate a gross disturbance of carpal relationships (Figs. 1, 2) (see also Chapter 13). In a dorsal perilunate dislocation, the lateral radiograph shows the longitudinal axis of the capitate dorsal to the longitudinal axis of the radius and the proximal pole of the scaphoid rotated dorsally. A scapholunate angle greater than 70° on the lateral is one accepted radiographic criterion for identifying an acute scapholunate dissociation. In the anteroposterior (AP) projection, the carpus is foreshortened. AP radiography reveals a scapholunate interval greater than 2 mm (Terry Thomas sign). The lunate is triangular, and Gilula's wrist arches are disrupted. In a lunate dislocation, the longitudinal axis of the capitate tends to be nearly or actually colinear with that of the radius, and the lunate is displaced palmarward ("spilled tea cup" sign) (15).

We believe that all acute perilunate dislocations require surgery. Closed anatomic reduction of acute perilunate dissociations is difficult to achieve and cannot be maintained reliably by external immobilization alone. Adkinson and Chapman

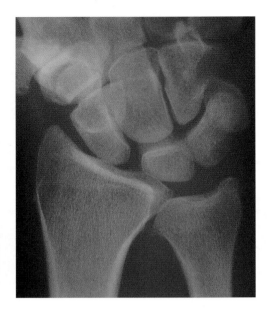

**FIGURE 1.** Anteroposterior radiograph of a patient with an acute scapholunate dissociation. Notice the scapholunate gap of 4 mm (Terry Thomas sign) and the triangular shape of the lunate.

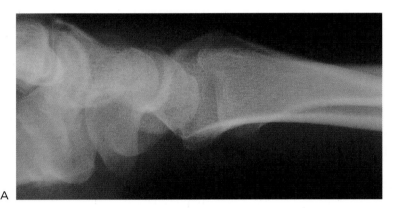

A

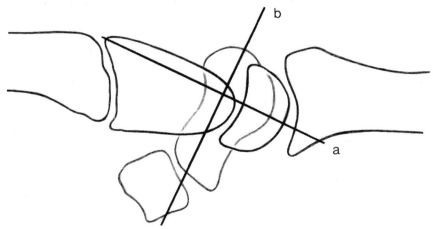

B

**FIGURE 2.  A:** Lateral radiograph of a patient with scapholunate dissociation. The lunate is dorsiflexed, and the scaphoid is palmar flexed—dorsiflexion intercalated segment instability pattern. The scapholunate angle is 90°. **B:** The scapholunate angle is measured on a true lateral radiograph by drawing a line through the longitudinal axis of the midportion of the lunate (a), and a second line through the longitudinal axis of the scaphoid (b). The angle created by the intersection of these two lines is the scapholunate angle. Although difficult to define precisely, the normal range for this angle is regarded to be 30° to 60°, with an average of 47°. Angles greater than 80°, however, are considered a definite indication of scapholunate dissociation.

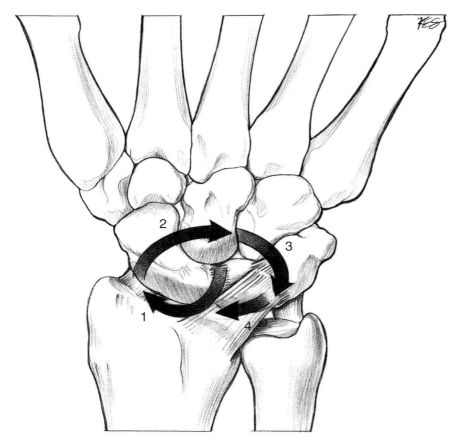

**FIGURE 3.** The spectrum of progressive lunate instability is simplified by Mayfield's scheme of four stages: Stage 1 begins with injury to the scapholunate interosseous ligament; stage 2 includes failure of the midcarpal portion of the radioscaphocapitate ligament, or the greater arc variant where the scaphoid and possibly the capitate is fractured; stage 3 includes failure of the lunotriquetral interosseous and ulnotriquetral ligaments; and stage 4 includes failure of the dorsal radioscapholunotriquetral ligament, thus allowing palmar dislocation of the lunate. (Modified from Mayfield, J. K.: Mechanism of carpal injuries. *Clin. Orthop.*, 149: 45–54, 1980, with permission.)

(1) noted that only 27% of acute perilunate dislocations managed by closed reduction and external immobilization retained their initial reduction.

After producing a series of scapholunate dislocations in cadavers, Mayfield (17–19) identified a predictable sequence of progressive failure of ligamentous restraints. He postulated a mechanism of injury involving wrist extension, ulnar deviation, and intercarpal supination in combination producing the various patterns of injury observed, and noted that hyperextension in pronation/supination neutral tended to produce a scaphoid fracture. The addition of ulnar deviation and intercarpal supination resulted in failure of the scapholunate interosseous ligament (SLIL) and radioscaphocapitate ligament (RSCL), or combined osseous and ligamentous injuries. The pattern of sequential failure begins on the radiopalmar wrist and extends to the ulnar and dorsal wrist.

While Mayfield noted structural heterogeneity of the palmar capsular ligaments, Kuhlmann et al. (13) further characterized the variability in the elastic modulus, elongation to failure, and ultimate tensile strength of these same ligaments. The heterogeneous nature of the ligamentous restraints and the multiple combinations of dorsiflexion, ulnar deviation, and intercarpal supination explain the wide spectrum of injuries seen clinically. Mayfield's proposal of greater and lesser arc injuries with four stages of severity is a useful classification for operative planning (Fig. 3).

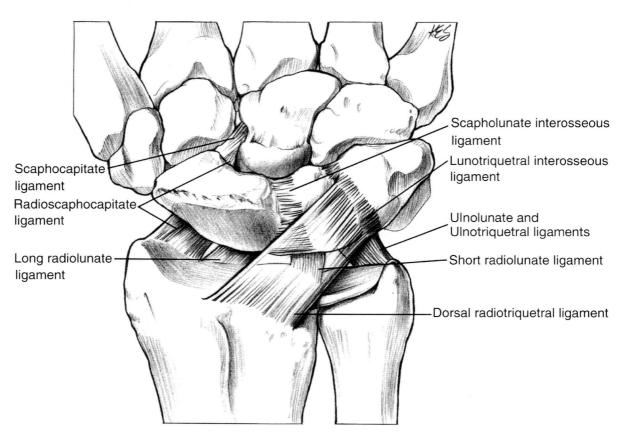

**FIGURE 4.** Dorsal perspective of the ligamentous anatomy of the wrist, viewed with a distraction load applied to demonstrate the dominant palmar capsular ligaments and intrinsic intercarpal ligaments.

Appreciation of ligamentous anatomy is fundamental to treating instability injuries (Fig. 4). The palmar radial carpal ligament consists of three strong components: the radioscaphocapitate, long radiolunate, and short radiolunate ligaments. The radioscaphocapitate ligament has three parts: radial collateral, radioscaphoid, and radiocapitate. These distinctions are made on the location of insertion, not on discrete anatomic divisions (3). The RSCL runs from the radial styloid through a groove in the waist of the scaphoid, ending in the palmar aspect of the capitate. This ligament acts as a fulcrum around which the scaphoid rotates. The RSCL is the only ligamentous connection between the radius and the scaphoid. The long radiolunate ligament is parallel to the radioscaphocapitate ligament from the palmar rim of the distal radius to the radial margin of the palmar horn of the lunate. As the central radiocarpal ligament, it augments the scapholunate interosseous ligament palmarly. The long radiolunate ligament and the palmar lunotriquetral interosseous ligament were thought to be in continuity, thus previously were called the *radiotriquetral ligament* (20).

Between the radioscaphocapitate and long radiolunate ligaments is an area of potential weakness over the capitate-lunate articulation, known as the *space of Poirier.* In a stage IV perilunate dislocation, the lunate becomes dislocated palmarly through this space. The short radiolunate ligament originates from the palmar margin of the distal radius in the area of the lunate facet and inserts into the proximal palmar surface of the lunate; it is contiguous with palmar fibers from the triangular fibrocartilage complex. The radioscapholunate ligament (ligament of Testut), previously thought to be an important stabilizer of the scaphoid, is found between the long and short radiolunate ligaments. It is actually a neurovascular pedicle to the scapholunate interosseous ligament derived from the anterior interosseous and radial arteries and the anterior interosseous nerve (4). The ulno-lunate and ulnotriquetral ligaments arise from the ulnar triangular meniscus of the wrist and insert on their respective carpal bones.

The dorsal radiocarpal ligament originates from the dorsal margin of the distal radius and extends ulnar obliquely and distally. Its radial fibers attach to the lunate and lunotriquetral interosseous ligament and the remainder inserts onto the dorsal tubercle of the triquetrum. The dorsal intercarpal ligament originates from the triquetrum, extends radially, and inserts onto the lunate, the dorsal groove of the scaphoid, and the trapezium (33).

## PREOPERATIVE PLANNING

Before focusing attention on the ligamentous injury, the surgeon carries out an examination of the neurovascular status. Assess the median nerve before and after any manipulative closed reduction. The onset of numbness and/or motor deficit at the time of injury without tense swelling in the carpal canal suggests contusion or traction rather than acute carpal tunnel syndrome. Carpal tunnel release is not indicated. Median nerve deficit that develops progressively after injury, along with tense swelling, probably indicates acute compression, and carpal tunnel release is necessary. If the history and physical examination are nondiagnostic, then measurement of carpal tunnel pressure can be very helpful to distinguish acute carpal tunnel syndrome from contusion (30).

Initial radiographs may reveal a palmar dislocation of the lunate. If so, undertake closed reduction under intravenous sedation. Place the hand in finger traps and apply 10 lb of countertraction. Extend the wrist with one hand, then gently push the lunate back into place with the thumb of the contralateral hand. Bring the wrist into neutral, remove the finger traps, and apply a plaster sugar-tong splint. Repeat radiographs to confirm reduction and evaluate the type and degree of injury. Measure the scapholunate interval on the AP film and the scapholunate angle on the lateral. Compare the films with views of the opposite wrist.

Distortion of the concentric arcs of the proximal and distal rows indicates that the injury has extended to the ulnar side of the carpus. Frank diastasis of the lunotriquetral interval may confirm this finding, but frequently the radiographic appearance of a stage III or IV injury is subtle, manifested by small avulsion fractures on the ulnar side of the carpus or an ulnar styloid fracture. A traction film can be helpful by exaggerating the displacement. Radiographs may reveal unusual variants of carpal ligamentous injury; for example, displacement of the proximal pole of the scaphoid from the scaphoid fossa is diagnostic of a scaphoid dislocation rather than perilunate dislocation. Palmar rather than dorsal perilunate dislocation is rarely encountered (2,9,27).

Transosseous variants (e.g., transscaphoid, transcapitate) are common, and are termed *greater arc injuries*. The combination of a radial styloid fracture and ulnar styloid fracture may be a greater arc injury; make every effort to identify the concomitant ligamentous injury. Fracture of the proximal pole of the capitate can be surprisingly subtle. This injury can be obscure, even though the proximal pole fragment is flipped 180° with the articular surface facing distally (32). Oblique films or tomograms are necessary if the head of the capitate cannot be visualized clearly (8). Palmar and radial displacement of the proximal pole of the scaphoid from the scaphoid fossa is diagnostic of a scaphoid dislocation rather than perilunate dislocation. The lack of an intact ligamentous hinge distally or interposition of soft tissue (torn ligaments) may prevent successful restoration of anatomy with closed reduction (31).

## SURGERY

Position the patient supine on the operating room table; place a tourniquet around the upper arm. Administer either general anesthesia or axillary block.

Whereas some advocate reduction and percutaneous pin fixation under direct arthroscopic visualization (25,26), open reduction with internal fixation is the preferred technique (1,6,12). The surgical approach for ligamentous injury alone can be dorsal or combined dorsal and palmar; it depends on the status of the median nerve. If the patient is neurologically intact (no signs of acute carpal tunnel syndrome), use a dorsal approach. If the median nerve is compromised or reduction cannot be obtained with a dorsal approach alone, use a combined dorsal and palmar approach. A transscaphoid perilunate dislocation may need only a palmar approach.

Once the fractured scaphoid is reduced and stabilized, examine intraoperative radiographs to confirm normal carpal relationships. At times, a small chondral fragment will block reduction and a dorsal approach will be needed to remove this fragment. It occurs predominantly between the capitate and lunate; look for colinearity of this articulation. Alternatively, internal fixation of the scaphoid may also be carried out with a compression screw that is inserted through a dorsal approach alone.

### Technique

**Dorsal Approach.** Make a dorsal longitudinal incision in the skin in line with Lister's tubercle. A 5- to 6-cm incision provides sufficient exposure (Fig. 5). Develop the interval between the third and fourth dorsal compartments by dividing the distal portion of the extensor retinaculum and the septum between the two compartments. Retract the tendons of the fourth compartment ulnarly and the extensor pollicis longus radially (Fig. 6). In a stage IV injury, the dorsal capsule may be torn. In such a case, extend the traumatic capsulotomy as needed for exposure. Otherwise, make a longitudinal capsulotomy in line with Lister's tubercle extending distally over the dorsum of the capitate. Elevate the capsular flaps by subperiosteal dissection, releasing dorsal attachments to the carpal bones until the scaphoid, lunate capitate, and triquetral articulations are well visualized (Fig. 7). Avoid dissection of the dorsal ridge portion of the scaphoid to prevent compromise to the blood supply to the proximal pole of the scaphoid (10,11).

We use a joystick to manipulate the scaphoid and lunate into anatomic relationship in the coronal and sagittal planes. Place a 0.062-in. K-wire in a dorsal-to-palmar direction into the lunate and another parallel K-wire into the proximal pole of the scaphoid. Place them close to the palmar cortex so that they can be used as levers to restore the scapholunate angle. Take care to close the scapholunate interval. Manipulate the scaphoid to reduce its palmar flexion and the lunate to reduce its dorsiflexion. While an assistant maintains this position, drill two 0.045-in. K-wires from the radial side of the carpus percutaneously through the proximal pole of the scaphoid into the lunate (Fig. 8). Place a third 0.045-in. K-wire percutaneously through the proximal pole of the scaphoid and into the capitate (Fig. 9). Inspect the midcarpal joint before placing this pin to make sure that there are no chondral fragments that block reduction of the capitolunate joint and that there is no capitate fracture.

Suture the dorsal portion of the scapholunate interosseous ligament if possible, using 4–0 braided nonabsorbable suture. If the tear is off the bone, drill parallel tunnels in either the proximal pole of the scaphoid or the lunate with a 0.035-in. K-wire. Place a horizontal mattress suture in the ligament, passing one end through each tunnel, and tying over bone (14).

Use percutaneous fixation of the lunate to the triquetrum and triquetrum to the capitate when injury is found to have propagated to the ulnar side of the carpus. Apply a palmar force to the dorsum of the triquetrum to reduce the triquetrum to

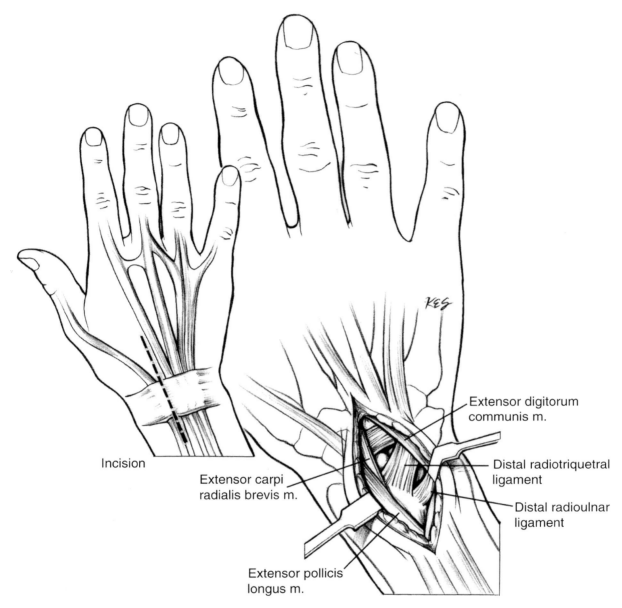

**FIGURE 5.** Dorsal exposure of the wrist capsule.

the lunate. Maintain this position while driving a K-wire from the ulnar side of the triquetrum into the lunate. Pass a second 0.045-in. K-wire from the triquetrum into the capitate.

Percutaneous pinning about the wrist puts the terminal branches of the radial sensory nerve and the dorsal sensory branch of the ulnar nerve at risk. The radial artery is located very close to pins passing into the proximal pole of the scaphoid. To minimize the risk of neurovascular injury, use the following technique:

Make a 3-mm skin incision. With a fine hemostat, spread the soft tissues until resistance of the capsule is encountered. Use a blunted 14-gauge angiocath between the tines of a hemostat as a guide, and pass the K-wire through the guide into the bone. Cut the wires beneath the skin. This skin incision usually does not require a suture.

Having secured anatomic intercarpal relationships with K-wires, position the wrist in slight flexion and radial deviation. We do not place pins across the radio-carpal joint; they are unnecessary.

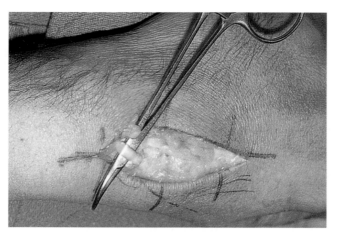

**FIGURE 6.** After the dorsal skin incision is made, the extensor pollicis longus tendon is identified so that the interval between the third and fourth dorsal compartments can be developed.

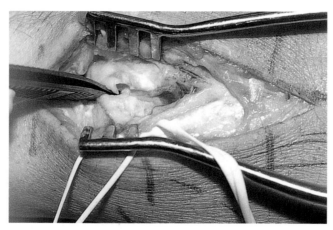

**FIGURE 7.** The torn scapholunate interosseous ligament is identified.

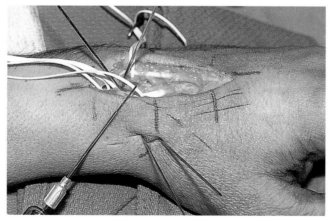

**FIGURE 8.** The two wires almost perpendicular to the dorsal wound are the joysticks used to reduce the scaphoid and lunate. The two wires inserted radially are maintaining the reduction. The placement of these two wires can be facilitated through a 14-gauge angiocath (shown on the wire driver) as a guide.

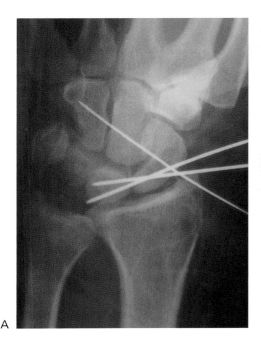

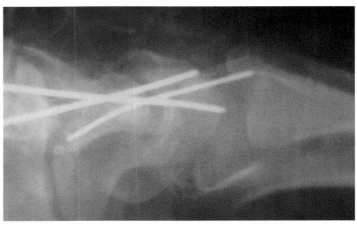

A

B

**FIGURE 9.** Radiographs demonstrating reduction and recommended internal fixation for a perilunate dislocation. **A:** Anteroposterior view. **B:** Lateral view.

Close the capsulotomy incision, any tears in the dorsal capsule, and the extensor retinaculum with 4–0 Teflon-coated braided Dacron suture. Approximate the skin edges with 4–0 nylon suture. A drain is usually not needed.

**Palmar Approach.** Recognizing that the palmar ligaments are torn, many surgeons prefer direct repair from the palmar side in all cases (29). We feel that this is unnecessary; a dorsal approach offers a superior perspective on carpal relationships and facilitates manipulation and pinning of the carpal bones. Sotereanos and colleagues compared the percentage of patients with satisfactory results from single-incision or two-incision approaches and found no statistically significant differences; the series analyzed was small (29). The palmar radiocarpal ligaments include distinct structures when viewed from within the joint. The presence of an overlying diffuse layer of capsule precludes the distinction of discrete capsular ligaments from the palmar approach (4). The distortion, which occurs with the acute trauma, compounds the problem, making it very unlikely that the ligaments can be sutured directly in the correct orientation and at the correct tension. Our experience has been that more motion is lost with direct repair of the palmar ligaments. We have never encountered late instability when these palmar ligaments have been left to heal without direct repair. The presence of rich vascular arches that traverse the palmar capsule suggests a superior healing potential when additional surgical trauma does not complicate the situation (11).

We reserve the addition of a palmar approach for a palmar lunate dislocation (stage IV), which cannot be reduced closed, and for an associated acute carpal tunnel syndrome. We use a standard carpal tunnel syndrome approach, extending the incision obliquely and ulnarly across the wrist crease for 1 cm.

We fix transscaphoid, transcapitate, and radial styloid fractures (greater arc injuries) with K-wires or an interfragmentary screw based on the size and degree of comminution of the fracture fragments (22,23,28). In greater arc injuries involving a scaphoid fracture, we most often employ a palmar approach for anatomic reduction and fixation of the scaphoid. Alternatively, a compression screw can be inserted retrograde from proximal to distal with a dorsal approach. Sometimes chondral fractures prevent complete reduction and a dorsal approach is added to inspect the midcarpal joint and remove loose fragments.

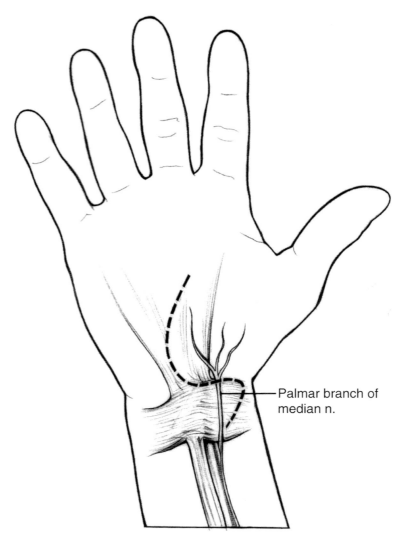

**FIGURE 10.** Incision used for combined approach to the scaphoid and carpal tunnel. Subcutaneous dissection *must* include identification of the palmar cutaneous branch of the median nerve.

Our customary palmar approach is that described by Russe; if the carpal tunnel needs to be released, however, we deviate the proximal extension of the incision radially and make the palmar portion of the incision along the thenar crease (Fig. 10). When the incision extends across the wrist, identify the palmar cutaneous nerve proximally before proceeding with subcutaneous dissection distally. We have used the Herbert screw for stabilization of the scaphoid fracture. Because recent data emphasize the importance of the palmar scaphotrapezial and scaphocapitate ligaments in providing stability to the distal pole of the scaphoid, we now prefer K-wires for stabilization of the scaphoid. They can be inserted without stripping the scaphotrapezial and scaphocapitate ligaments. With comminution at the waist, it is sometimes necessary to use distal radial or iliac crest bone graft acutely. Although it is possible to use a dorsal approach on a scaphoid fracture, we continue to use the palmar approach for stabilization of the scaphoid to avoid potential injury to the dorsal ridge vessels and because the dorsal approach prevents us from addressing the palmar comminution.

To begin the palmar approach, center a palmar incision over the flexor carpi radialis (FCR) tendon. Cross the wrist crease at a 45° angle paralleling the ulnar border of the shaft of the thumb metacarpal (Fig. 11). Identify the palmar cuta-

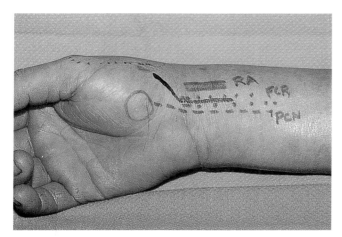

**FIGURE 11.** FCR, flexor carpi radialis tendon; PCN, palmar cutaneous nerve; RA, radial artery.

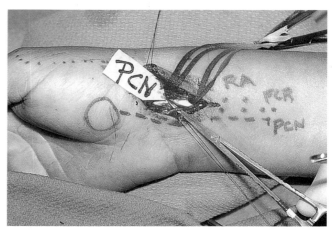

**FIGURE 12.** The palmar cutaneous branch of the median nerve is identified ulnar to the flexor carpi radialis tendon. FCR, flexor carpi radialis tendon; PCN, palmar cutaneous nerve; RA, radial artery.

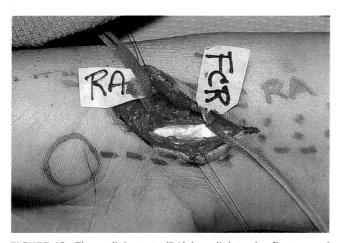

**FIGURE 13.** The radial artery (RA) is radial to the flexor carpi radialis tendon (FCR) and tagged with umbilical tape.

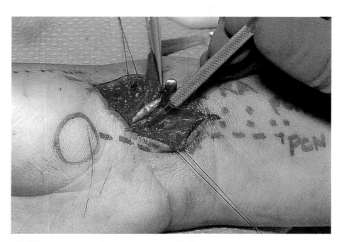

**FIGURE 14.** The flexor carpi radialis tendon is retracted radially and an incision is made in the posterior tendon sheath and palmar ligaments to enter the radiocarpal joint.

neous branch of the median nerve, which is ulnar to the FCR tendon (Fig. 12). Identify the radial artery radial to the FCR tendon and tag it with umbilical tape (Fig. 13). Retract the FCR tendon radially and make an incision in the posterior tendon sheath and palmar ligaments to enter the radiocarpal joint. Take care to make this incision perpendicular to the long axis of the radius and not to slant off ulnarly, which will cause injury to the median nerve or its palmar cutaneous branch (Fig. 14).

With the palmar ligaments retracted, the scaphoid fracture is well visualized (Fig. 15). Insert a 0.045-in. smooth K-wire perpendicular to each of the two main fragments of the scaphoid (Fig. 16). Once these wires are inserted use them like joysticks to manipulate and reduce the scaphoid fracture (Fig. 17). Once the fracture is reduced, place a Freer elevator in the radioscaphoid joint to maintain reduction and apply counterforce while an assistant drives two smooth 0.045-in. K-wires parallel across the fracture (Fig. 18). Check fracture reduction, wire placement, and carpal relationships with fluoroscopy (Fig. 19). Suture the palmar ligaments using interrupted 4–0 Teflon-coated braided Dacron horizontal mattress sutures (Fig. 20). Close the incision using 5–0 interrupted horizontal mattress nylon sutures (Fig. 21).

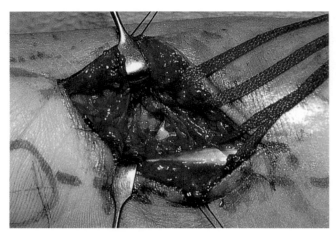

**FIGURE 15.** With the palmar ligaments retracted, the scaphoid fracture is well visualized.

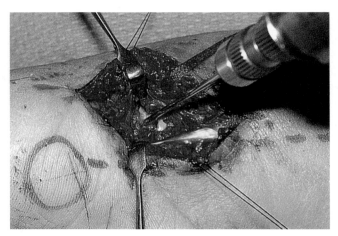

**FIGURE 16.** A 0.045-in. smooth K-wire is inserted perpendicular to each of the two main fragments of the scaphoid.

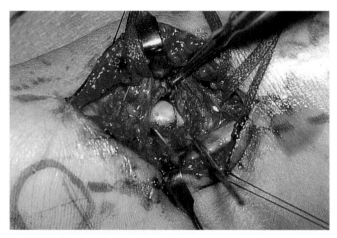

**FIGURE 17.** Once inserted, the wires are used like joysticks to manipulate and reduce the scaphoid fracture.

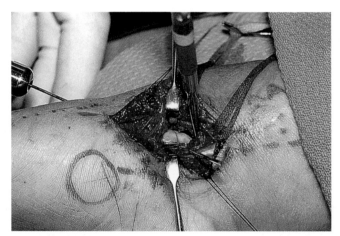

**FIGURE 18.** Once the fracture is reduced, a Freer elevator is placed in the radioscaphoid joint to maintain reduction and apply counterforce while two smooth 0.045-in. K-wires are driven parallel across the fracture.

Acute palmar perilunate dislocation is encountered rarely. Simulated injuries in cadavers emphasize the importance of the dorsal radiocarpal ligament (18). Acute management is similar to that of the more common dorsal perilunate dislocation.

## POSTOPERATIVE MANAGEMENT

Apply a long-arm bulky splint with the forearm in neutral, and the wrist in 15° of flexion and 10° of radial deviation. If the carpal tunnel has been released, immobilize the wrist in neutral. Convert to a long-arm thumb spica cast at 10 days when the sutures are removed. At 6 weeks apply a short-arm thumb spica cast. Remove the intercarpal pins at 8 weeks; leave the pins stabilizing a scaphoid fracture or other associated fractures in place, however, until union is documented radiographically. Discontinue immobilization at 12 weeks. Provide a removable palmar wrist splint for comfort for an additional 2 weeks. Patients with scaphoid fractures may need additional immobilization.

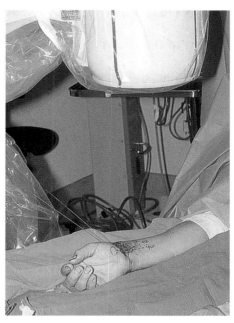

**FIGURE 19.** Fluoroscopy is used to check fracture reduction, wire placement, and carpal relationships.

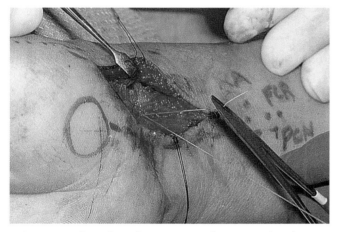

**FIGURE 20.** The palmar ligaments are then sutured with interrupted 4–0 Teflon-coated braided Dacron horizontal mattress sutures.

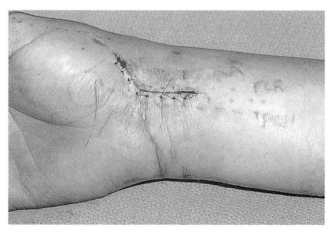

**FIGURE 21.** The incision is closed with 5–0 interrupted horizontal mattress nylon sutures.

Encourage active finger motion throughout the period of immobilization. At 12 weeks, encourage active motion of the wrist, ideally supervised by a hand therapist who employs local modalities to alleviate stiffness, provide pain relief, and control swelling. Prescribe progressive resistive exercises for grip strengthening as range of motion improves, usually at 16 weeks. Check radiographs at 2 weeks; 1, 3, and 6 months; and at 1 year.

Expectations for restoration of motion, grip strength, pain-free function, and return to previous employment and sports are determined case by case and tend to parallel the severity of initial injury and the adequacy of initial reduction (5,21). Individual tendencies toward stiffness, occupational demands, motivation, and compliance with rehabilitation may influence outcome. Prognosis is improved with early identification of these problems and individualization of the rehabilitation program. In general, some limitation of motion persists.

## COMPLICATIONS

### Failure of Diagnosis

The authors of a multicenter study of 166 perilunate dislocations and fracture dislocations found that open injury and delay in treatment had an adverse effect on outcome. Frequent oversight led to many missed diagnoses (25%) (12). Failure to appreciate small chondral fragments blocking reduction can lead to rapid deterioration of the radiocarpal or midcarpal joints. Similarly, failure to appreciate and treat the dorsal subluxation of the triquetrum on the lunate will lead to persistent instability, pain, and loss of motion.

### Pin-Related Complications

Adhering to a technique of percutaneous pinning, which includes spreading dissection down to the capsule, should avoid most complications related to transfixation of tendons or sensory nerves. Attention to appropriate percutaneous pin technique avoiding any transfixation of tendons will facilitate the recovery of finger motion. Cut intercarpal pins that remain *in situ* for 2 months beneath the skin to lessen the chance of infection. Counsel the patient carefully regarding appropriate actions to take to ensure prompt attention in the event of pin-site infection. Remove or replace loose or migrating pins if necessary.

### Carpal Tunnel Syndrome

Acute carpal tunnel syndrome requires carpal tunnel release, with its attending possible complications. Postoperatively the wrist is immobilized in neutral. Persistent median nerve deficits may indicate additional nerve contusion. The palmar cutaneous nerve is at particular risk, and should be identified and protected to avoid its injury.

### Reflex Sympathetic Dystrophy

As with any upper extremity injury, the healing process may be complicated by sympathetic mediated pain. Diffuse excessive pain and stiffness should lead to early consideration of sympathetic block, hand therapy, and counseling of the patient to encourage active patient participation in the recovery process. Unrecognized carpal tunnel syndrome may contribute to this problem.

### Persistent Ligamentous Instability

The best insurance against chronic instability following surgery in the acute setting is to achieve anatomic reduction. K-wire stabilization for 8 weeks, followed by immobilization for a total of 12 weeks, results in a very low incidence of lost reduction or chronic instability.

Inadequate reduction is best avoided by ensuring adequate exposure and obtaining intraoperative plain films; C-arm images can be misleading. Even plain films can be difficult to evaluate, especially with respect to the restoration of the radioscaphoid and radiolunate angles. Loss of reduction can occur if the ligaments have failed to heal by the time of pin removal.

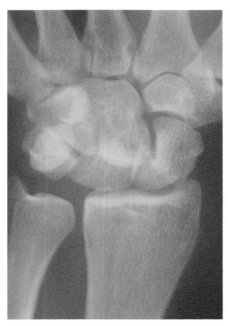

**FIGURE 22.** Anteroposterior radiograph of the transscaphoid perilunate dislocation.

## Malunion and Nonunion

Associated fractures, especially scaphoid fractures, may go on to become delayed union or nonunion. Confirm fracture union with plain radiographs or tomograms before removing pins. Bridging trabeculae should be present before immobilization is discontinued. Malunion is avoidable by obtaining adequate exposure to judge the quality of reduction and careful evaluation of intraoperative radiographs. Comminution of the palmar cortex of the scaphoid may lead to loss of reduction and development of a humpback deformity. Primary bone grafting may avoid this situation. Should loss of reduction result in a humpback deformity, proceed with open reduction and insertion of a trapezoidal wedge-shaped bone graft rather than waiting for union in a malreduced position (7). Scaphoid nonunion or malunion may lead to degenerative arthritis of the carpus (16,24). The time frame is quite variable. Mack described the average early changes to occur 8 years after injury with progression of advanced arthritis noted on the average of 31 years after injury (16).

## Stiffness

Stiffness can be expected after any severe ligamentous injury to the wrist. It is a far more common problem than is chronic instability. Ligaments heal with scar. Because the mechanical properties of scar are not the same as those of the original ligament, some loss of motion is unavoidable.

## Arthritis

Direct cartilage injury occurs in varying degrees in association with these ligamentous injuries and can result in posttraumatic arthritis. Repeated passage of K-wires through the joint surfaces and forced vigorous reduction maneuvers may

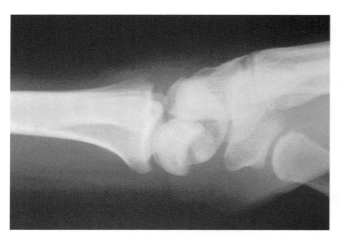

**FIGURE 23.** Lateral radiograph of the transscaphoid perilunate dislocation. Note the carpus dislocates with the distal pole of the scaphoid, leaving the proximal pole and lunate reduced in relationship to the radius.

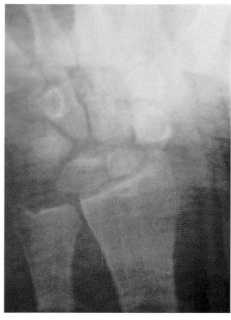

**FIGURE 24.** The dislocation was reduced by placing the hand in finger traps with 7 lb of countertraction; a dorsal and palmar plaster slab was applied. Note that the scaphoid fracture is still displaced, indicating persistent instability.

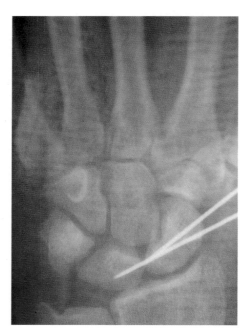

**FIGURE 25.** Anteroposterior radiograph obtained after the dressing was applied. In this case, one wire crosses the scapholunate joint. This adds some stability but is not essential.

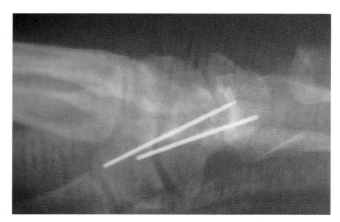

**FIGURE 26.** Lateral radiograph after the dressing is applied. Note the reduction of the scaphoid fracture as well as the carpal dislocation.

contribute iatrogenic injury. Additional wear on the cartilage due to abnormal mechanics or noncongruous reduction can explain posttraumatic arthritis following acute lunate and perilunate dislocation (5). The incidence of posttraumatic arthritis despite surgical treatment was high (56%) in one multicenter study (12).

## ILLUSTRATIVE CASE FOR TECHNIQUE

A 26-year-old right-hand-dominant man sustained a transscaphoid perilunate dislocation to his dominant hand in a high-speed motor vehicle accident. AP (Fig. 22) and lateral (Fig. 23) radiographs of his initial injury show a displaced scaphoid fracture and carpus dislocating dorsally with the distal pole of the scaphoid. The proximal pole remains at the radius with the lunate.

Closed reduction was accomplished by placing the hand in fingertraps with 7 lb of countertraction; a dorsal and palmar plaster slab was applied. The scaphoid fracture remained displaced. This is best seen in the AP radiograph (Fig. 24), which indicates persistent instability.

Open reduction and internal fixation of the scaphoid was performed by a palmar approach (see the Surgery section).

AP (Fig. 25) and lateral (Fig. 26) radiographs were obtained after the dressing was applied. The scaphoid was reduced and stabilized by K-wires, and all carpal relationships were restored. In this case one wire crossed the scapholunate joint. This adds a little more stability, but is not essential.

## RECOMMENDED READING

1.  Adkison, J., Chapman, M.: Treatment of acute lunate and perilunate dislocations. *Clin. Orthop.*, 164: 199–207, 1982.
2.  Aitken, A., Nalebuff, E.: Volar transnavicular perilunar dislocation of the carpus. *J. Bone Joint Surg.*, 42A: 1051–1057, 1960.
3.  Berger, R. A., Landsmeer, J. M.: The palmar radiocarpal ligaments: a study of adult and fetal human wrist joints. *J. Hand Surg.*, 15A(6): 847–854, 1990.
4.  Berger, R. A., Kauer, J. M., Landsmeer, J. M.: Radioscapholunate ligament: a gross anatomic and histologic study of fetal and adult wrists. *J. Hand Surg.*, 16A(2): 350–355, 1991.
5.  Burgess, R. C.: The effect of rotatory subluxation of the scaphoid on radio-scaphoid contact. *J. Hand Surg.*, 12A: 771–774, 1987.
6.  Campbell, R. Jr., Thompson, T., Lance, E, Adler, JB. Indications for open reduction of lunate and perilunate dislocations of the carpal bones. *J. Bone Joint Surg.*, 47A: 915–937, 1965.
7.  Cooney, W. P., Bussey, R., Dobyns, J. H., Linschied, R. L.: Difficult wrist fractures. *Clin. Orthop.*, 214(Jan): 136–147, 1987.
8.  Daffner, R. H., Emmerling, E. W., Buterbabaugh, G. A.: Proximal and distal oblique radiography of the wrist: value in occult injuries. *J. Hand Surg.*, 17A: 499–503, 1992.
9.  Fernandes, H. J., Koberle, G., Ferreira, G. H., Camargo, J. Jr.: Volar transscaphoid perilunar dislocation. *Hand*, 15(3): 276–280, 1983.
10. Gelberman, R. H., Menon, J.: The vascularity of the scaphoid bone. *J. Hand Surg.*, 5A: 508–513, 1980.
11. Gelberman, R. H., Panagis, J. S., Taleisnik, J., Baumgaertner, M.: The arterial anatomy of the human carpus. Part 1: The extraosseous vascularity. *J. Hand Surg.*, 8A(4): 367–374, 1983.
12. Herzberg, G., Comtet, J. J., Linscheid, R. L., Amadio, P. C., Cooney, W. P., Stalder, J.: Perilunate dislocations and fracture-dislocations: a multicenter study. *J. Hand Surg.*, 18A: 768–779, 1993.
13. Kuhlmann, J. N., Luboinski, J., Laudet, C., Boabighi, A., Landjerit, B., Guerin, S. H., et al.: Properties of the fibrous structures of the wrist. *J. Hand Surg.*, 15B(3): 335–341, 1990.
14. Lavernia, C. J., Cohen, M. S., Taleisnik, J.: Treatment of scapholunate dissociation by ligamentous repair and capsulodesis. *J. Hand Surg.*, 17(2): 354–359, 1992.
15. Linscheid, R. L., Dobyns, J. H., Beabout, J. W., Bryan, R. S.: Traumatic instability of the wrist. Diagnosis, classification, and pathomechanics. *J. Bone Joint Surg.*, 54A: 1612–1632, 1972.
16. Mack, G., Bosse, M., Gelberman, R., Yu, E.: The natural history of scaphoid nonunion. *J. Bone Joint Surg.*, 66A: 504–509, 1984.
17. Mayfield, J. K.: Patterns of injury to carpal ligaments. *J. Hand Surg.*, 187A: 36–42, 1984.
18. Mayfield, J. K.: Mechanism of carpal injuries. *Clin. Orthop.*, 149: 45–54, 1980.
19. Mayfield, J. K., Johnson, R. P., Kilcoyne, R. K.: Carpal dislocations: pathomechanics and progressive perilunar instability. *J. Hand Surg.*, 5A(3): 226–241, 1980.
20. Mayfield, J. K., Johnson, R. P., Kilcoyne, R. F.: The ligaments of the human wrist and their functional significance. *Anat. Rec.*, 186(3): 417–428, 1976.
21. Minami, A., Ogino, T., Ohshio, I., Minami, M.: Correlation between clinical results and carpal instabilities in patients after reduction of lunate and perilunar dislocations. *J. Hand Surg.*, 11B(2): 213–220, 1986.
22. Moneim, M. S., Hofammann, K. E. I., Omer, G. E.: Transscaphoid perilunate fracture-dislocation. Result of open reduction and pin fixation. *Clin. Orthop.*, 190: 227–235, 1984.
23. Moneim, M. S.: Management of greater arc carpal fractures. *Hand Clin.*, 4(3): 457–467, 1988.
24. Ruby, L., Stinson, J., Belsky, M.: The natural history of scaphoid nonunion. A review of fifty-five cases. *J. Bone Joint Surg.*, 67A: 428–432, 1985.
25. Ruch, D. S., Bowling, J.: Arthroscopic assessment of carpal instability. *Arthroscopy*, 14(7): 675–681, 1998.
26. Ruch, D., Poehling, G.: Arthroscopic management of partial scapholunate and lunotriquetral injuries of the wrist. *J. Hand Surg.*, 21A: 412–417, 1996.
27. Saunier, J., Chamay, A.: Volar perilunar dislocation of the wrist. *Clin. Orthop.*, 157: 139–142, 1981.

28. Schranz, P. J., Fagg, P. S.: Trans-radial styloid, trans-scaphoid, trans-triquetral perilunate dislocation. *J. R. Army Med. Corps.*, 137(3): 146–148, 1991.

29. Sotereanos, D. G., Mitsionis, G. J., Giannakopoulos, P. N., Tomaino, M. M., Herndon, J. H.: Perilunate dislocation and fracture dislocation: a critical analysis of the volar-dorsal approach. *J. Hand Surg.*, 22A(1): 49–56, 1997.

30. Szabo, R. M., Gelberman, R. H.: Peripheral nerve compression—etiology, critical pressure threshold and clinical assessment. *Orthopedics*, 7: 1461–1466, 1984.

31. Szabo, R. M., Newland, C. C., Johnson, P. G., Steinberg, D. R., Tortosa, R.: Spectrum of injury and treatment options for isolated dislocation of the scaphoid. A report of three cases. *J. Bone Joint Surg.*, 77A(4): 608–615, 1995.

32. Vance, R., Gelberman, R. H., Evans, E.: Scaphocapitate fractures: patterns of dislocation, mechanism of injury, and preliminary results of treatment. *J. Bone Joint Surg.*, 62A: 271–276, 1980.

33. Viegas, S.: The dorsal ligaments of the wrist: anatomy, mechanical properties and function. *J. Hand Surg.*, 24A: 456–468, 1999.

# 16

# Triscaphe Arthrodesis

H. Kirk Watson, Jeffrey Weinzweig,
and Duffield Ashmead IV

## INDICATIONS/CONTRAINDICATIONS

Triscaphe arthrodesis addresses a diverse spectrum of carpal abnormalities. It provides a stable radial column for load transfer across the wrist to the radius and permits the unloading of carpal units no longer capable of bearing load, such as the lunate in Kienböck's disease. In addition, it provides stability and strength to a wrist with rotary subluxation of the scaphoid (RSS) or midcarpal instability.

Other procedures, such as scapholunate ligamentous reconstruction, joint leveling procedures, and scaphocapitate arthrodesis, have been advocated for the management of the diverse group of carpal disorders for which we advocate triscaphe arthrodesis. Nonetheless, we believe that the latter type of limited wrist arthrodesis provides the most reliable and enduring means of stabilizing the scaphoid and permitting efficient load transfer across the wrist.

Long-term radiographic follow-up has revealed only rare instances of progressive radioscaphoid or intercarpal degenerative change. It happens almost exclusively in those patients who had some evidence of disease in these joints at the time of original surgery (8–10,13).

Indications for triscaphe arthrodesis include dynamic or static RSS, persistent symptomatic predynamic RSS with instability, degenerative disease of the triscaphe joint, nonunion of the scaphoid, Kienböck's disease, scapholunate dissociation, traumatic dislocations, midcarpal instability, and congenital synchondrosis of the triscaphe joint (3–5,7,9,11,12,14–16,18).

Triscaphe arthrodesis is contraindicated if significant degenerative change is found at the radioscaphoid joint (1,2).

## PREOPERATIVE PLANNING

Preoperative evaluation of patients with a carpal abnormality involving the scapho-trapezio-trapezoid (triscaphe) joint and radial side of the wrist should include physical examination and plain radiographic assessment. Patients with this pathology usually have an extended history of wrist-related complaints, including pain, loss of strength, and considerable restriction of motion. The patient may or may not have a specific history of previous wrist trauma.

Physical examination generally reveals periscaphoid swelling and synovitis as well as restricted flexion and extension. We have found the scaphoid shift maneuver to be extremely sensitive in identifying scaphoid and periscaphoid pathology, although our radial wrist examination consists of several additional maneuvers (17). Clinical suspicion of pathology involving the radial wrist is often confirmed radiographically. With the exception of predynamic rotary subluxation of the scaphoid (a clinical diagnosis of periscaphoid instability derived from physical examination alone), all other forms of carpal pathology requiring triscaphe limited wrist arthrodesis, such as Kienböck's disease, triscaphe joint arthritis, and scapholunate dissociation, are usually apparent on radiographic evaluation. Plain radiographs obviate the need for tomograms, arthrograms, computed tomography scans, or arthroscopy.

During preoperative radiographic evaluation the integrity of the radioscaphoid articulation is assessed. Radiographic evidence of degenerative change invariably predicts dramatic findings at surgery that usually will preclude triscaphe arthrodesis as an appropriate reconstructive technique.

## SURGERY

To perform triscaphe limited wrist arthrodesis, position the patient supine, and use standard prepping and draping. Apply an upper-arm tourniquet. We generally do not administer perioperative antibiotics. The procedure is performed under general anesthesia in most cases, although regional block would be equally effective. With the arm fully abducted and pronated on the hand table, the surgeon can perform the procedure most comfortably seated on the axillary side of the wrist.

### Technique

Approach the triscaphe joint through a 4-cm transverse dorsal wrist incision just distal to the radial styloid (Fig. 1). Use spreading technique to preserve dorsal veins and branches of the superficial branch of the radial nerve. Expose the radial styloid through an incision in the capsule overlying the radial styloid-scaphoid junction; remove the distal 5 mm of the styloid with a rongeur, sloping volarly from distal to proximal (Figs. 2, 3). Make a transverse incision in the dorsal capsule and inspect the radioscaphoid joint. If significant degenerative disease is found despite the absence of preoperative radiographic evidence, our procedure of choice is scapholunate advanced collapse (SLAC) reconstruction rather than triscaphe arthrodesis. Open the distal aspect of the extensor retinaculum along the extensor pollicis longus and approach the triscaphe joint through a transverse capsular incision between the extensor carpi radialis longus and brevis tendons (Fig. 4).

Remove the entire articular surfaces of the scaphoid, trapezium, and trapezoid with a rongeur, taking care to remove the proximal one-half of the trapezium-trapezoid articulation only. It is mandatory that the hard subchondral bone be removed and the softer cancellous surfaces exposed. Also remove the cortex dorsal to the articular cartilage on the trapezium and trapezoid to broaden the surface

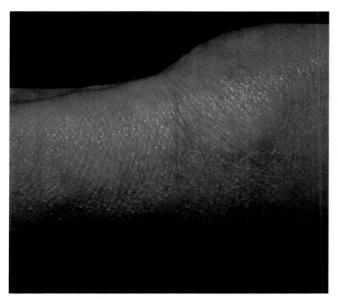

**FIGURE 1.** Wrist surgery, with few exceptions, is carried out most efficiently through transverse incisions. These are the recently healed transverse incisions used for triscaphe limited wrist arthrodesis. Proximally on the radius, the transverse incision for the bone graft donor site can be seen. The bone graft can be obtained through the distal wrist incision used to perform the arthrodesis; however, the degree of traction necessary to harvest bone graft through this incision usually causes a greater cosmetic defect in the transverse wrist incision than that resulting from two transverse incisions properly handled to produce minimal cosmetic deficit.

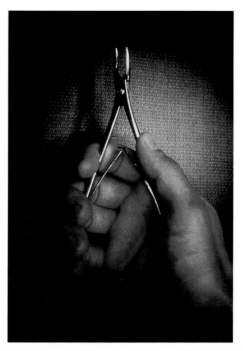

**FIGURE 2.** An essential instrument for performing a limited wrist arthrodesis is the dental rongeur. Placing the instrument deep along the distal articular surface of the scaphoid and levering the handle distally allows excision of the cartilage and subchondral bone from even the volar aspect of the distal articular surface of the scaphoid.

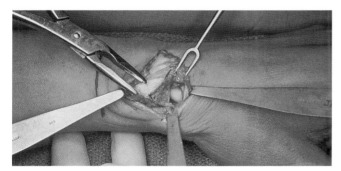

**FIGURE 3.** A limited radial styloidectomy has been performed with the dental rongeur. This method provides broader access to the radioscaphoid joint and prevents postoperative radial styloid impingement. The smooth proximal pole of the scaphoid can be visualized easily.

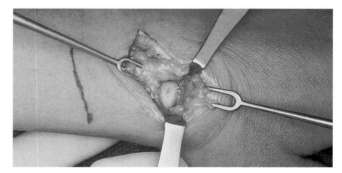

**FIGURE 4.** The triscaphe joint is visualized best between the two radial wrist extensors. The distal pole of the scaphoid and proximal articular surfaces of the trapezium and trapezoid are shown (fingers are pointing to the right).

area for grafting (Figs. 5, 6). The volar lip of the scaphoid is rongeured by inserting a dental rongeur deep into the joint and levering the handle distally. Harvest cancellous bone graft from the distal radius.

Drive two 0.045-in. K-wires percutaneously in preset fashion from the distal aspect of the dorsal trapezoid proximally. Pass the first radially positioned K-wire to the point of just touching the surface of the scaphoid. Pass the second ulnarly positioned K-wire proximally to the point of entering the scapho-trapezoid space. In large individuals, one or both of these K-wires may be a 0.062-in. wire.

Place a 5-mm spacer, usually the handle of a small hook, into the scapho-trapezoid space to maintain the original external dimensions of the triscaphe joint, and drive the radial K-wire into the scaphoid, avoiding placement into the radioscaphoid

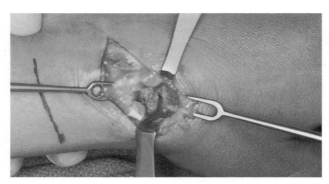

**FIGURE 5.** Bony resection commences with rongeur excision of the dorsal nonarticular surface of the distal scaphoid, which provides a broader cancellous surface for fusion.

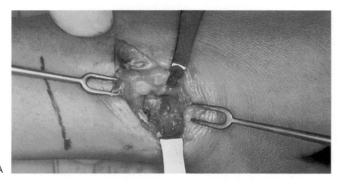

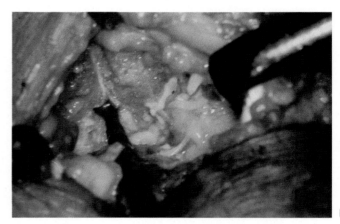

A                                                                                            B

**FIGURE 6. A:** The scapho-trapezio-trapezoid joint, as well as the trapezoid-trapezium interspace, have been excavated using both rongeur and curette to create a broad space for cancellous grafting. The preset K-wires are then driven from trapezoid to scaphoid, and the open space is densely packed with cancellous bone graft. **B:** A curette is used to remove the proximal half of the articular cartilage and subchondral bone between the trapezium and trapezoid.

joint. Then place the wrist in full radial deviation and 45° of dorsiflexion; use your thumb to reduce the scaphoid tuberosity to prevent scaphoid overcorrection (Fig. 7 A–C).

Remove the spacer and drive the ulnar K-wire into the scaphoid. Take care when driving the pins proximally into the scaphoid to avoid placing the K-wires into the radioscaphoid joint space or the radius itself (Fig. 8). After pinning, the scaphoid should lie at approximately 55° to 60° of palmar flexion relative to the long axis of the radius when seen from the lateral view.

This positioning ensures optimal radioscaphoid congruity and maximizes postoperative range of motion. It is not necessary to correct any abnormal rotation of the lunate. Do not overcorrect the scaphoid by placing its long axis in line with the forearm, thus markedly decreasing the scapholunate angle. This juxtaposition will limit the motion obtained after surgery and run the risk of cartilage destruction on the proximal pole of the scaphoid.

It cannot be overemphasized that the major concern in triscaphe arthrodesis is overcorrection. The neutral scaphoid normally lies 47° to the long axis of the radius; following triscaphe arthrodesis, the mechanics of load transfer change. The radial styloid must be removed and the scaphoid must lie significantly more flexed than normal (i.e., 55° to 60°) in relation to the long axis of the radius (Fig. 9).

Harvest cancellous bone from the distal radius, and pack it densely into the spaces between scaphoid, trapezium, and trapezoid using a dental amalgam

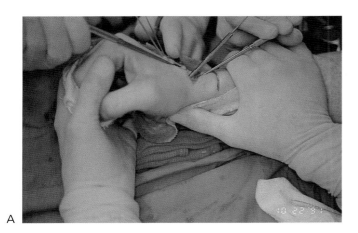

A

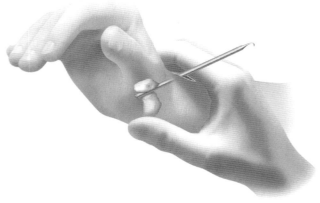

B

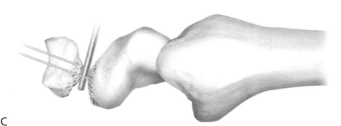

C

**FIGURE 7. A** and **B:** The key to triscaphe limited wrist arthrodesis is scaphoid position. This is easily accomplished with an automated technique by placing a 5-mm spacer between the scaphoid and trapezoid. The wrist is then fully radially deviated and dorsiflexed 45°. The surgeon's thumb maintains the scaphoid within these constraints. **C:** The assistant or scrub nurse can run the preset pins, which are aligned to cross into the scaphoid. The scaphoid should lie more flexed than in a normal wrist at 55° to 60° to the long axis of the forearm.

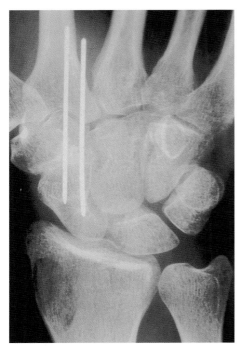

**FIGURE 8.** The relatively parallel pins from the trapezoid to the scaphoid allow muscular tone to maintain compression on the bone grafts until healing is complete at 6 weeks. The pins are removed in the office with small puncture incisions. Note the lucency at the site of distal radius bone graft donor site.

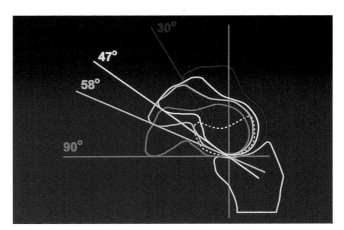

**FIGURE 9.** The normal scaphoid lies at an approximate angle of 47° to the long axis of the forearm. With rotary subluxation of the scaphoid, that angle can reach 90° or greater. There is a temptation to overcorrect the scaphoid during the triscaphe limited wrist procedure, bringing it up into a position less than 47° (*white*), such as the 30° shown here (*red*). This is unacceptable and will result in highly limited motion and early degenerative change on the apex of that scaphoid against the radius. Ideally, the scaphoid should be fused between 55° and 60° of flexion (*yellow*). This is more flexion than normal and is necessary because of the change in wrist mechanics.

tamp. Maintenance of the original external dimensions of the triscaphe joint usually translates to a 4- to 8-mm gap between the three bones, which is filled with the cancellous bone graft. Cut the pins beneath the skin level and close the skin incisions with a single-layer, subcuticular monofilament suture (stainless steel or Prolene). Realign the wrist capsule and extensor retinaculum without suturing.

The postoperative dressing consists of a bulky noncompressive wrap incorporating a long-arm plaster splint. Place the hand in a protected position with the wrist in slight extension and radial deviation, the forearm neutral, and the elbow at 90°.

## POSTOPERATIVE MANAGEMENT

Our postoperative management is similar for most intercarpal arthrodeses. Maximum initial immobilization is mandatory for these small-bone fusions. Three to 5 days following surgery, remove the bulky dressing and apply a long-arm thumb spica cast.

Although the proximal carpal row is immobilized easily by casting the forearm and arm, it is difficult to maintain the position of the distal carpal row adequately. Therefore, the metacarpophalangeal joints of the index and middle fingers are flexed to 80° to 90° and included in the long-arm cast, whereas the interphalangeal joints are left free.

The index and middle metacarpals are mortised into the carpals as the "fixed unit" of the hand. Thus, their immobilization tends to maintain the position of the distal carpal row. Since there is relatively free motion at the base of the ring and little metacarpals, they are not included in the cast. As with any thumb spica cast, the thumb is immobilized to the tip. We refer to this type of immobilization as a "Groucho Marx" cast, as it is reminiscent of the comedian's classic pose holding a cigar.

Three weeks following limited wrist arthrodesis, remove the long-arm cast and the intracuticular sutures. Apply a short-arm thumb spica cast for an additional 3 weeks. Only the thumb is included in this cast.

Six weeks postoperatively, remove the short-arm cast and take radiographs. If radiographic evidence of union is seen, remove the pins in the office and refer the patient for hand therapy for full wrist mobilization. Patients occasionally may be splinted for an additional week or two if there is any doubt as to the status of bony healing, especially in large individuals who smoke.

In our experience, triscaphe limited wrist arthrodesis has yielded excellent functional results and pain-free, stable wrists. After 4 to 6 weeks of hand therapy, the average range of motion is usually 50% to 70% that of the contralateral normal wrist, increasing to an average of 80% one year following surgery (Fig. 10A, B). Grip strength has averaged 90% of the unaffected wrist.

## COMPLICATIONS

Triscaphe arthrodesis has been an extremely reliable procedure with relatively few complications. More than 900 of these procedures have been performed. Triscaphe arthrodesis has been performed for symptomatic rotary subluxation of the scaphoid in 68% of the patients who underwent this procedure. Other indications have included Kienböck's disease (10%), triscaphe degenerative disease (8%), and scaphoid nonunion (2%). Additional indications have included midcarpal instability, avascular necrosis of the scaphoid, and symptomatic congenital synchondrosis of the triscaphe joint. The mean postoperative immobilization,

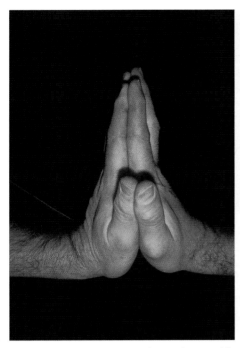 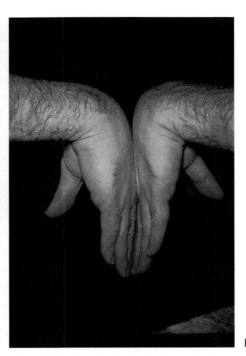

A                                                                                       B

**FIGURE 10.** Over 25 years of experience with more than 900 triscaphe limited wrist arthrodeses demonstrates average dorsiflexion **(A)** and palmar flexion **(B)** arcs of just under 80% that of the normal untreated wrist.

used as a measure of time to bony fusion, was 48 days (range from 30 to 294 days).

In early cases there was a significant postoperative incidence of radial styloid impaction. The stabilized scaphoid is unable to flex and avoid abutting the styloid in radial deviation. Among these early cases, approximately 20% required a subsequent styloidectomy, achieving an improvement in radial deviation and relief of impaction symptoms. Since 1987, radial styloidectomy has been routinely performed as part of the triscaphe arthrodesis procedure to avoid this problem (1).

Nonunion has been extremely uncommon, with a rate of 1% to 3% depending on the indication for limited wrist arthrodesis. We believe that this rate of nonunion is kept low by the broad cancellous surface created at the time of articular resection and the large volume of cancellous graft used in performing the fusion. Infection, hematoma, and transient neurapraxias have been exceedingly rare in our experience and should be completely avoidable. One patient required drainage and antibiotics for a postoperative wound infection. Fifteen patients (2%) were treated for postoperative reflex sympathetic dystrophy with a stress-loading regimen consisting of compression (scrubbing tasks) and traction (carrying weights) modalities referred to as a *dystrophile* program (6).

Although degenerative change at the radioscaphoid joint, consistent with SLAC wrist, occurred in 1.5% of patients following triscaphe arthrodesis, necessitating subsequent SLAC reconstruction, radiolunate degenerative change was not observed in any cases. One and a half percent of triscaphe arthrodeses thus required conversion to SLAC reconstruction. This entailed osteotomy through the triscaphe fusion, carpectomy of the scaphoid, and arthrodesis of the capitate, lunate, hamate, and triquetrum. Pain was the usual indication, but radioscaphoid degenerative joint disease occurred in patients in whom some degenerative joint disease was present at the time of the original surgery.

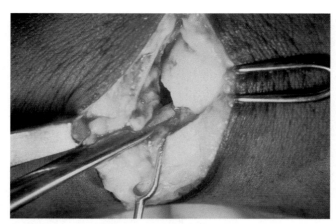

**FIGURE 11.** A professional basketball player with rotary subluxation of the scaphoid demonstrates a central area of destruction in the proximal pole articular surface, actually placing this in the realm of scapholunate advanced collapse. The triscaphe arthrodesis places this destroyed area of the scaphoid in the normal cartilage in the center of the radial fossa and provides a functionally asymptomatic wrist for many years. This may be converted to a scapholunate advanced collapse reconstruction following an osteotomy of the triscaphe fusion at a later date. Professional athletes with high earning capacities of short duration warrant this approach.

There were several cases in which patients were willing to accept expected future degenerative arthritis in exchange for shorter-term, full-power, asymptomatic function with increased range of motion. This tradeoff allowed them to finish out careers during their exceptional remuneration years. Several professional athletes and one world-class wrestler demonstrated eburnated bone with complete cartilage loss involving the proximal scaphoid pole (Fig. 11). This approach is successful because the central portion of the scaphoid pole is destroyed while the periphery of the scaphoid fossa of the radius is preserved. Triscaphe arthrodesis places the damaged proximal pole back in the center of the preserved cartilage of the scaphoid fossa.

## ILLUSTRATIVE CASE

A 46-year-old male baseball player, while sliding into third-base, either reinjured his scapholunate ligament or completely ruptured a previously intact scapholunate interosseous system. Immediately after the injury, he experienced marked pain and significant postactivity ache, and was unable to use the hand for any load capacity. Radiographic evaluation confirmed disruption of the scaphoid (Fig. 12A, B). Triscape limited wrist arthrodesis was performed (Fig. 12C) with solid bony fusion achieved 6 weeks postoperatively (Fig. 12D).

After scapho-trapezium-trapezoid arthrodesis, a greater than normal degree of scaphoid flexion was maintained. The result was a painless wrist with full power and 80% flexion/extension compared with the opposite normal wrist. At surgical follow-up 23 years later, there was continued full functional capacity of the wrist and no secondary degenerative arthritis.

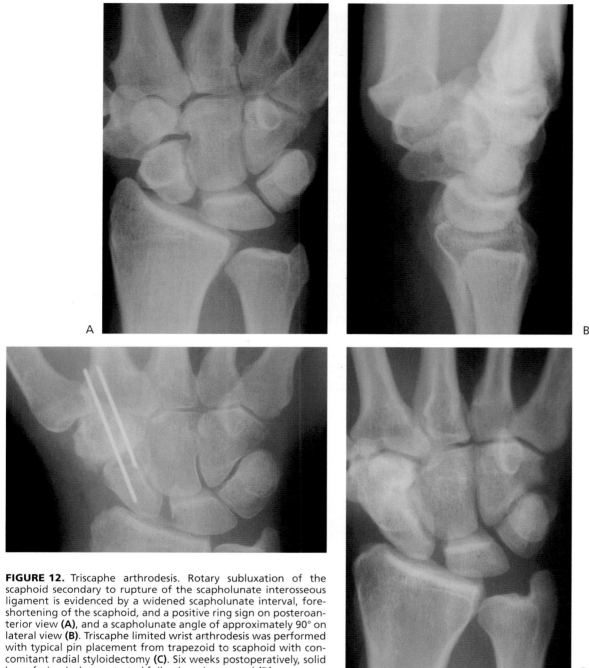

**FIGURE 12.** Triscaphe arthrodesis. Rotary subluxation of the scaphoid secondary to rupture of the scapholunate interosseous ligament is evidenced by a widened scapholunate interval, fore-shortening of the scaphoid, and a positive ring sign on posteroan-terior view **(A)**, and a scapholunate angle of approximately 90° on lateral view **(B)**. Triscaphe limited wrist arthrodesis was performed with typical pin placement from trapezoid to scaphoid with con-comitant radial styloidectomy **(C)**. Six weeks postoperatively, solid bony fusion is demonstrated following pin removal **(D)**.

## RECOMMENDED READING

1. Rogers, W. D., Watson, H. K.: Radial styloid impingement after triscaphe arthrodesis. *J. Hand Surg.*, 14A: 297–301, 1989.
2. Trumble, T., Bour, C., Smith, R., Edwards, G.: Intercarpal arthrodesis for static and dynamic volar intercalated segment instability. *J. Hand Surg.*, 13A: 396–402, 1988.
3. Vender, M. I., Watson, H. K., Wiener, B. D., Black, D. M.: Degenerative change in symptomatic scaphoid nonunion. *J. Hand Surg.*, 12A: 514–519, 1987.
4. Viegas, S. F., Patterson, R. M., Peterson, P. D., Pogue, D. J., Jenkins, D. K., Sweo, T. D., Hokan-

son, J. A.: Evaluation of the biomechanical efficacy of limited intercarpal fusions for the treatment of scapho-lunate dissociation. *J. Hand Surg.*, 15A: 120–128, 1990.

5. Watson, H. K., Ashmead, D.: Triscaphe Fusion for Chronic Scapholunate Instability. In: *Master Techniques in Orthopaedic Surgery: The Wrist*, edited by R. H. Gelberman, Raven Press, New York, pp. 183–194, 1994.
6. Watson, H. K., Carlson, L.: Treatment of reflex sympathetic dystrophy of the hand with an active "stress loading" program. *J. Hand Surg.*, 12A: 779, 1987.
7. Watson, H. K., Fink, J. A., Monacelli, D. M.: Use of triscaphe fusion in the treatment of Kienbock's disease. *Hand Clin.*, 9(3): 493–499, 1993.
8. Watson, H. K., Goodman, M. L., Johnson, T. R.: Limited wrist arthrodesis. Part II: Intercarpal and radiocarpal combinations. *J. Hand Surg.*, 6: 223–232, 1981.
9. Watson, H. K., Hempton, R. E.: Limited wrist arthrodesis. Part I: The triscaphoid joint. *J. Hand Surg.*, 5: 320–327, 1980.
10. Watson, H. K., Ottoni, L., Pitts, E. C., Handal, A. G.: Rotary subluxation of the scaphoid: a spectrum of instability. *J. Hand Surg.*, 18B: 62–64, 1993.
11. Watson, H. K., Ryu, J., DiBella, A.: An approach to Kienbock's disease: triscaphe arthrodesis. *J. Hand Surg.*, 10A: 179–187, 1985.
12. Watson, H. K., Ryu, J., Akelman, E.: Limited triscaphoid intercarpal arthrodesis for rotary subluxation of the scaphoid. *J. Bone Joint Surg.*, 68A: 345–349, 1986.
13. Watson, H. K., Weinzweig, J., Guidera, P., Zeppieri, J., Ashmead, D.: One thousand intercarpal arthrodeses. *J. Hand Surg.*, 24B: 320–330, 1999.
14. Watson, H. K., Weinzweig, J.: Intercarpal Arthrodesis. In: *Operative Hand Surgery*, 4th ed., edited by D. P. Green, R. N. Hotchkiss, W. C. Pederson, Churchill Livingstone, New York, pp. 108–130, 1999.
15. Watson, H. K., Weinzweig, J., Zeppieri, J.: The natural progression of scaphoid instability. *Hand Clin.*, 13(1): 39–50, 1997.
16. Watson, H. K., Weinzweig, J.: Treatment of Kienbock's Disease with Triscaphe Arthrodesis. In: *Proceedings of the 6th Congress of the International Federation of Societies for Surgery of the Hand*, edited by M. Vastamaki, S. Vilkki, H. Goransson, H. Jaroma, T. Raatikainen, T. Viljakka, Monduzzi Editore, Bologna, Italy, pp. 347–349, 1995.
17. Watson, H. K., Weinzweig, J.: Physical examination of the wrist. *Hand Clin.*, 13(1): 17–34, 1997.
18. Weinzweig, J., Watson, H. K., Herbert, T. J., Shaer, J.: Congenital synchondrosis of the scaphotrapezio-trapezoid joint. *J. Hand Surg.*, 22A: 74–77, 1997.

PART **VIII**

# Osteoarthritis

# 17

# SLAC Wrist: Scaphoid Excision and Four-Corner Arthrodesis

Duffield Ashmead IV, Jeffrey Weinzweig, and H. Kirk Watson

## INDICATIONS/CONTRAINDICATIONS

Scapholunate advanced collapse (SLAC) is the most common pattern of degenerative arthritis in the wrist. The invariably intact radiolunate articulation provides the basis for reconstructing a wrist with useful motion. We perform this reconstruction by excising the scaphoid and doing a limited wrist arthrodesis incorporating capitate, lunate, hamate, and triquetrum.

The key to reconstruction of the SLAC wrist lies in the radiolunate articulation, which is preserved at all stages of the SLAC sequence. Virtually all patients with SLAC wrist are candidates for this form of reconstruction, whatever the primary etiology of the degenerative process, be it chronic rotary subluxation of the scaphoid or chronic scaphoid nonunion (the two most common causes). The SLAC reconstructive procedure also may be appropriate for patients with isolated midcarpal degenerative change.

Patients who have lunate or radiolunate abnormalities are *not* candidates for this type of reconstruction. Contraindications include Kienböck's disease as well as established radiolunate degenerative change or ulnar translocation of the carpus. The reconstruction depends upon a normal radiolunate articulation; if this cannot be ensured, consider an alternative means of reconstruction.

## PREOPERATIVE PLANNING

Preoperative history, physical examination, and plain radiographs form the basis for patient evaluation and preoperative planning in SLAC wrist. Because SLAC represents a final common pathway for a variety of primary wrist processes, patient histories may be quite variable; most patients have many years of wrist-related difficulty. Those with chronic static rotary subluxation of the scaphoid may have undergone previous attempts at ligamentous reconstruction or scaphoid stabilization. Those with chronic scaphoid nonunion may have undergone bone graft or may have been in a cast for extended periods. Less common causes of SLAC wrist include avascular necrosis of the scaphoid (Preiser's disease) and distal radial fracture involving the radioscaphoid articulation. Despite these widely divergent histories, however, the physical examination is likely to be consistent.

Patients present with dorsal wrist swelling and tenderness (synovitis in a periscaphoid distribution). Extension/flexion is likely to be extremely restricted and quite painful. A "scaphoid shift maneuver" is also quite painful, with a virtually immobile scaphoid (see Chapter 16).

Plain radiographs confirm the diagnosis with the classic pattern of degenerative change. In stage I, degenerative change is limited to the radioscaphoid articulation, although there may be evidence of midcarpal instability. With progressive collapse, the degenerative process extends to the midcarpal (capitate-lunate, hamate-lunate) articulations, which constitutes stage II. Radiographs should be examined carefully for any evidence of accompanying radiolunate degenerative change or ulnar translocation of the carpus; either condition would preclude reliable salvage by this technique.

We do not see any role for complex radiologic evaluation or for invasive procedures in the evaluation of patients with SLAC wrist.

## SURGERY

Patient positioning, prepping, draping, and the use of an upper arm tourniquet are standard. The surgeon generally sits in the axilla with assistant(s) facing across the hand table and a scrub nurse at the patient's fingertips. The procedure usually is performed under general anesthesia, although regional block would be equally acceptable.

### Technique

The surgical approach is identical to that used for triscaphe limited wrist arthrodesis (see Chapter 16). Make two parallel incisions—one overlying the radiocarpal joint dorsally and one proximally over the distal radial aspect of the radius—for harvest of radial bone graft (Fig. 1).

Begin the procedure with the distal incision; carry out dissection using a blunt spread technique to avoid injury to dorsal veins and nerve branches. Identify the extensor retinaculum and incise along the third compartment, providing access to the wrist capsule. Approach the scaphoid in the interval between the extensors carpi radialis longus and brevis. Incise the wrist capsule transversely, and remove the scaphoid in a piecemeal fashion with a dental rongeur (Fig. 2). Take care to protect adjacent radial and palmar capsular structures.

At this time, longitudinal traction on the fingers allows wide exposure of the radial lunate joint space and confirmation that this is well preserved (Fig. 3). Shift your attention ulnarly, and identify the capitate, lunate, hamate, and triquetrum; remove their adjoining cartilaginous surfaces with a dental rongeur, down to cancellous matrix (Figs. 4–6). Once again, longitudinal traction may prove helpful in providing access to the intercarpal joints.

Harvest cancellous bone graft from the distal radius through the separate proximal parallel incision, using a standard technique detailed in the chapter on triscaphe arthrodesis. Insert fixation pins (generally 0.045- or 0.062-in.) percutaneously as follows: one pin each in the capitate, hamate, and triquetrum, directed toward the lunate; and one additional pin from the triquetrum toward the capitate (Fig. 7 A, B). Place part of the cancellous graft deep in the interval between the

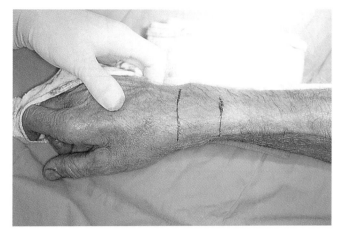

**FIGURE 1.** Skin incisions.

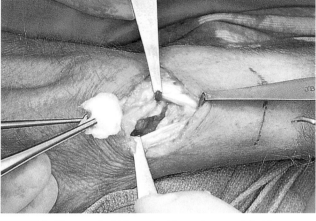

**FIGURE 2.** The scaphoid is excised in a piecemeal fashion.

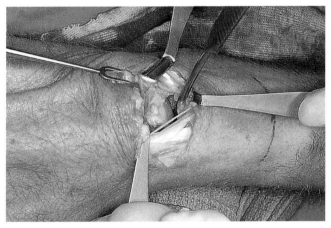

**FIGURE 3.** With distal traction on the hand, the proximal articular surface of the lunate can be visualized between the third and fourth extensor compartments. Here it is found to be well preserved (as was the corresponding articular surface of the radius).

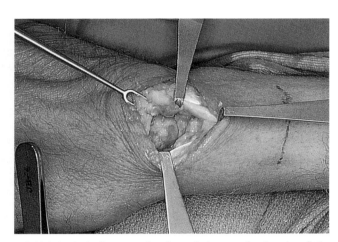

**FIGURE 4.** A similar examination of the proximal pole of the capitate revealed destruction of articular cartilage with exposed subchondral bone (typical of advanced, stage II, SLAC wrist).

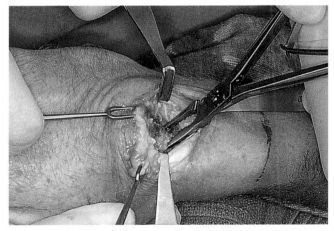

**FIGURE 5.** With dental rongeur, facing articular surfaces of capitate, lunate, hamate, and triquetrum are removed down to cancellous bone.

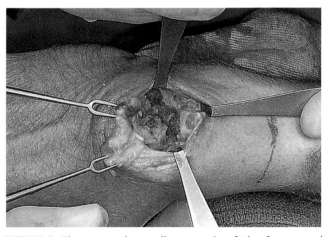

**FIGURE 6.** The exposed cancellous matrix of the four carpal bones to be fused.

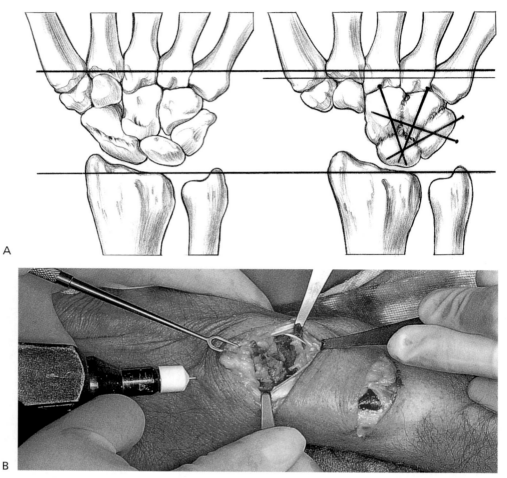

**FIGURE 7.** **A** and **B**: K-wires are preset (the proximal incision represents the bone graft donor site).

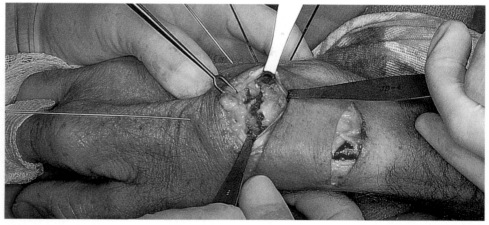

**FIGURE 8.** The lunate dorsal intercalated segment instability posture is reduced (note a visible portion of the proximal articular surface), and K-wires are driven across to maintain carpal alignment.

capitate and lunate, and, after achieving optimal bony alignment, drive the fixation pins across (Fig. 8).

The most important component of the SLAC wrist reconstructive procedure is bony alignment. The capitate is displaced palmarly on the lunate, reducing the nearly universal tendency for dorsiflexion intercalated segment instability of the

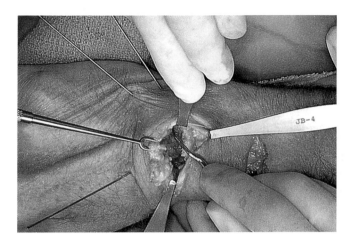

**FIGURE 9.** Intercarpal spaces are filled with cancellous graft using a dental tamp.

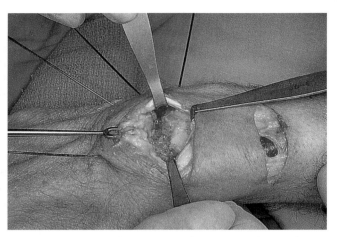

**FIGURE 10.** All available intercarpal space is packed with cancellous graft.

lunate. Fusion in uncorrected alignment will lead to impingement of the capitate on the radius in wrist extension, markedly reducing the ultimate range of motion and leading to wrist pain. Slight lunate volar intercalated segment instability (VISI) positioning is desirable. It is occasionally necessary to fix the lunate to the radius temporarily, allowing the capitate to be brought into proper alignment with the lunate before cross-pinning.

Drive all long-term pins so as to avoid crossing the radial lunate articulation; cut them off below skin level. Pack all available bone graft densely into the intercarpal crevices using a dental tamp (Figs. 9, 10). Some surgeons may wish to obtain intraoperative radiographs to confirm adequate capitate-lunate alignment. In our experience, visual inspection is at least as accurate as, if not more helpful than, fluoroscopy or plain films.

Ordinarily, in limited wrist arthrodesis, carpal spacing must be maintained to preserve the external dimensions of the fusion block. In SLAC reconstruction, some collapse of the capitate and hamate onto the lunate and triquetrum may be allowed because no other joints are affected by the altered external height of the four-bone unit (Fig. 7A).

For many years, we inserted a Silastic scaphoid replacement. It was employed as a spacer and was not intended to participate in load transfer across the wrist. It became clear, however, that load transfer and fragmentation of the prosthesis *did* occur, and, in a significant number of patients, led to particulate synovitis. Many of these early patients subsequently have undergone removal of the implant with no complications. It is currently our policy not to use any form of scaphoid replacement in SLAC wrist reconstruction.

The wrist capsule and extensor retinaculum are allowed to close without suturing; use a single-layer intracuticular monofilament closure for the skin. Apply a long-arm bulky hand dressing.

## POSTOPERATIVE MANAGEMENT

At the first postoperative visit, 1 week after surgery, remove the long-arm dressing and replace it with a long-arm thumb spica cast, extended to incorporate the fingers in metacarpophalangeal flexion. The long-arm cast is intended to provide better stabilization of the metacarpals than that afforded by a standard thumb spica cast.

Four weeks after surgery, remove the long-arm cast, assess the wounds, and remove sutures. Apply a short-arm thumb spica for an additional 2 weeks. Radiographs at 6 weeks usually demonstrate evidence of early trabecular bridging between the four fused carpal bones. In this case, remove pins in the office and refer the patient for hand therapy. In smokers or patients whose radiographic evidence of bony healing is scant, an additional week or two of immobilization may be indicated.

Recent review of 100 SLAC wrist reconstructions has revealed remarkably consistent functional results. Ninety percent of patients experience either complete relief of pain (40%) or minimal pain only with extremes of heavy work (50%). Eighty percent have been able to return to their original employment, whether executive, clerical, or manual labor. In addition, 80% have resumed wrist-related recreational activities, including golf and bowling.

Range of motion has averaged 50% that of the normal opposite wrist, both in flexion/extension and in radial/ulnar deviation (when a normal opposite wrist was available for comparison). Grip strength has averaged approximately 80%. While some critics have expressed concern over the long-term durability of a wrist run exclusively on the radial lunate joint, objective measures of function have shown improvement when comparison is made between patients less than 2 years postoperative and patients more than 4 years postoperative. Radiolunate degenerative change has been seen only in extremely rare cases, and always in the context of ulnar translocation. In these cases, our recommendation has been to proceed with total wrist fusion.

## REHABILITATION

All SLAC reconstructive patients are seen by the hand therapist at the time of the initial postoperative visit. Following removal of the operative dressing and construction of a long-arm cast, the patients are referred for shoulder range-of-motion exercises. At 4 weeks after surgery, when they are changed to a short-arm cast, have them begin elbow and finger exercises.

Immediately after pin removal, the patients are seen for construction of a thermoplastic resting splint, which they should wear at all times for the first several days, until the inflammation of pin removal has subsided. It may be worn intermittently thereafter for patient comfort between range-of-motion exercises.

Have the patient begin progressive resistive exercise at 8 to 9 weeks. Depending on the patient's functional needs, begin work hardening and job simulation at 9 to 10 weeks and continue into the twelfth postoperative week as needed. Address any early symptoms of reflex sympathetic dystrophy immediately with a stress-loading protocol. Even if the patient is still in a cast, a modified or "towel scrub" program works nicely. Soft tissue scarring is managed with wound massage and occasionally pressure garments.

## COMPLICATIONS

Among our earlier patients, a significant number developed a postoperative impingement between the dorsal rim of the radius and the capitate as range of motion improved. While this condition can be addressed with dorsal radial resection arthroplasty (resulting in improved extension amplitude), the complication can be avoided by proper alignment of capitate and lunate at the time of surgery. It cannot be overemphasized that the lunate and capitate must be in axial alignment, fully correcting any preexisting lunate dorsiflexion intercalated segment instability posture. This alignment maintains maximal carpal height and maximizes the available extension arc (Figs. 11, 12).

In our earlier cases, it was our practice to replace the scaphoid with a silicone implant. While it was intended simply as a spacer, the implant clearly participated

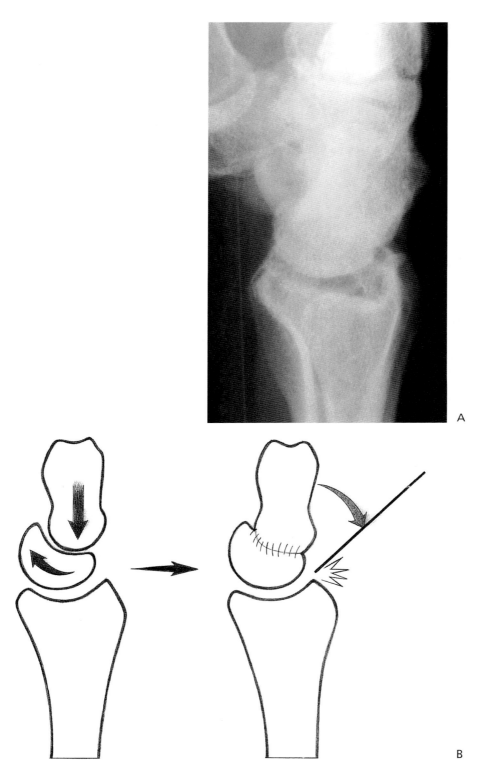

**FIGURE 11. A and B:** Suboptimal capitate lunate alignment within the fusion block. The lunate remains in approximately 30° of dorsiflexion intercalated segment instability, and the capitate is displaced dorsally. This results in impingement of the proximal capitate on the dorsal radius as extension amplitude improves.

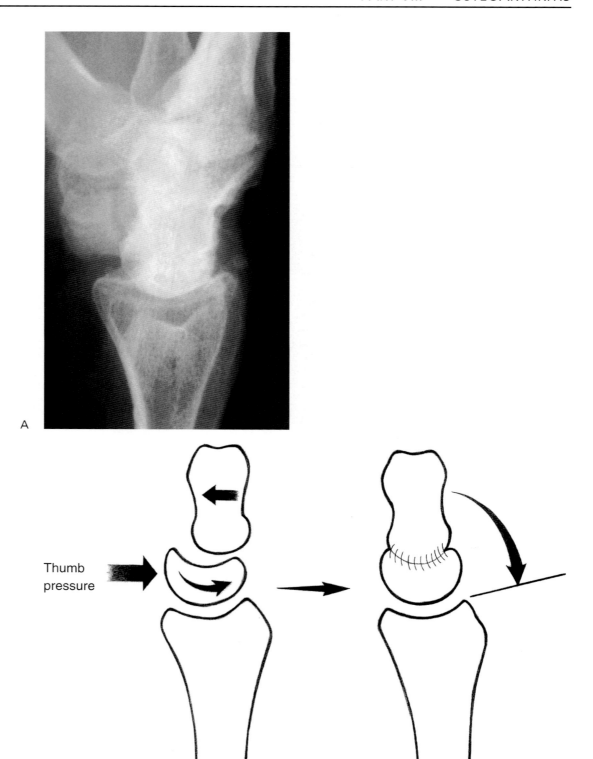

**FIGURE 12.** **A** and **B:** Optimal coaxial alignment of capitate and lunate. This maximizes preservation of carpal height and avoids a dorsal impingement phenomenon. Extension arc also is improved.

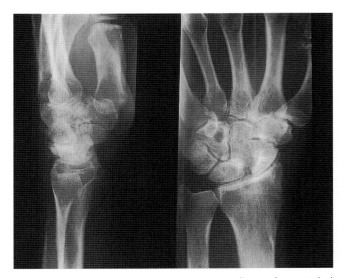

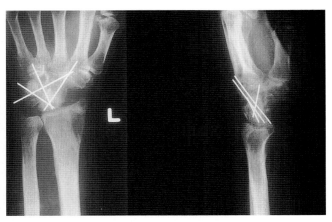

**FIGURE 13.** Lateral and posteroanterior radiographs revealed stage II scapholunate advanced collapse. There is static rotary subluxation of the scaphoid with augmentation of scapholunate interval and scapholunate angle. Both the radioscaphoid and capitolunate articular intervals have been obliterated, with adjacent sclerotic change. There appear to be degenerative cysts in the distal radius and hamate. The radiolunate interval, however, remains well preserved.

**FIGURE 14.** Six weeks after wrist salvage by scapholunate advanced collapse reconstruction, pins are seen in their standard configuration. Intercarpal spaces within the fusion block have been filled with bone graft and/or obliterated by early bone healing. Pins were removed at this time and the patient referred to hand therapy for mobilization.

in load transfer and we had an alarming rate of particulate synovitis (10% to 15%) at greater than 4 years postoperative. As a result, we no longer use any form of scaphoid replacement. Functional outcome has been indistinguishable from that in patients with scaphoid replacement.

Nonunion has been rare with the four-bone block fusion (less than 2%). A broad cancellous contact surface and large volume of cancellous bone graft contribute to making this an extremely reliable limited wrist arthrodesis.

## ILLUSTRATIVE CASES FOR TECHNIQUE

### Case History 1

A 66-year-old right-dominant male retiree presented for evaluation of his left wrist. He described several years of progressively more severe discomfort, including pain symptoms at rest as well as during and after activity. He recalled an ill-defined wrist injury some 20 years before, but indicated that his symptoms had developed over at most 5 years.

Examination revealed demonstrable swelling about the radial and dorsal side of the wrist, with extension/flexion restricted at 49/58. Manipulative examination suggested significant periscaphoid synovitis.

Radiographs (Fig. 13) revealed scapholunate advanced collapse stage II, attributed to static rotary subluxation of the scaphoid. In addition to augmentation of scapholunate interval and scapholunate angle, there was obliteration of both radiocarpal and midcarpal joint spaces. The radiolunate articulation, however, was well preserved.

The patient subsequently underwent SLAC wrist reconstruction as described, including scaphoid excision and capitate-hamate-lunate-triquetrum limited wrist arthrodesis with internal K-wire fixation. At 6 weeks follow-up, x-rays revealed evidence of early bony consolidation (Fig. 14) and pins were removed in the office setting. The patient subsequently was referred for hand therapy. His recovery and rehabilitation were uneventful.

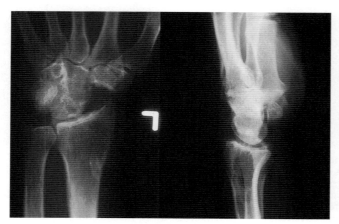

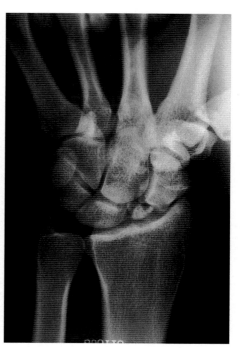

**FIGURE 15.** Thirty-two months after reconstruction. Posteroanterior and lateral radiographs demonstrate a solid four-bone fusion block with a well-preserved radiolunate interval. The patient feels he is "much better."

**FIGURE 16.** Posteroanterior radiograph of this 32-year-old laborer reveals an established scaphoid nonunion. There is sclerosis and resorption of the proximal pole fragment, as well as narrowing of the articular interval between the distal scaphoid fragment and the radius.

At most recent follow-up, 2.5 years after reconstruction, the patient denied experiencing residual symptoms of pain. He had resumed use of the wrist for recreational activities, including athletics and gardening. He described pain symptoms as "much better" than preoperatively and strength as "better." Although he felt his motion was "worse," his overall assessment was "much better," and he would undergo the same reconstruction if faced with the decision again.

Examination revealed acceptable soft tissue healing without residual swelling. Wrist extension/flexion was reasonable at 50/30 (50/55 on the opposite side). Grip strength was 72 lb bilaterally. Follow-up x-rays (Fig. 15) confirmed a solid arthrodesis with a well-preserved radiolunate articular interval.

### Case History 2

SLAC wrist reconstruction also is appropriate when the primary etiology is scaphoid nonunion (referred to by some as *scaphoid nonunion advanced collapse* or *SNAC*). Such a patient is illustrated by this case (Fig. 16).

A 32-year-old right-dominant male presented 1 month after a hyperextension injury to his left wrist that had left him with ongoing pain, particularly in the context and aftermath of activity. Clinical examination demonstrated limited wrist extension/flexion (35/65 versus 58/80) with periscaphoid tenderness and pain on scaphoid shift maneuver.

X-rays revealed an established scaphoid proximal pole nonunion with osteophyte formation and bone resorption, suggesting a substantially older injury. Based on radiographic findings, the patient was not viewed as a reasonable candidate for scaphoid bone grafting; at surgical exploration, considerable degenerative change was confirmed. The scaphoid was removed in its entirety and a SLAC wrist reconstruction completed using distal radial bone graft for the limited wrist arthrodesis.

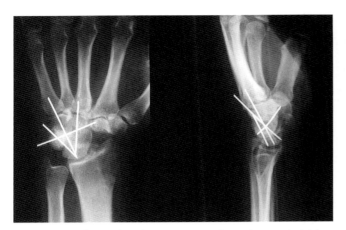

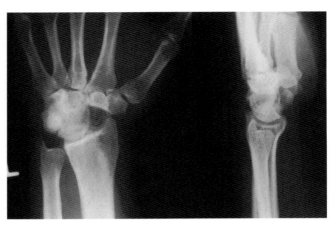

**FIGURE 17.** Six weeks after reconstruction; the scaphoid has been removed in its entirety, and early radiographic union of a limited wrist arthrodesis is apparent. The distal radial bone graft donor site is also visualized.

**FIGURE 18.** Twenty-nine months after reconstruction, the limited wrist arthrodesis is seen to be well healed. The radiolunate articular interval remains well preserved.

At 6 weeks postoperative, x-rays revealed reasonable early bone healing; pins were removed the following week in the operating room (Fig. 17). By 3 months after reconstruction, the patient had regained reasonable wrist mobility and grip strength exceeding 50% of the opposite side. At long-term follow-up, 2.5 years after reconstruction, wrist extension/flexion was 40/18 (versus 46/62) and grip strength was 88 lb (versus 125 lb). The patient had resumed his preinjury employment as a plumber as well as previous recreational activities. Although he described his mobility as "worse," pain, strength, and overall assessment were "much better" (Fig. 18).

## RECOMMENDED READING

1. Ashmead, D., Watson, H. K., et al.: The scapholunate advanced collapse wrist salvage. *J Hand Surg.*, 19A: 741–750, 1994.
2. Watson, H. K., Ballet, F.: The SLAC wrist: scapholunate advanced collapse pattern of degenerative arthritis. *J. Hand Surg.*, 9A(3): 358–365, 1984.
3. Watson, H. K., Carlson, L.: Treatment of reflex sympathetic dystrophy of the hand with an active "stress loading" program. *J. Hand Surg.*, 12A(5): 779–785, 1987.
4. Watson, H. K., Goodman, M. L., Johnson, T. R.: Limited wrist arthrodesis. Part II: Intercarpal and radiocarpal combinations. *J. Hand Surg.*, 6(3): 223–233, 1981.
5. Watson, H. K., Weinzweig, J., et al.: One thousand intercarpal arthrodeses. *J. Hand Surg.*, 24B(3): 307–315, 1999.

# 18

# SLAC Wrist: Capitolunate Fusion with Scaphoid and Triquetrum Excision

James H. Calandruccio and Richard H. Gelberman

## INDICATIONS/CONTRAINDICATIONS

Capitolunate fusion combined with excision of the scaphoid and triquetrum (CLF) is an alternative motion-preserving procedure for certain posttraumatic and degenerative arthritic wrist disorders. Indications for use of this technique include scapholunate advanced collapse (SLAC) and scaphoid nonunion advanced collapse wrist degenerative disease with significant midcarpal arthritis. Posttraumatic osteochondral capitate head defects, which may accompany such injuries as non-reconstructible transscaphoid perilunar injuries, also may be successfully managed by this technique.

Contraindications to use of CLF include degeneration of the distal radius lunate facet, Kienböck's disease, and conditions precluding secure screw purchase in the capitolunate complex, such as multicystic carpal disease involving the capitate or lunate. Relative contraindications include osteopenia, recent or remote infection in the operative area, and personality disorders that preclude compliance with the postoperative immobilization and rehabilitation protocols.

## PREOPERATIVE PLANNING

SLAC is the most common form of wrist arthritis and evolves in a predictable sequence (3). The radial styloid and the adjacent scaphoid waist are involved in stage I disease. Progression to stage II occurs when degenerative changes develop between the proximal pole of the scaphoid and the elliptical fossa of the radius, and capitolunate joint arthritis marks stage III.

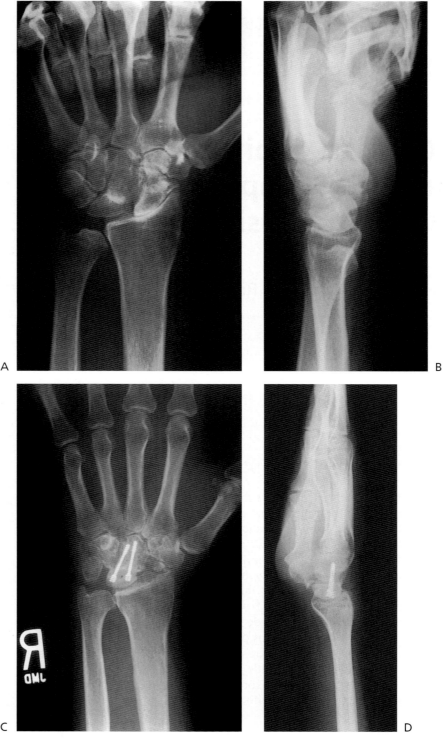

**FIGURE 1.** **A** and **B:** Anteroposterior and lateral preoperative wrist radiographs of a 30-year-old forester with a history of several remote wrist traumas. He was diagnosed with a scaphoid nonunion with proximal pole avascular necrosis. **C** and **D:** Three years after scaphoid and triquetrum excision and capitolunate fusion, he continued normal activities with no pain.

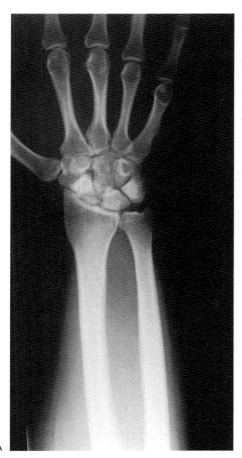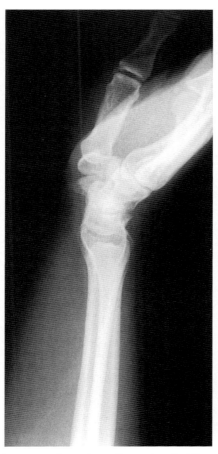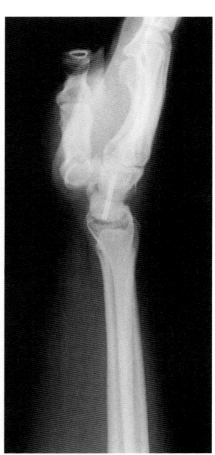

A                                                                                                                                    B,C

**FIGURE 2.** **A** and **B:** Anteroposterior and lateral preoperative wrist radiographs of a 70-year-old retired male office worker with scapholunate advanced collapse wrist deformity who recalled no previous trauma. He underwent a capitolunate fusion following scaphoid and triquetrum excision. **C:** Four years after surgery, he had minimal discomfort with jarring motions; x-rays revealed no radiolunate degeneration. His motion was the same as preoperatively, and his grip strength improved from 50 to 90 lb.

The radiolunate joint surfaces are rarely involved. Patients with SLAC wrists may be unable to recall an injury to the wrist, because the SLAC process often develops insidiously (Fig. 1). Specific episodes of wrist trauma, however, usually can be documented in scaphoid nonunion advanced collapse wrists or in those patients with perilunar fractures or fracture-dislocations of the wrist.

Regardless of the specific etiology of the wrist condition, hallmarks of significant radioscaphoid degeneration include localized swelling and tenderness, crepitation, and painful wrist motion, most notable in extension and radial deviation. Posteroanterior (PA) and lateral plain x-rays are sufficient to evaluate most wrist conditions. The degree of capitolunate joint involvement often is difficult to evaluate on plain x-rays; the radiolunate joint, however, is predictably spared in these disorders (1–3).

The goal of the CLF is to eliminate the radioscaphoid degenerative articulation by excision of the scaphoid. The midcarpal arthritic component is treated with capitolunate fusion, which can be achieved by compression arthrodesis through mating cancellous surfaces by excision of the triquetrum (Fig. 2).

## SURGERY

A standard dorsal approach to the wrist through a longitudinal dorsal skin incision is preferable to a cosmetic transverse incision. Curvilinear or straight dorsal

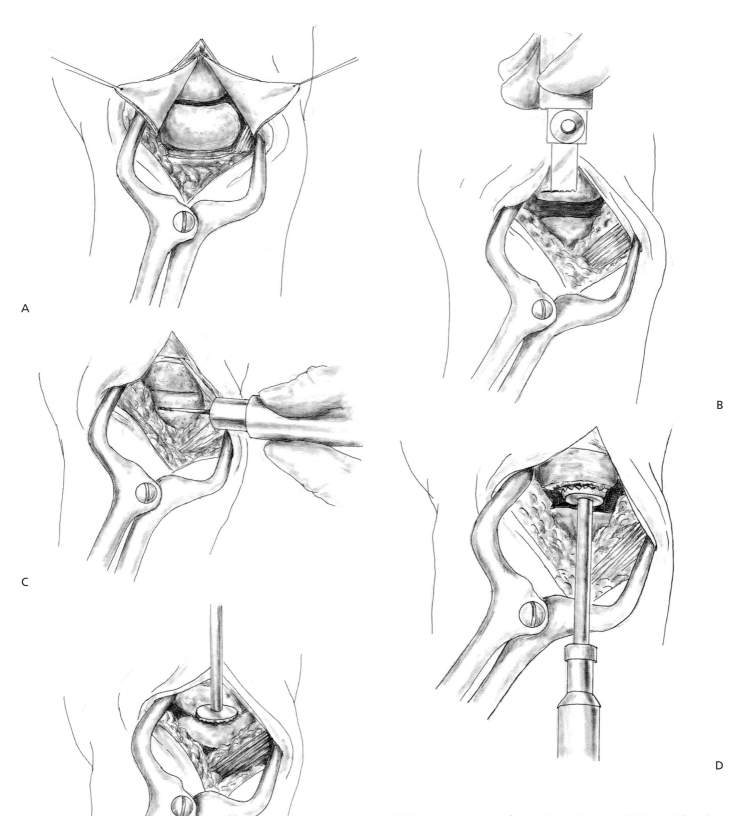

**FIGURE 3. A:** Exposure of wrist through inverted T-shaped dorsal capsular approach. **B:** Remove the head of the capitate at the level of the proximal pole of the hamate perpendicular to the axis of the capitate. **C:** Remove the distal surface of lunate to the cancellous surface perpendicular to the axis of the lunate. **D** and **E:** Prepare opposing surfaces of the capitate and lunate by matching concavo-convex reamers. (*continued.*)

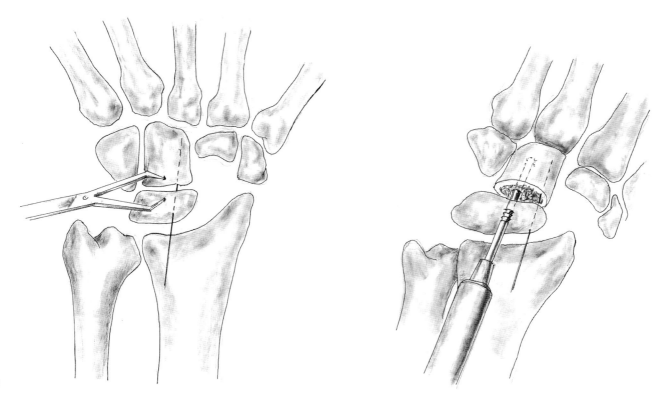

F

G

**FIGURE 3. *(continued.)* F:** Use Kirschner wire and forceps to provisionally stabilize the capitolunate complex. **G:** Position the subchondral screw with an antirotation Kirschner wire in place.

longitudinal incisions are extensile, and, if indicated, total wrist arthrodesis can readily be performed through this approach.

Isolate the dorsal sensory branches of the radial nerve and retract them to clearly expose the extensor retinaculum from the level of the carpometacarpal joints to the metaphyseal region of the distal radius. Cauterize and divide perforating vessels into the extensor retinaculum. Locate the extensor pollicis longus over the thumb metacarpal, expose it along its ulnar border, and follow it proximally over the radial wrist extensor tendons to the level of the radiocarpal joint.

Retract the extensor pollicis longus and radial wrist extensor tendons radially. Next, retract the fourth dorsal compartment ulnarward by reflection of the extensor infratendinous retinaculum from the underlying extrinsic radiocarpal ligaments and dorsal capsule. The extrinsic radiocarpal ligaments and dorsal capsule are reflected from the radius in the form of an inverted T (Fig. 3A). Assessment of the extent of the degenerative joint disease can easily be made at this time.

After verifying that the radiolunate joint cartilage is in good condition, transect the remaining scapholunate and lunatotriquetral ligaments. Remove the scaphoid and triquetrum piecemeal, using a rongeur. Denude the proximal capitate and distal lunate articular surfaces of articular cartilage to the level of subchondral bone.

Prepare the mating surfaces of the capitate and lunate in one of two ways. One method is to transect the surfaces of each bone, using an oscillating saw or rongeur, so that the cut surfaces are perpendicular to the longitudinal axes of both bones (Fig. 3B, C). Another method makes use of matched concavo-convex curvature reamers (Coughlin Howmedica, Inc., Rutherford, NJ), which allow precise machining of the opposing capitate and lunate surfaces (Fig. 3D, E). Approximate the capitolunate complex and maintain it in place by means of either a modified towel clamp or a smooth 0.045-in. Kirschner wire placed longitudinally in the dorsal one-third of the two bones (Fig. 3F). Confirm the alignment of the carpal bones with biplanar intraoperative fluoroscopy. The longitudinal axes of the capitate and lunate should be collinear on both PA and lateral projections.

Once proper alignment is achieved, equal amounts (3 to 4 mm) of distal lunate cancellous surface will be volar and dorsal to the capitate neck. Flex the wrist and insert a small blunt elevator into the radiolunate joint to elevate and expose the proximal surface of the lunate for antegrade screw placement across the arthrodesis site (Fig. 3G). Capitolunate complex screw fixation can be achieved with cannulated or noncannulated Herbert screws (Zimmer Inc, Warsaw, IN), 3.0-mm cannulated screws (Synthes USA, Paoli, PA), or Acutrak screws (Acumed, Beaverton, OR). Insert the screws in a direction that is 10° radial to the longitudinal axis of the capitate; this screw orientation helps avoid penetration into the capitohamate joint.

A partial radial styloidectomy can be carried out if abutment of the radial styloid and remaining carpus occurs with radial deviation of the wrist. Confirm final alignment and screw positions with intraoperative x-rays before closing the wound, placing the drains, and applying a sugar-tong splint.

## POSTOPERATIVE MANAGEMENT

If drains have been used, they usually can be removed within 24 to 48 hours by the patient or family. The first postoperative clinic visit at 10 to 14 days is for wound inspection, suture removal, and repeat x-ray examination. Apply a sugar-tong splint or short-arm cast that the patient will wear for an additional 4 weeks.

The second postoperative visit is at 6 weeks, at which time the radiographic union is assessed. If there is evidence of trabecular bridging across the arthrodesis site, prescribe a removable wrist splint and initiate a home active-wrist-motion program. Progressive strengthening exercises are allowed at 8 weeks after surgery, and full activity is encouraged at 3 months. Continue sugar-tong or short-arm cast immobilization until there is clinical and x-ray evidence of fusion, if a solid fusion has not been noted on x-ray at 6 weeks after surgery.

## COMPLICATIONS

An incorrectly placed screw across the capitolunate complex may penetrate the capitohamate joint. Avoid such an error by placing a Kirschner wire in the intended screw direction and checking its position on intraoperative x-rays or fluoroscopy. Screw redirection is recommended; the screw can be left in place, however, if alignment of the capitolunate complex is satisfactory and stable. The capitohamate joint should be fused as well, and cancellous graft from the scaphoid or triquetrum can be used for this purpose. Additional fixation is usually not necessary if decortication of the capitohamate joint does not destabilize the capitolunate-hamate unit.

Malposition of the capitolunate complex can result from two technical errors. The first error pertains to preparing the mating surfaces of the capitate and lunate. Oscillating saw cuts that do not allow collinear alignment of the capitolunate complex are difficult to correct. If the error is in the capitate cut, more bone can be removed perpendicular to the long capitate axis in the PA and lateral planes. This procedure may require partial removal of the proximal pole of the hamate. The lunate cut cannot be compensated for by additional cuts because they may shorten the lunate enough to compromise the screw purchase. The best possible alignment should then be secured with a screw.

Another error in capitolunate alignment can occur when the dorsal neck of the capitate is located too far dorsally on the lunate. This error can be corrected before screw placement by volar translation of the capitate. Both of these errors can be avoided if a cup-and-cone reamer is used to prepare the bone ends. This method of bone preparation will not permit dorsal translation of the capitate neck because the capitate neck essentially sits into the machined concave fossa of the distal lunate. Furthermore, the matching cup-and-cone reamers allow angular adjustment in both PA and lateral planes.

Patients with poor bone quality for which vascularization is equivocal are not candidates for this procedure. Lunate fragmentation and collapse can occur in individuals with factors compromising bone union.

## RECOMMENDED READING

1. Kirschenbaum, O., Schneider, L. H., Kirkpatrick, W. H.: Scaphoid excision and capitolunate arthrodesis for radioscaphoid arthritis. *J. Hand Surg.*, 18A: 780–785, 1993.
2. Watson, H. K., Ballet, F. L.: The SLAC wrist: scapholunate advanced collapse pattern of degenerative arthritis. *J. Hand Surg.*, 9A: 358–365, 1984.
3. Watson, H. K., Ryu, J.: Evaluation of arthritis of the wrist. *Clin. Orthop.*, 202: 57–67, 1986.

# 19

# Proximal Row Carpectomy

Ann E. Van Heest and James H. House

## INDICATIONS/CONTRAINDICATIONS

The majority of candidates for a proximal row carpectomy have a severely disabled, painful wrist with a limited arc of motion and decreased grip strength. Removal of the diseased proximal carpal bones with careful capsular repair provides capitoradial articulation with adequate soft tissue stability to allow a functional range of motion (4–8). By comparison with fusion procedures, early mobilization is possible with proximal row carpectomy. A variety of specific conditions for which a proximal row carpectomy are indicated are described.

### Scapholunate Advanced Collapse

Degenerative arthritis secondary to scapholunate instability develops in a progressive pattern, as Watson and Ballet have documented (12). Degenerative changes most commonly originate between the tip of the radial styloid and the scaphoid, progressing along the scaphoradial joint. The capitolunate articulation is next affected, and the radiolunate joint is spared. Even in advanced cases, the articular cartilage of the lunate fossa remains unaffected, so that proximal row carpectomy is an ideal option.

The articular cartilage of the capitate may be affected to varying degrees in advanced cases. In our experience, even if the capitate has some fissuring or thinning, proximal row carpectomy results are not compromised. When there is severe midcarpal arthritis with significant degenerative changes in the head of the capitate, proximal row carpectomy is contraindicated.

In our opinion, proximal row carpectomy is a superior option to either intercarpal fusion or wrist arthrodesis for the scapholunate advanced collapse (SLAC) wrist for the following reasons. Intercarpal arthrodesis (four-bone fusion) alters the biomechanics of the wrist, producing a ball-and-socket joint the way the proximal row carpectomy does (see Chapter 17). The prolonged immobilization necessary for intercarpal fusion, however, further stiffens the wrist. Wrist arthrodesis also requires prolonged immobilization and has the further disadvantages of a high reoperation rate and significant functional impairment inherent in a wrist that has undergone arthrodesis.

### Kienböck's Disease

Alexander and Lichtman (1) consider proximal row carpectomy a salvage procedure suitable only for stage IV Kienböck's disease (carpal collapse with associated degenerative changes). In our experience, however, stage II (lunate fracturing) and stage III (carpal collapse without degenerative changes) disease are equally suitable for proximal row carpectomy treatment in patients who are not candidates for "joint leveling" by osteotomy (see Chapter 33). If the disease process is treated in its earlier stages, the articular cartilage of the lunate fossa and capitate head are intact, a condition that theoretically allows greater longevity for the proximal row carpectomy.

### Scaphoid Nonunions

Persistent scaphoid nonunions following surgical intervention are amenable to effective treatment with a proximal row carpectomy. Nonunions with small proximal pole fragments, unrecognized nonunions presenting with dorsal intercalated segmental instability, and secondary radioscaphoid degenerative changes are also treatable in this way.

### Acute/Subacute Carpal Dislocations/Fracture Dislocations

Acute injuries to the proximal carpal row on occasion can be severe. In open (2) or closed injuries, especially with devascularized scaphoid or lunate fragments or multiple proximal carpal fractures, proximal row carpectomy provides simple and effective definitive management. Additionally, dislocations and ligamentous disruptions, especially those initially unrecognized and unreduced, can be effectively treated subacutely with proximal row carpectomy. In our experience, this patient group achieves the best postoperative results, manifested by near-normal grip strength, improved range of motion, and excellent pain relief.

### Failed Silicone Implants

Patients who have undergone revision of *scaphoid* silicone arthroplasty to proximal row carpectomy have fared better than those with failed silicone *lunate* implants. Proximal row carpectomy in our experience offers pain relief as well as preservation of motion following removal of scaphoid implants.

### Avascular Necrosis of the Scaphoid

Patients with idiopathic or posttraumatic avascular necrosis of the scaphoid are excellent candidates for proximal carpectomy.

### Severe Flexion Contractures Associated with Arthrogryposis, Cerebral Palsy, or Other Spastic Conditions

When a patient has severe functional deficits due to a flexion posture that is rigid or not amenable to tendon transfer alone, proximal row carpectomy shortens the carpal segment, allowing more functional positioning (10,13). This procedure is also a useful adjunct to wrist arthrodesis for patients with chronic wrist flexion contractures who have sufficient digital control to function with an immobile wrist.

### Other Proximal Carpal Disorders

Proximal row carpectomy can be used in a variety of difficult clinical situations as an alternative to wrist fusion, especially when a patient has a strong occupational or avocational need to preserve wrist motion. It can be used, for example, to salvage failed scapholunate ligament reconstructions or capsulodesis procedures. Similarly, persistent scaphoid nonunions despite internal fixation or bone grafting can be salvaged with a proximal row carpectomy without precluding later wrist arthrodesis. In our experience, however, the wrist that has undergone multiple previous procedures obtains inferior clinical results compared with primary proximal row carpectomy.

In our opinion, three relative contraindications to proximal row carpectomy exist. First, Ferlic et al. reported unsatisfactory results in 75% of patients with rheumatoid arthritis (3). Next, in our experience, patients with failed lunate silicone implants have had variable clinical results with proximal row carpectomy. Although some patients, after having a Silastic lunate, have done well with proximal row carpectomy as a salvage procedure, in general, clinical results are unpredictable. Finally, significant capitate articular damage is a contraindication to proximal row carpectomy. In a patient with SLAC wrist, we often opt before surgery for either four-bone intercarpal fusion or proximal row carpectomy; we make an intraoperative decision depending on the condition of the head of the capitate.

## PREOPERATIVE PLANNING

Candidates for proximal row carpectomy have a variety of proximal carpal diseases, as previously discussed. Consistent physical findings include limited and painful range of motion in the wrist and decreased grip strength.

It is important for the physician to accurately record preoperative motion and strength values for postoperative comparison. Obtain routine radiographs as well as appropriate special imaging studies to accurately diagnose and stage the patient's condition.

## SURGERY

After regional or general anesthesia has been administered, position the patient supine and place a tourniquet on the proximal arm. After routine surgical scrubbing and limb draping, elevate the limb, exsanguinate it using a Martin bandage, and inflate the tourniquet to a pressure of 250 mm Hg.

### Technique

Make an oblique longitudinal incision, centered over the radiocarpal joint, from the ulnar side of the radius proximally to the base of the second metacarpal distally (Fig. 1). Dissect the subcutaneous tissue to the extensor retinaculum, taking special care to preserve subcutaneous nerves and vessels (Fig. 2). Identify the proximal and distal extents of the extensor retinaculum (Fig. 3).

Make an oblique incision, starting distally at the radial border of the third dorsal compartment, dissecting the retinaculum off the septum between the third and fourth compartments, and ending proximally at the ulnar border of the fourth compartment (Fig. 4). Leave a rim of retinaculum proximally. Identify the poste-

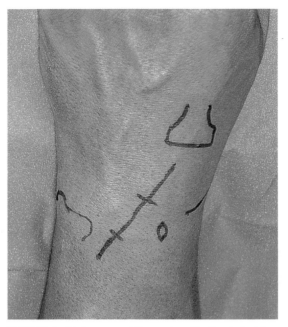

**FIGURE 1.** Make an oblique longitudinal incision centered over the radiocarpal joint from the ulnar side of the radius proximally to the second metacarpal base distally, as demonstrated in this patient's left wrist. (The ulnar head, Lister's tubercle, and the radial styloid are also marked on the skin.)

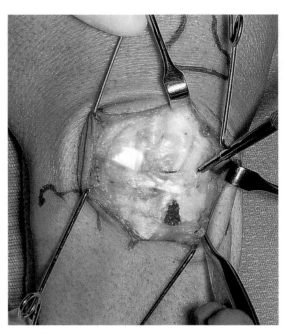

**FIGURE 2.** Identify the proximal and distal extents of the extensor retinaculum. The dental probe distally is under the extensor pollicis longus tendon.

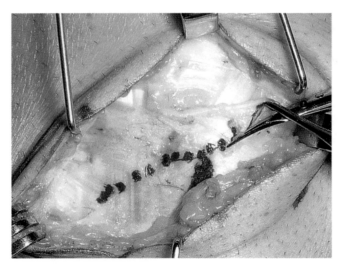

**FIGURE 3.** Plan an oblique incision through the extensor retinaculum from the radial border of the third dorsal compartment extending proximally to the ulnar border of the fourth dorsal compartment.

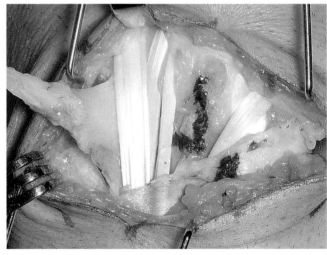

**FIGURE 4.** Dissect the retinaculum free and reflect it to the ulnar side, leaving a proximal rim of retinaculum in place.

rior interosseous nerve in the floor of the fourth compartment and sharply transect it proximally (Fig. 5).

Plan a T-capsulotomy several millimeters distal to the end of the radius with a distal limb extending over the scapholunate interval (Fig. 6). Opening of the wrist joint (Fig. 7) reveals complete dissociation of the scapholunate ligament with resultant degenerative changes on the radioscaphoid articulation, consistent findings in SLAC. The head of the capitate is well preserved (Fig. 7).

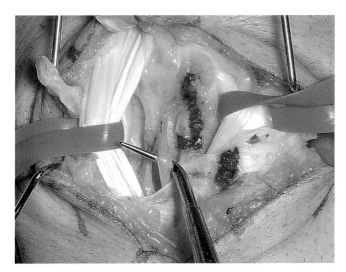

**FIGURE 5.** Identify the posterior interosseous nerve (dental probe) and then transect it proximally.

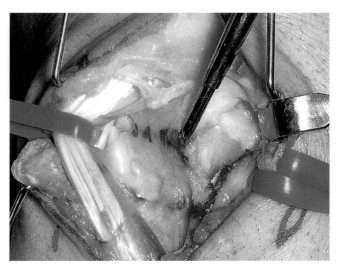

**FIGURE 6.** Perform a T-capsulotomy with the distal limb at the level of the scapholunate junction. The probe shows the scapholunate interval.

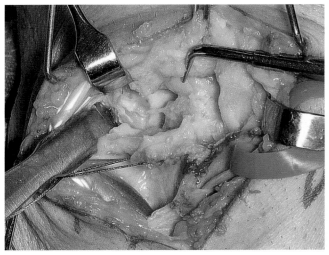

**FIGURE 7.** Opening the wrist joint shows this patient's complete scapholunate dissociation and radioscaphoid arthrosis, with a well-preserved capitate articular surface (dental probe); consistent findings in a scapholunate advanced collapse wrist.

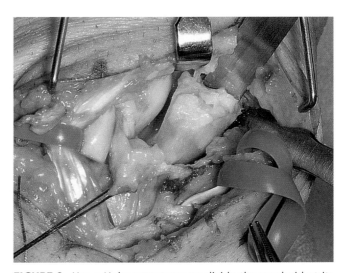

**FIGURE 8.** Use a Hoke osteotome to divide the scaphoid at its waist, facilitating removal of the proximal pole.

Use a Hoke osteotome to divide the diseased scaphoid at its waist (Fig. 8), and resect the proximal pole. Place an external fixator or threaded Steinmann pin into the distal fragment and use it as a joystick (Fig. 9); dissect its capsular attachments free using curved periosteal elevators, a #15 blade, or curved #66 Beaver blades. Carefully dissect the soft tissue attachments directly at their bone insertions.

Patience is imperative and will be rewarded by a well-preserved capsular and ligamentous envelope with no articular damage to adjacent bones. Identify the radioscaphocapitate ("sling") ligament on the palmar capsule and verify its integrity (Fig. 10). This ligament is crucial as a radial support for the capitate when it later rests in the lunate fossa.

Mark the external fixator pin for the anticipated depth of insertion (Fig. 11) to avoid penetration through the palmar capsule into the carpal canal. Place the external fixator pin in the lunate as a joystick (Fig. 12) to aid in sharp dissection

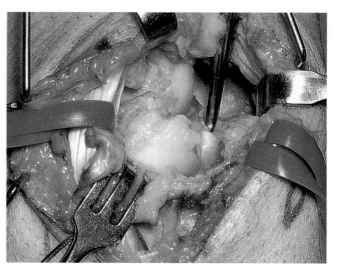

**FIGURE 9.** Place an external fixator pin into the distal scaphoid and use it as a joystick to carefully dissect the capsular attachments free subperiosteally.

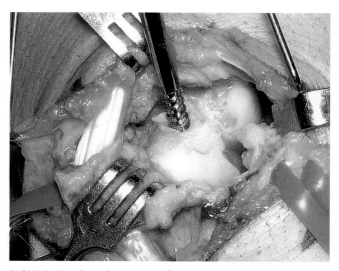

**FIGURE 10.** Inspect the palmar wrist capsule to verify the preservation of the radioscaphocapitate ("sling") ligament, held up by the dental probe.

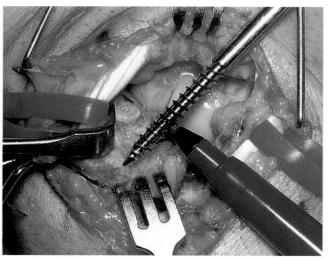

**FIGURE 11.** Mark the threaded external fixator pin for the anticipated depth of insertion into the lunate to avoid penetration into the carpal canal.

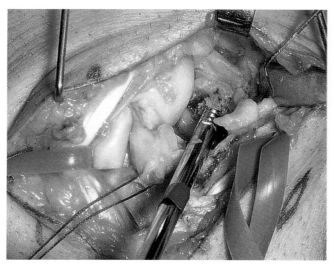

**FIGURE 12.** Place the external fixator pin in the lunate to serve as a joystick and aid in sharp dissection and removal of the lunate.

and removal of the lunate (Fig. 13). Carefully protect the lunate fossa and capitate head. Finally, dissect the triquetrum free, after placing the joystick to aid exposure (Fig. 14). Excise the proximal row (Fig. 15).

When it is appropriate to perform a radial styloidectomy it can be done through the same skin incision. Carry down dissection between the first and second dorsal compartment to the radial styloid (Fig. 16). Dissect the distal 5 to 7 mm of radial styloid free of its dorsal and palmar attachments (Fig. 17); carefully preserve the radioscaphocapitate ligament. Transect the distal 5 to 7 mm of radial styloid (Fig. 18) and remove it.

Again inspect the capitate articular cartilage (Fig. 19). It naturally rests proximally into the lunate fossa because of the length of the intact radiocapitate ligament (Fig. 20). Maintain this position by careful repair of both limbs of the dorsal T-capsulotomy (Fig. 21). Test the wrist in flexion and extension and in radial and ulnar deviation for stability. Then repair the retinaculum (Fig. 22).

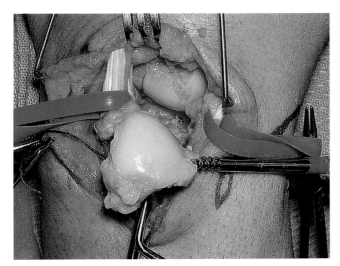

**FIGURE 13.** Remove the lunate by careful sharp dissection of its ligament attachments.

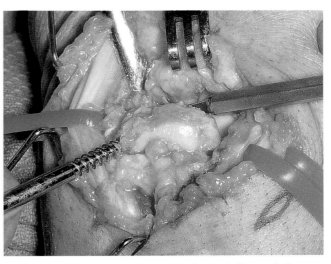

**FIGURE 14.** Remove the triquetrum by a similar technique; a Beaver blade is very useful for this dissection.

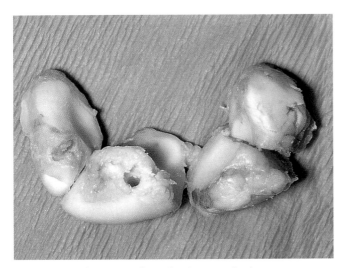

**FIGURE 15.** The proximal row has been excised.

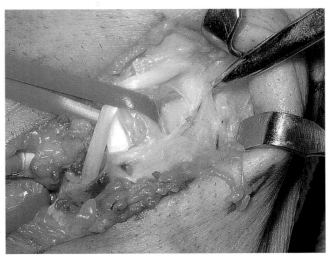

**FIGURE 16.** Preparing for a radial styloidectomy, carry dissection down through the same incision between the first and second dorsal compartments.

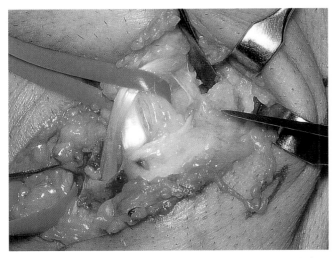

**FIGURE 17.** Dissect the distal 5 to 7 mm of radial styloid free and remove it, using a Hoke osteotome.

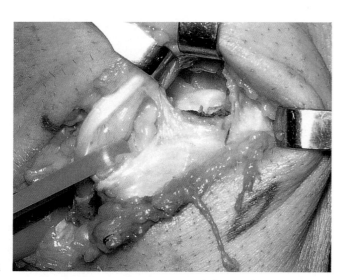

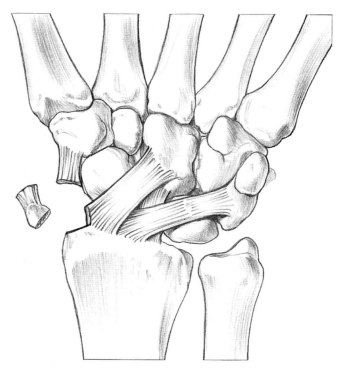

A                                                                                                B

**FIGURE 18. A:** Inspection reveals a carefully preserved radioscaphocapitate ligament. **B:** Viewed from the palmar aspect, the radial styloid is resected, preserving the radioscaphocapitate ligament. Carefully preserve the palmar aspect of the radiolunotriquetral ligament by careful lunate excision.

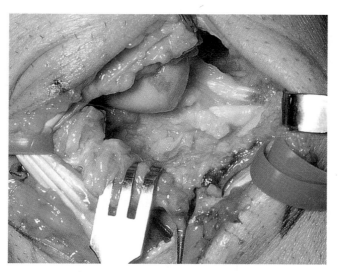

**FIGURE 19.** The articular cartilage of the capitate is again inspected and remains undamaged.

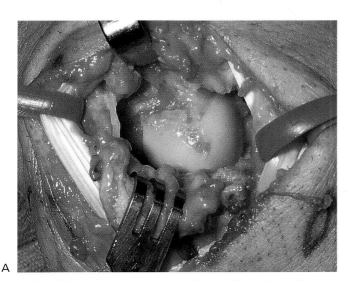

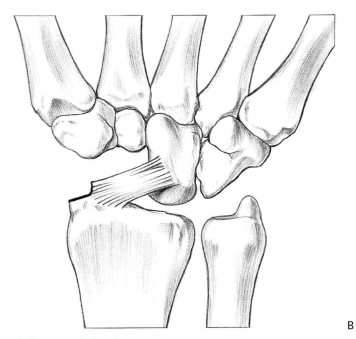

A                                                                                    B

**FIGURE 20. A:** Using the tension of the radioscaphocapitate ligament, the capitate head naturally rests in the lunate fossa. **B:** In this palmar view, the intact radioscaphocapitate ligament is of a proper length to control seating of the capitate into the lunate fossa of the radius.

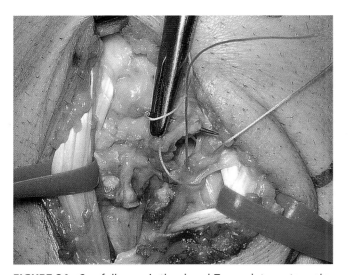

**FIGURE 21.** Carefully repair the dorsal T-capsulotomy to maintain this position.

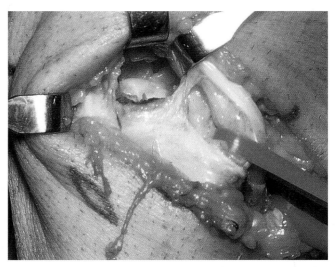

**FIGURE 22.** The retinaculum is repaired reconstructing the third compartment septum.

Deflate the tourniquet and obtain hemostasis. A drain is optional. Close the subcutaneous layer with 2–0 absorbable suture, and close the skin with 4–0 nylon. Apply a well-padded postoperative dressing with longitudinal plaster splints; carefully mold it in a neutral position.

## POSTOPERATIVE MANAGEMENT

Most patients are hospitalized overnight for analgesia, although on rare occasions this procedure has been done on an outpatient basis. The patient returns in

10 to 14 days for removal of the postoperative dressing and placement of a short-arm cast. The cast is bivalved or removed 1 to 2 weeks later. At this time, encourage the patient to begin range-of-motion exercises, light strength training, and functional use of the limb.

Continue part-time protection with a removable orthosis if necessary until approximately 6 weeks postoperatively as the patient regains strength. Depending upon the patient's hand dominance and the nature of his or her work, return to sedentary work is possible in 1 to 2 weeks postoperatively, to light duty in 6 to 8 weeks, and to manual labor as soon as adequate strength is demonstrated, usually 3 to 6 months.

A recent review of 42 consecutive cases done between 1979 and 1994 at the University of Minnesota (J. H. House, unpublished data) showed the following clinical results.

The average total wrist motion (dorsi/palmar flexion, radial/ulnar deviation) was 115° preoperatively and 109° postoperatively. Thus, a functional arc of wrist motion was maintained but not improved. Preoperatively the affected limb averaged 54% of the grip strength of the unaffected limb; postoperatively, it improved to 69%. Two manual laborers who had had proximal row carpectomies in their dominant wrists achieved grip strengths of 113 lb and 104 lb, respectively, in the surgically treated limbs!

All patients had relief of their preoperative pain. At final follow-up, one-fourth of the patients reported no pain, one-fourth reported cold-weather symptoms only, one-fourth reported mild pain not affecting their activity, and one-fourth reported moderate pain affecting some activities. No patients had severe pain. All employed patients returned to work. One patient doing manual labor was retrained to lighter work; eight patients had some work limitations, and the remainder returned to previous employment without limitation. All patients except one were satisfied with surgery and said they would repeat the surgery for the condition if it recurred.

No patients required subsequent wrist fusion. One patient required a subsequent radial styloidectomy.

## COMPLICATIONS

1. *Radial styloidectomy*: After reviewing our clinical results, we no longer recommend routine radial styloidectomy. In the case of a prominent radial styloid or when extensive radioscaphoid osteophytes exist, a radial styloidectomy is recommended. Preservation of the radioscaphocapitate ("sling") ligament is crucial. If too much of the radial styloid is resected the origin of this ligament is removed and the capitate is destabilized (11). Although other authors have recommended a more extensive radial styloidectomy (9), we recommend excision only of the prominent 5 to 7 mm of radial styloid in order to preserve the sling ligament. The ligament allows the capitate to rest into the lunate fossa and provides crucial radial stability.
2. *Incomplete excision of the distal pole of the scaphoid*: Although removal of the distal pole of the scaphoid has previously been optional, we have seen several cases in long-term follow-up with radiographic progression of impingement between the distal pole of the scaphoid and the radial styloid. We now recommend routine complete excision of the scaphoid.
3. *Pin complications*: It is acceptable—although in our experience unnecessary—to place pins judiciously through the scaphoid fossa into the nonarticular capitate. Follow-up cases have shown progressive cyst formation from pins in the lunate fossa or into the capitate head, as well as avascular necrosis of the capitate from crossed Steinmann pins. Because of the many potential problems and no apparent benefit from the use of pins, we recommend avoiding use of pins altogether, relying instead on a careful capsular closure.

4. *Excessive immobilization*: Complications such as reflex sympathetic dystrophy and stiffness can be avoided by early functional mobilization of the wrist and hand. Encourage use of the fingers immediately after surgery. Initiate use of the wrist 2 to 4 weeks postoperatively, depending on the condition of the wound.

## RECOMMENDED READING

1. Alexander, A. H., Lichtman, D. M.: Kienbock's disease. *Orthop. Clin. North Am.*, 17(3): 461–472, 1986.
2. Ferenz, C. C., Freundlich, B. D.: Proximal row carpectomy for open fracture-dislocation of the carpus. *J. Trauma*, 27(1): 85–88, 1987.
3. Ferlic, D. C., Clayton, M. L., Mills, M. F.: Proximal row carpectomy: review of rheumatoid and nonrheumatoid wrists. *J. Hand Surg.*, 16(A): 420–424, 1991.
4. Green, D. P.: Proximal row carpectomy. *Hand Clin.*, 3(1): 163–168, 1987.
5. Imbriglia, J. E., Broudy, A. S., Hagberg, W. C., McKernan, D.: Proximal row carpectomy: clinical evaluation. *J. Hand Surg.*, 15(A): 426–430, 1990.
6. Inglis, A. E., Jones, E. C.: Proximal row carpectomy for diseases of the proximal row. *J. Bone Joint Surg.*, 59A: 460–463, 1977.
7. Jorgenson, E. C.: Proximal row carpectomy. *J. Bone Joint Surg.*, 51A: 1104–1111, 1969.
8. Neviaser, R. J.: Proximal row carpectomy for posttraumatic disorders of the carpus. *J. Hand Surg.*, 8: 301–305, 1983.
9. Neviaser, R. J.: On resection of the proximal carpal row. *Clin. Orthop.*, 202: 12–15, 1986.
10. Omer, G. E., Capen, D. A.: Proximal row carpectomy with muscle transfers for spastic paralysis. *J. Hand Surg.*, 1: 197–204, 1976.
11. Siegel, D. B., Gelberman, R. H.: Radial styloidectomy: an anatomical study with special reference to radiocarpal intracapsular ligamentous morphology. *J. Hand Surg.*, 16(A): 40–44, 1991.
12. Watson, H. K., Ballet, F. L.: The SLAC wrist: scapholunate advance collapse pattern of degenerative arthritis. *J. Hand Surg.*, 9A: 358–365, 1984.
13. Wenner, S. M., Sapieria, B. S.: Proximal row carpectomy in arthrogrypotic wrist deformity. *J. Hand Surg.*, 12(A): 523–525, 1987.

# 20

# Arthrodesis of the Osteoarthritic Wrist

Robin R. Richards

## INDICATIONS/CONTRAINDICATIONS

The most common indication for wrist arthrodesis is posttraumatic arthritis of the radiocarpal and midcarpal joints. For example, a chronically nonunited scaphoid fracture or scapholunate dissociation with advanced carpal collapse and secondary degenerative arthritis can be treated effectively by wrist arthrodesis. When posttraumatic arthritis involves only the radiocarpal joint or midcarpal joint, wrist arthrodesis is an alternative to limited arthrodesis. Wrist arthrodesis often is required to salvage a failed previous more limited arthrodesis or wrist arthroplasty (4,12). It is unlikely that any wrist reconstruction will improve motion. For this reason, wrist arthrodesis is recommended as the preferred initial treatment in cases of limited disease when wrist dorsiflexion and palmar flexion are less than 30° (Algorithm 1).

Less frequent indications for wrist arthrodesis include diseases that cause significant instability, such as rheumatoid arthritis or infection. Segmental bone loss involving the distal radius and carpus resulting from severe crush is another indication, as well as mutilating open injuries inflicted by gunshot blasts, saws, press injuries, or other industrial trauma (Fig. 1). Paralytic disorders may cause a wrist deformity interfering with hand function that is corrected most effectively by arthrodesis of the wrist in a position of stable alignment. At times hand reconstruction for combined nerve palsy requires use of a single residual functioning wrist motor, which is possible only by stabilization of the wrist. Wrist arthrodesis can be indicated as a method of reconstruction following tumor resection (7).

The primary contraindication to wrist arthrodesis is the rare situation in which motion is essential to perform a highly important or dependent activity. For example, a tetraplegic patient must have wrist dorsiflexion preserved to be capable of body transfer. A second contraindication is the necessity for wrist motion to provide for or to augment digital motion by tenodesis effect.

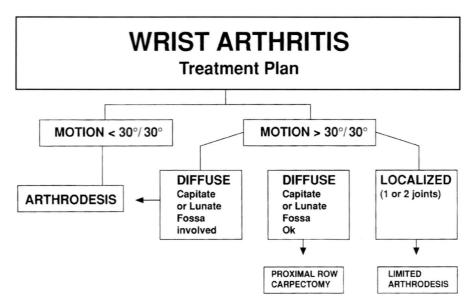

**ALGORITHM 1.** Treatment plan for wrist arthritis.

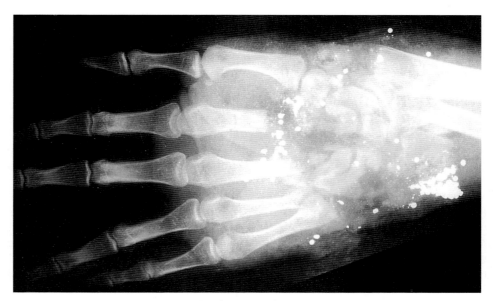

**FIGURE 1.** Anteroposterior radiograph of 34-year-old man who sustained a severely comminuted and contaminated gunshot wound to carpus with segmental bone loss across carpus and metacarpus.

## PREOPERATIVE PLANNING

Most patients considered for wrist arthrodesis have pain with use, limited wrist motion, and weakness. Physical findings vary with the location and extent of arthritis. It is important to note the presence and location of swelling, crepitus, and tenderness. It is desirable to record preoperative grip and range-of-motion measurements accurately. The distal radioulnar joint is examined to detect potential problems such as pain, instability, or restriction of forearm rotation that may require surgical treatment in addition to wrist arthrodesis.

Many patients with long-standing arthritis or deformity of the wrist also have symptoms of carpal tunnel syndrome. Even if the symptoms initially are mild, they can become clinically significant following surgery. All patients scheduled to undergo wrist arthrodesis are examined for the presence of carpal tunnel syndrome by Phalen's test (8) and sensory testing. The symptoms of carpal tunnel syndrome can increase following wrist arthrodesis due to perioperative edema formation. Carpal tunnel release should be considered prior to, or concomitant with, wrist arthrodesis when clinical evaluation is positive and the presence of a compressive neuropathy affecting the median nerve is confirmed by electrodiagnostic testing.

Appropriate radiographic evaluation includes an anteroposterior and lateral view as well as two oblique views. The oblique view best shows the extent of arthritic involvement. The ulnar midcarpal joint (triquetral-hamate and capitohamate) is evaluated carefully to determine if it is free of clinical and radiographic deformity or if it is arthritic and therefore requires inclusion within the fusion. The lateral view is helpful in evaluating the capitolunate and distal radioulnar joints.

Additional studies may be indicated based on the findings of the routine radiographs. An ulnar deviated posteroanterior view often is needed to evaluate the scaphotrapeziotrapezoid joint for arthritic deformity. Trispiral tomograms or a computed tomographic scan provides the best assessment for the capitolunate joint, which may be difficult to evaluate for arthritic deformity using routine radiographs.

## SURGERY

Surgery can be performed under axillary block or general anesthesia. A general anesthetic is required if an iliac crest bone graft is to be used. The involved extremity and the opposite iliac crest are prepared and draped if an iliac crest bone graft is to be performed.

### Technique

A brachial tourniquet is inflated 50 to 100 mm Hg above systolic pressure. The wrist is placed in neutral position with respect to radioulnar deviation and a straight incision is made beginning at the distal third of the index-middle interosseous space, proceeding across Lister's tubercle, and ending over the radius at the proximal border of the abductor pollicis longus muscle (Fig. 2). One or two crossing veins may require division and suture ligature (Fig. 3).

A radially based skin and subcutaneous flap containing the dorsal sensory radial nerve is elevated off the extensor retinaculum. The extensor retinaculum is stepcut to allow for its repair at the conclusion of the procedure. The third dorsal compartment is opened and the extensor pollicis longus tendon and muscle are elevated (Fig. 4). The sheath distal to the retinaculum must be incised to allow adequate retraction of the extensor pollicis longus tendon (Figs. 5, 6). Umbilical tapes are placed around the extensor tendons so that they can be retracted as the procedure progresses.

The periosteum over the long finger metacarpal is incised after retraction of the overlying extensor tendons and the dorsal aspect of the metacarpal is exposed subperiosteally. The radial and ulnar borders of the metacarpal are left undisturbed. An incision is made through the dorsal wrist capsule and extended proximally to the radius along its dorsal surface. With sharp dissection the capsule and second dorsal compartment are elevated radially and the capsule and fourth dorsal compartment are elevated ulnarly, taking care not to enter the undersurface of the compartment.

The joint surfaces to be included in the fusion are exposed and decorticated down to cancellous bone. The carpometacarpal joints of the long and index fingers, scaphocapitate joint, capitolunate joint, radioscaphoid joint, and the radiolu-

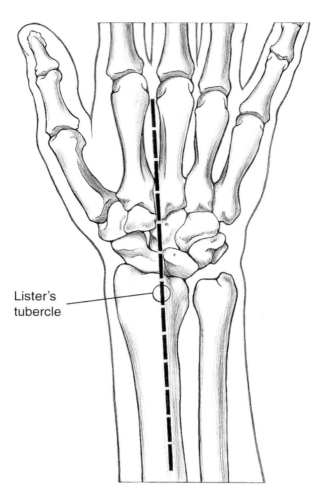

Lister's tubercle

**FIGURE 2.** A straight dorsal incision is centered from the radial aspect of the third metacarpal, across Lister's tubercle, and across the dorsal distal radius.

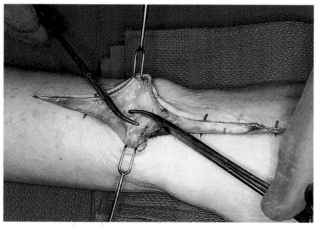

**FIGURE 3.** Surgical approach is through a straight dorsal incision. One or more large crossing veins require division and suture ligature.

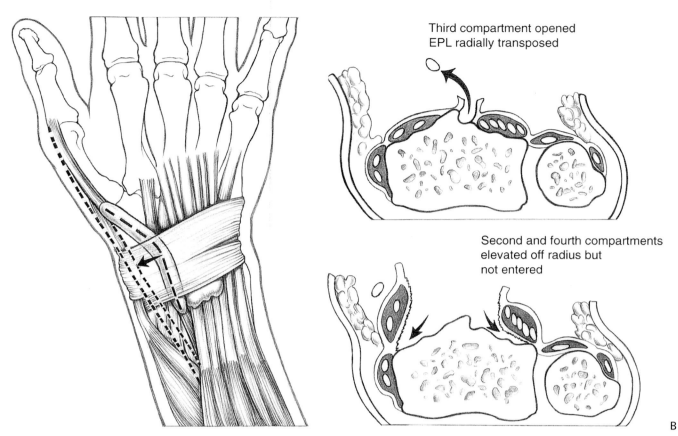

**Third compartment opened**
**EPL radially transposed**

**Second and fourth compartments**
**elevated off radius but**
**not entered**

A                                                                                                                B

**FIGURE 4.** **A:** Incision through third dorsal compartment to remove and radially transpose the extensor pollicis longus (EPL). **B:** Coronal sections show opening of the third dorsal compartment. Alternatively, the retinaculum is step-cut, the tendons are retracted using moistened umbilical tapes, and the retinaculum repaired at the conclusion of the procedure. Care must be taken to prevent bowstringing of the extensor tendons by keeping the retinaculum intact or repairing it at the end of the procedure.

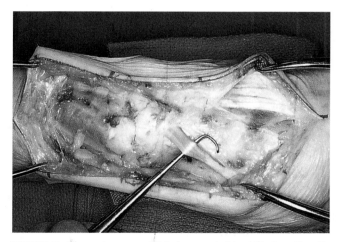

**FIGURE 5.** The extensor pollicis longus is identified as it exits from the third dorsal compartment.

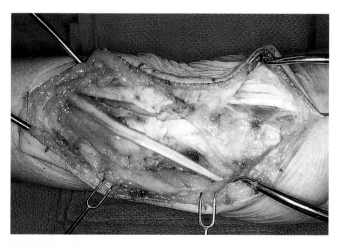

**FIGURE 6.** The third dorsal compartment is opened and the extensor pollicis longus reflected radially.

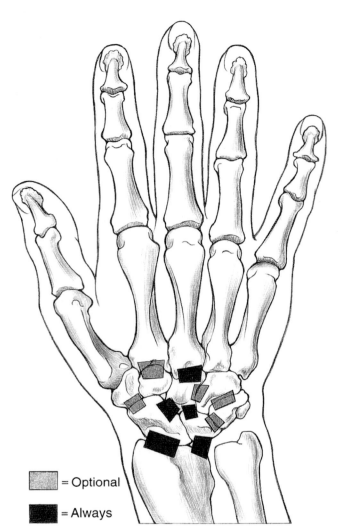

= Optional

= Always

**FIGURE 7.** Joints always to be included in a wrist arthrodesis are as follows: (1) the third carpometacarpal, (2) the scaphocapi-tate, (3) the capitolunate, (4) the radioscaphoid, and (5) the radiolunate. Optional joints depend on whether deformity and arthritis are present on examination of radiographs prior to wrist arthrodesis. These joints include triquetral-lunate, trique-tral-hamate, capitohamate, scaphotrapeziotrapezoid, and trap-ezoid-second metacarpal.

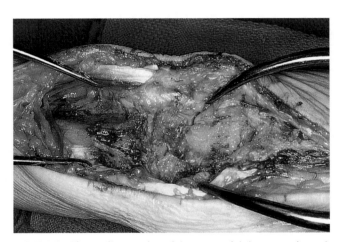

**FIGURE 8.** The radiocarpal and intercarpal joints are decorti-cated down to cancellous bone.

nate joint are included as a rule. The ulnar carpus is left undisturbed to preserve supple motion of the ulnar hand. When preoperative radiographic and clinical examinations have shown symptomatic arthritic involvement of other joints, these are included as well (Figs. 7, 8).

Exposure of the base of the index and long finger carpometacarpal joints is obtained most expediently by removal of the dorsal surface of the capitate and trapezoid with an osteotome. The dorsal surfaces of the scaphoid and lunate are removed down to cancellous bone by serially shaving each with an osteotome (Figs. 9, 10) and removing up to 60% of the anteroposterior diameter. Some of these dorsal shavings can be used as additional cancellous bone graft. All remaining joint surfaces, including the articular surface of the distal radius, are decorticated with osteotomes, rongeurs, or curettes. I have found use of osteotomes to be the quickest method of decortication. A transverse slot is cut in the bases of the index and long finger metacarpals to receive a bone graft. Care is taken to leave

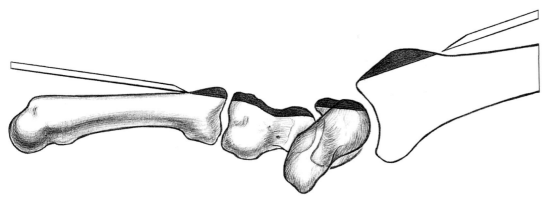

**FIGURE 9.** Osteotomy of Lister's tubercle and distal radial metaphysis—osteotomy of dorsal aspect of third carpometacarpal joint along with dorsal aspect of scaphoid, lunate, and capitate.

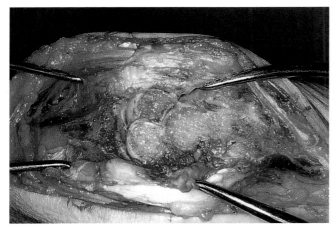

**FIGURE 10.** The dorsal aspects of the scaphoid, lunate, and capitate have been decorticated down to cancellous bone.

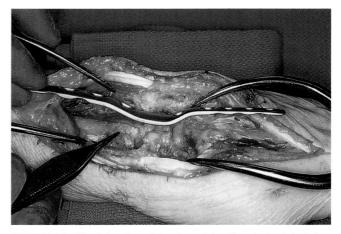

**FIGURE 11.** The lateral profile of a wrist arthrodesis plate takes into consideration the resulting profile after removal of Lister's tubercle and hump.

the palmar aspects of the carpometacarpal joints intact to prevent the creation of rotational deformity after plate fixation.

**Technique Using Iliac Crest Bone Graft.** Iliac crest bone graft can be used as an alternative to a dorsal sliding radial bone graft. If iliac crest bone graft is used, there is some increase in the morbidity of the procedure. It has always been my practice to harvest bone graft from the inner aspect of the iliac crest in the form of a corticocancellous slab when using iliac crest bone graft for this procedure. Use of a gelatin sponge can be helpful to reduce the likelihood of postoperative hematoma formation. In recent years, I have not used iliac crest bone graft because patient discharge usually is delayed by at least one day due to postoperative discomfort and impaired ambulatory ability.

Specially designed implants are useful when performing wrist arthrodesis (9). A titanium, low contact, dynamic compression plate has been designed and produced by Synthes (Paoli, PA) specifically for this operation (Fig. 11). To avoid prominence, edges of the implant are tapered and the screw heads are recessed. Three versions are available. One version with a precontoured short carpal bend is chosen for a small carpus or when arthrodesis follows a failed proximal row carpectomy. A second version with a longer carpal bend is used in larger individuals. A straight version is chosen when a corticocancellous intercalary bone graft is needed. These plates expedite the procedure by eliminating the need for precontouring and providing an automatic 10° of dorsiflexion (Fig. 12). Each plate uses

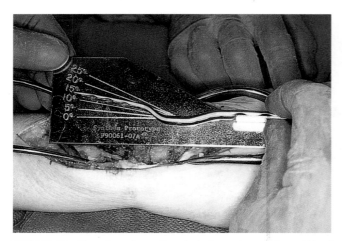

**FIGURE 12.** The plate for arthrodesis is contoured into 10° of dorsiflexion. This custom plate automatically builds in 10° of dorsiflexion.

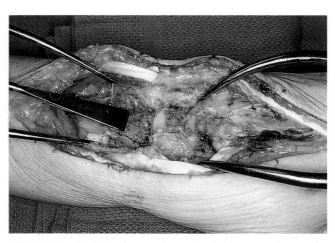

**FIGURE 13.** Additional cancellous local bone graft can be obtained through dorsal cancellous shavings from the distal radius.

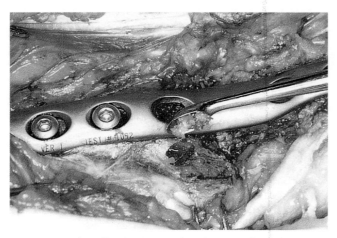

**FIGURE 14.** Plate fixation is completed proximally with 3.5-mm cortical screws. A window then can be made radial to the plate to harvest additional cancellous bone graft.

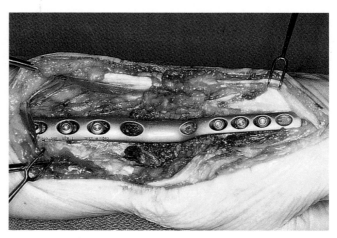

**FIGURE 15.** Completion of harvesting of bone graft from proximal metaphysis preserving at least 1 cm of metaphyseal and subchondral bone.

three 2.7-mm screws in the metacarpal, one 2.7-mm screw in the capitate, and four 3.5-mm screws in the radius. These plates usually are used in conjunction with an iliac crest bone graft.

**Technique Using Sliding Distal Radial Bone Graft.** A sliding bone graft can be harvested from the dorsal aspect of the distal radius (11). To use this technique, a plate must be selected that is long enough to extend two screw holes proximal to the donor site. A sagittal saw is used to cut a rectangular corticocancellous bone graft from the dorsal aspect of the distal radius. The bone graft is slid distally to fit into the slot previously cut in the bases of the index and long finger metacarpals. Cancellous bone shavings can be obtained from the adjacent dorsal carpal bones (Figs. 9,12–15).

A straight plate of adequate length is chosen and contoured to follow the dorsal radius, carpal sulcus, and contour of the third carpometacarpal joint. In a large individual a ten-hole, 3.5-mm low contact dynamic compression plate is chosen. However, this presents a palpable prominence at the metacarpal level that may require implant removal later due to tenderness over the plate (9). The plate is contoured into the desired amount of dorsiflexion, usually approximately 15°.

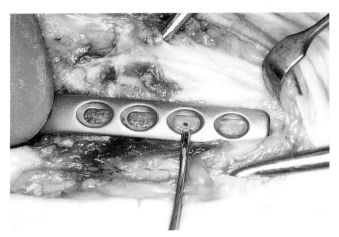

**FIGURE 16.** The plate is affixed to metacarpal distally first by marking the very central aspect of the plate hole.

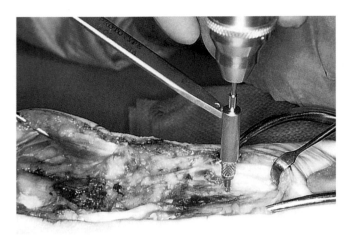

**FIGURE 17.** The plate is removed to facilitate direct visualization of the metacarpal as a 2.0-mm drill is passed directly dorsal to palmar.

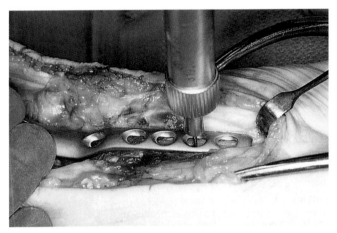

**FIGURE 18.** The plate is reapplied temporarily to allow for correct depth measurement through bone and plate.

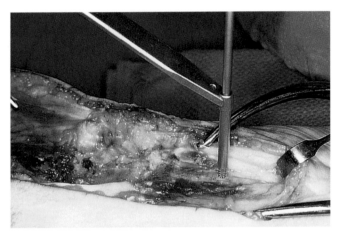

**FIGURE 19.** The distal metacarpal hole is tapped with a 2.7-mm tap with protective sleeve.

Bone graft is inserted into the joints to be fused. The plate is positioned over the dorsal third metacarpal and the center of the distalmost hole marked on bone (Fig. 16). A hole is drilled with a 2.0-mm drill for use of a 2.7-mm screw, or a 2.5-mm drill for use of a 3.5-mm screw. It is critical that the drill pass exactly dorsal to palmar in the sagittal plane (Fig. 17). If not, the plate will lie out of the frontal plane and subsequent radius fixation can induce a rotational deformity of the middle finger. The plate is repositioned temporarily to allow accurate screw length measurement through it (Fig. 18). When an AO wrist arthrodesis plate is utilized, the metacarpal holes are tapped with a 2.7-mm tap (Fig. 19) and 2.7-mm screws are used, which lie flush with the dorsal plate surface (Fig. 20).

The proximal plate should be aligned over the mid-dorsal aspect of the radius. The plate is secured to the radius by placing the screws in the neutral position on the plate. Care is taken not to shorten the carpus, which would alter the normal length-tension relationship of the muscle-tendon units and possibly lead to iatrogenic loss of grip strength. Fixation begins in the secondmost distal radius hole, drilling with a 2.5-mm drill eccentrically placed away from the wrist joint (Fig. 21). The depth is measured and drill hole tapped with a 3.5-mm cortical tap. An appropriate length screw is inserted. Completed fixation includes one screw in the distal metaphyseal region and three more proximal cortical screws.

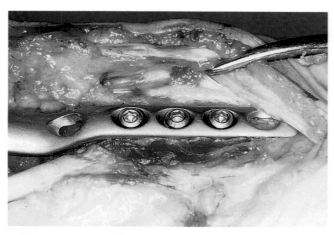

**FIGURE 20.** Bone graft is applied to the third carpometacarpal joint and distal plate fixation accomplished with 2.7-mm screws.

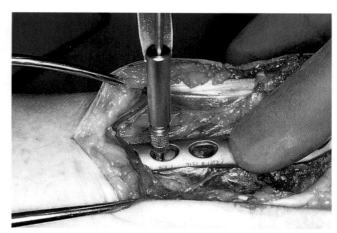

**FIGURE 21.** Cancellous bone graft is packed into the radiocarpal and metacarpal joints. The wrist is compressed and aligned into slight ulnar deviation. Further compression is achieved by proximally eccentric drilling of the first hole proximal to metaphysis in cortical bone.

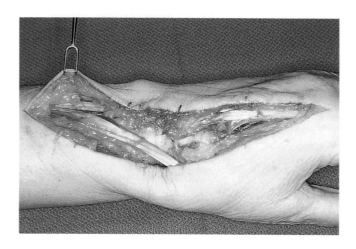

**FIGURE 22.** Additional local cancellous or distal cancellous bone graft is packed into the arthrodesis areas. Capsular closure has been completed, completely covering the plate, and leaving the extensor pollicis longus radially transposed.

Wound closure is accomplished over a suction drain. Coverage of the distal plate with soft tissue is not essential but usually can be accomplished with the dorsal fascia and periosteum. The extensor pollicis longus is left radially transposed (Fig. 22). The extensor retinaculum is repaired with interrupted 2–0 polyglycolic acid sutures. The dermis is closed with a resorbable 3–0 suture and skin closed with interrupted nylon or staples. A bulky dressing incorporating a plaster slab extending above the elbow aids elevation of the limb when the patient is recumbent and helps to control swelling. Elastic digital socks or wraps are applied to prevent digital edema while allowing continued motion. There is no need for rigid splinting.

## POSTOPERATIVE MANAGEMENT

The suction drain is removed at 24 hours. Active and passive range of finger and thumb motion is encouraged. At 10 to 14 days, sutures are removed. A short-arm cast allowing free motion of the fingers and thumb is applied. Alternatively, a light compressive dressing or elastic sleeve and a thermoplastic molded splint are applied, as a protective reminder that only light use of the hand and wrist is permissible.

Putty for light strengthening is given at 4 weeks. Normally, by 6 weeks, fusion is adequate to allow discontinuation of the splint and formal progressive strengthening. Full, unrestricted use is permitted by 10 to 12 weeks, providing there is no radiographic sign of screw loosening.

## Outcome Expectations

Patients undergoing wrist arthrodesis by AO technique for posttraumatic conditions were compared with a closely matched group who underwent wrist arthrodesis by non-AO technique. Solid arthrodesis occurred on the first surgical attempt in 56 of 57 (98%) fusions using AO technique compared to 26 of 33 (78%) fusions using other techniques. This difference was statistically significant ($p = .009$; Fisher exact test). Mean time to union was 10.3 weeks (3).

In a comparison review of two fairly evenly matched groups of patients (group 1, wrist arthrodesis; group 2, motion-preserving procedure), fusion patients were found to be more satisfied (91% versus 83%), equally willing to have the same procedure again (96% versus 96%), and more eager to have had the procedure sooner (91% versus 83%).

## Physical Examination

Following wrist arthrodesis, grip strength was 77% to 83% of the opposite hand in the dominant extremity and 56% to 82% of the nondominant hand (1).

## Activities of Daily Living Skills

Weiss undertook a comprehensive functional evaluation of 23 patients who underwent wrist arthrodesis for posttraumatic conditions (13). Follow-up evaluation averaged 54 months and consisted of a clinical questionnaire, the Jebsen hand function test, and a functional rating devised by Buck-Gramcko/Lohmann. Fifteen of 23 patients returned to their regular jobs. The most difficult tasks for patients following wrist arthrodesis involved perineal care and manipulating the hand in tight spaces. The Jebsen hand function test demonstrated a 64% task completion rate compared to a 78% task completion rate for the normal wrist. The Buck-Gramcko/Lohmann evaluations demonstrated an average score of 8.3 out of a possible 10.

Moneim et al. also found that patients with fused wrists adapted their activities but still had some difficulties such as getting the hand into tight places, heavy lifting, and positioning the hand for some specific tasks (5). Patients who have undergone wrist arthrodesis can accomplish most activities of daily living and other functional requirements, although some adaptation to accomplish these tasks is required.

## Pain Relief

Sagerman and Palmer reviewed 17 patients who had undergone wrist arthrodesis (10). Fourteen patients had undergone previous procedures. Mean follow-up was 48 months. All but one patient reported considerable pain relief and were satisfied with the results of the procedure. Moneim et al. reported wrist arthrodesis to provide satisfactory results in the 24 patients they reviewed following the procedure (5). Bolano and Green reported that failure to fuse the index and long finger carpometacarpal joints might result in residual pain, requiring a second procedure (1). They recommended that index and long finger carpometacarpal joint arthrodesis be performed at the time of wrist arthrodesis for patients with heavy labor jobs. The author routinely fuses these joints when performing wrist arthrodesis. O'Bierne et al. reported satisfactory clinical outcome in 26 of 32 wrists following arthrodesis (6). Complete pain relief cannot be achieved in all cases following wrist arthrodesis for patients who have undergone multiple prior surgical procedures, although significant improvement usually is achieved.

### Return to Work

Most patients can return to work following wrist arthrodesis, although often some modification to their work is required. Patients with wrist arthrodesis often have to avoid impact-type activities such as hammering and forceful or repetitive use of their hand against resistance. Activities requiring a full range of wrist motion are not possible as well, although the vast majority of the normal activities of daily living are performed with the wrist in some extension, which is the position recommended for arthrodesis.

## COMPLICATIONS

Complications are frequent following wrist arthrodesis, although most can be treated successfully. Hastings found that complications were less frequent when a plate was used to obtain arthrodesis (3).

### Flexor/Extensor Adhesions Requiring Tenolysis

Adhesions can be caused by excessively long screws within the carpal canal, requiring subsequent screw removal. Avoidance of this complication depends on careful depth measurement and a check that the screw chosen is the correct length. A custom wrist arthrodesis plate is desirable in this regard because the metacarpal screws do not project above the surface of the plate and the distal edge, and sides of the plate are contoured to present a smooth gliding surface. Tendon adherence also can develop if patients do not move their digits early in the postoperative period due to digital edema and/or poor motivation. All patients require close supervision and firm guidance in the immediate postoperative period so that hand stiffness does not develop.

### Subsequent Arthritis of Adjacent Joint

There has been no consensus within the literature as to which joints to include when performing wrist arthrodesis. When the carpometacarpal joints of the index and long finger metacarpals are not included in the arthrodesis and removal of the plate is required later, these joints can become symptomatic. Subsequent related arthritis of adjacent previously normal joints has not been seen post-arthrodesis, but can occur if initially abnormal and not included in the arthrodesis. I recommend that the ulnar midcarpal joint not be included in the former wrist arthrodesis if normal preoperatively. If clinically or radiographically abnormal, the arthrodesis should include the ulnar midcarpal joint.

### Persistent Unexplained Pain Postunion

Wrist arthrodesis is extremely predictable in providing pain relief. Patients who have undergone multiple prior surgical procedures occasionally have persistent pain post-arthrodesis for unexplained reasons despite inclusion of all symptomatic joints and proper arthrodesis. Zachary and Stern found that 8 of the 73 wrist arthrodeses they reviewed had chronic, unexplained pain (14). If this is seen, selective wrist nerve block may be indicated. Buck-Gramcko has described a wrist denervation procedure for recalcitrant pain (2).

## Iliac Crest Fracture

Fracture of the anterior superior iliac spine can occur after harvesting a large corticocancellous graft. Hernia formation has been reported if the iliac wing fragment does not unite and is excised. Iliac crest bone graft should be harvested posterior to the anterior superior iliac spine and from the inner aspect of the iliac crest. Complications related to the harvest of iliac crest bone graft can be avoided by the use of a sliding bone graft obtained from the dorsal aspect of the distal radius.

## Reflex Sympathetic Dystrophy

Any upper extremity reconstructive procedure carries a very slight risk for development of reflex sympathetic dystrophy. Arthrodesis with a plate avoids cast immobilization and provides for stability that contributes to comfort. Early finger and thumb motion postoperatively is encouraged. The dorsal incision is protective of the dorsal sensory branches of the radial nerve.

## Plate Tenderness

The soft tissue over the distal plates is often tender following wrist arthrodesis. Plate removal due to chronic tenderness may be required. It is believed that the new wrist arthrodesis plate design will reduce the frequency of subsequent plate removal. The distal and lateral edges of the plate are thin in comparison to the body of the plate. The metacarpal screws are recessed flush with the dorsal plate surface.

## Carpal Tunnel Syndrome

Some patients may exhibit signs of carpal tunnel syndrome following wrist arthrodesis. The surgeon must be careful to rule out preoperative carpal tunnel symptoms that might go unrecognized and become symptomatic with swelling postoperatively. The overall three-dimensional architecture of the carpal canal should not be disturbed by wrist arthrodesis if the plate is adapted to the normal contour of the carpus and the surgeon avoids translation of the carpus as the fixation is applied.

## Wound Healing Problems

Wound healing problems can occur following wrist arthrodesis. Great care must be taken to prevent hematoma formation by the use of a suction drain in the initial postoperative period. Previous incisions may be incorporated partially in the incision if they do not lead to creation of extensive flap elevation. If a hematoma forms postoperatively, it should be drained surgically. Wound breakdown over the dorsum of the wrist is problematic due to the presence of the extensor tendons and the need to maintain their excursion.

## ILLUSTRATIVE CASE FOR TECHNIQUE

Mr. J. L. had sustained an occupational injury in 1986. He had undergone a left wrist arthrodesis in 1993. He complained of some ongoing dorsal discomfort and prominence of the plate used to fuse the left wrist. The plate was removed, after which painful motion was noted at the base of the long finger metacarpal. This problem was treated successfully by arthrodesis of the carpometacarpal joint of the long finger using a dorsal seven-hole one-third tubular plate (Fig. 23).

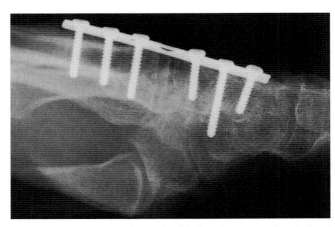

**FIGURE 23.** Lateral radiograph of left wrist post-arthrodesis of the carpometacarpal joint of the long finger using dorsal seven-hole plate.

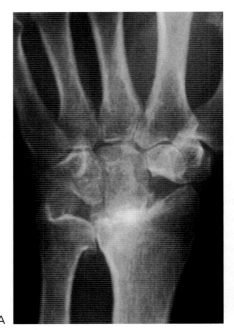

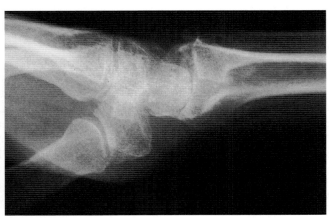

A                                                                                                                                 B

**FIGURE 24.** Anteroposterior **(A)** and lateral **(B)** radiographs post-proximal row carpectomy. Degenerative change has developed between the proximal pole of the capitate and the radius. The patient has ongoing symptoms of wrist pain related to activity.

In April 1995, the right wrist became symptomatic with diffuse dorsal wrist pain aggravated by activity.

On examination, the left wrist was fused. On the right side, dorsiflexion was 80°; volar flexion, 40°; ulnar deviation, 30°; radial deviation, 10°; pronation, 80°; and supination, 80°. Grip was 6 kg on the right side and 24 kg on the left side.

Radiographs of the right wrist demonstrated advanced radiocarpal osteoarthritis, particularly between the scaphoid and the radius. The pros and cons of a proximal row carpectomy were discussed with Mr. J. L. It was felt that with or without surgical treatment, Mr. J. L. was disabled for his regular occupation as a mechanic.

Mr. J. L. was admitted to the hospital in July of 1995 and underwent a proximal row carpectomy. The redundant dorsal capsule was interposed and sutured to the

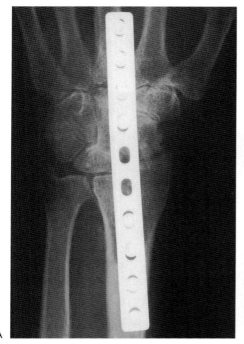

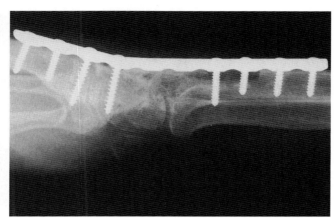

A                                                                                             B

**FIGURE 25.** Anteroposterior **(A)** and lateral **(B)** radiographs post-arthrodesis of the right wrist with a dorsal ten-hole low contact dynamic compression plate and a sliding bone graft harvested from the distal radius. The plate is contoured into the desired amount of dorsiflexion. The bone graft is slid into a slot created at the base of the index and long finger metacarpals. The distal radial articular surface has been resected. The plate extends proximal to the donor site of the bone graft by two screw holes in order to bridge the area of stress concentration created by harvest of the bone.

volar capsule, and the dorsal radiocarpal ligaments were repaired with interrupted sutures.

Postoperatively, Mr. J. L. underwent a program of rehabilitation and noted a short period of relief from pain. Radiographs showed progressive narrowing of the joint space between the capitate and the radius (Fig. 24). His ongoing symptoms led him to consider further surgical treatment in the form of a wrist arthrodesis. He was readmitted to the hospital in April of 1998. A wrist arthrodesis was performed using a dorsal sliding radial bone graft and a ten-hole 3.5 dynamic compression plate (Fig. 25). Postoperatively, he was kept in a cast for 6 weeks, followed by an ongoing course of physiotherapy.

When most recently seen, Mr. J. L. had recovered a grip strength of 20 kg on the left side and 24 kg on the right side. He had reasonably good pain relief and was able to use both hands for most of the normal activities of daily living. Radiographs showed solid arthrodesis (Fig. 26).

This case is illustrative for the following reasons:

- It demonstrates the importance of including the carpal metacarpal joints of the index and long fingers in the wrist arthrodesis as well as the need for revision surgery if painful mobility persists at the carpal metacarpal joints.
- It demonstrates the role of wrist arthrodesis if motion-preserving reconstructive procedures are not successful in relieving pain.
- It demonstrates the role of the sliding dorsal radial bone graft in performing wrist arthrodesis.
- It demonstrates the potential for wrist arthrodesis as a form of definitive treatment for bilateral wrist pathology.

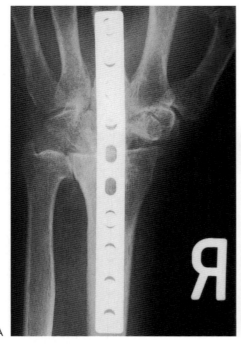
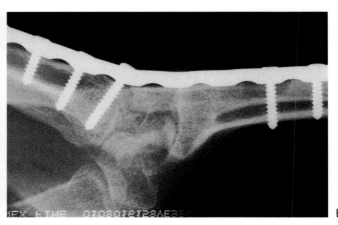

**FIGURE 26.** Anteroposterior **(A)** and lateral **(B)** radiographs taken 1 year after arthrodesis. The bone graft has now solidly incorporated, and the wrist is fused. The patient has good pain relief.

## ACKNOWLEDGMENT

In the first edition, this chapter was written by Hill Hastings, M. D., Indiana University Medical Center, Indianapolis, Indiana. I have used much of Dr. Hasting's material for this edition, and I acknowledge his significant contribution in this regard.

## RECOMMENDED READING

1. Bolano, L. E., Green, D. P.: Wrist arthrodesis in posttraumatic arthritis: a comparison of two methods. *J. Hand Surg.*, 18: 786, 1993.
2. Buck-Gramcko, D.: Denervation of the wrist joint. *J. Hand Surg.*, 2: 54–61, 1977.
3. Hastings, H., Weiss, A. P., Quenzer, D., Wiedeman, G. P., Hanington, K. R., Strickland, J. W.: Arthrodesis of the wrist for post-traumatic disorders. *J. Bone Joint Surg.*, 78: 897, 1996.
4. Lorei, M. P., Figgie, M. P., Ranawat, C. S., Inglis, A. E.: Failed total wrist arthroplasty. Analysis of failures and results of operative management. *Clin. Orthop.*, 342: 84, 1997.
5. Moneim, M. S., Pribyl, C. R., Garst, J. R.: Wrist arthrodesis. Technique and functional evaluation. *Clin. Orthop.*, 341: 23, 1997.
6. O'Bierne, J., Boyer, M. I., Axelrod, T. S.: Wrist arthrodesis using a dynamic compression plate. *J. Bone Joint Surg. [Br.]*, 77: 700, 1995.
7. Ono, H., Yajima, H., Mizumoto, S., Miyauchi, Y., Mii, Y., Tamai, S.: Vascularized fibular graft for reconstruction of the wrist after excision of giant cell tumor. *Plast. Reconstr. Surg.*, 99: 1086, 1997.
8. Phalen, G. S.: The carpal tunnel syndrome: seventeen year's experience in diagnosis and treatment of 654 hands. *J. Bone Joint Surg.*, 48A: 211–228, 1966.
9. Richards, R. R., Patterson, S. D., Hearn, T. C.: A special plate for arthrodesis of the wrist: design considerations and biomechanical testing. *J. Hand Surg.*, 18: 476, 1993.
10. Sagerman, S. D., Palmer, A. K.: Wrist arthrodesis using a dynamic compression plate. *J. Hand Surg. [Br.]*, 21: 437, 1996.
11. Sorial, R., Tonkin, M. A., Gschwind, C.: Wrist arthrodesis using a sliding radial graft and plate fixation. *J. Hand Surg. [Br.]*, 19: 217, 1994.
12. Tomaino, M. M., Miller, R. J., Cole, I., Burton, R. I.: Scapholunate advanced collapse wrist: proximal row carpectomy or limited wrist arthrodesis with scaphoid excision? *J. Hand Surg.*, 19: 134, 1994.
13. Weiss, A. C., Wiedeman, G. Jr., Quenzer, D., Hanington, K. R., Hastings, H., Strickland: Upper extremity function following wrist arthrodesis. *J. Hand Surg.*, 20: 813, 1995.
14. Zachary, S. V., Stern, P. J.: Complications following AO/ASIF wrist arthrodesis. *J. Hand Surg.*, 20: 339, 1995.

# PART IX

# Distal Radioulnar Joint Instability

# 21

# Operative Reconstruction of the Distal Radioulnar Joint

Ronald L. Linscheid

## INDICATIONS/CONTRAINDICATIONS

Instability of the distal radioulnar joint (DRUJ) may cause pain, weakness, snapping, and loss of forearm rotation. Instability is usually the result of a sprain or dislocation, or a healed malalignment of one of the forearm bones. It also may be noted in patients with synovitis of the DRUJ or in patients with ligamentous laxity. A few patients also seem to have excessive curvature of the distal ulna as a congenital or developmental finding. This abnormality may cause the instability, although it is more accurate to consider this as a palmar radiocarpal subluxation.

Normal forearm rotation is dependent on smooth synergistic rotation of the radius about the ulna, depending on the maintenance of the normal complex curvature of the radius and ulna as well as the integrity of the proximal and distal radioulnar joint articulations (4,5). The static stability of the DRUJ is provided by the shallow concavity of the sigmoid notch, the dorsal and palmar radioulnar ligaments that are components of the triangular fibrocartilage (TFC), the interosseous membrane, and the dorsal retinaculum. Dynamic stability is provided by the pronator quadratus, extensor carpi ulnaris, and flexor carpi ulnaris. There is also a close interrelation of the carpus with the radioulnar joint. The carpus is tethered to the radius by the dorsal and palmar radiocarpal ligaments, and therefore rotates with the radius around the ulnar head during pronosupination.

The position of the ulnar head relative to the sigmoid notch moves from the palmar to the dorsal rim as one moves from supination to pronation (Fig. 1). At the same time, the ulna also translates from proximal to distal. Although this latter movement is only a millimeter in distance, the combined displacement aligns the ulnar head dorsal to the proximal lunotriquetral surface in full pronation (2). Approximately 10% of the joint compressive force is transmitted to the ulnar head through the TFC. A sprain or dislocation of the ulnar head dorsally usually occurs when the forearm is pronated. Increasing pronation, wrist extension, and radial

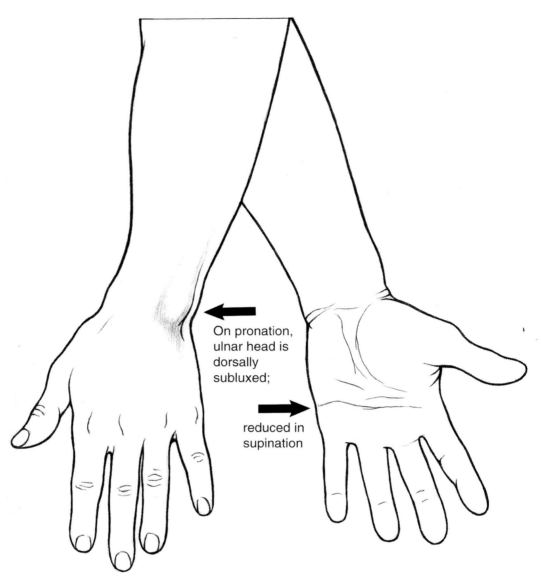

On pronation, ulnar head is dorsally subluxed;

reduced in supination

**FIGURE 1.** Dorsoulnar subluxation and ulnocarpal dissociation are recognized most often on pronation of the forearm if the ulnar head is normal and more prominent in pronation.

deviation increase the tension in the dorsal radioulnar, the ulnotriquetral, and the ulnar collateral ligaments, forcing the ulnar head dorsally out of the sigmoid notch and attenuating the above restraints. In full pronation, the ulnar head is then acted on by an oblique force that tends to displace it proximodorsally. Dynamic ulnar translation of the carpus augments this mechanism.

It is common for the radiocarpal complex to develop a supination deformity as the DRUJ develops dorsal instability (1). There is usually a common pathomechanical etiology. Dorsal instability of the DRUJ of this nature is the most common instability pattern. From a traumatic standpoint, it usually is induced by an energetic extension pronation loading of the wrist, such as that which occurs in a fall.

The purpose of the reconstructive technique described in this chapter is to correct both dorsal displacement of the ulnar head on the radius and supinated angulation of the carpus on the radius in cases of chronic dorsal instability. The primary indications are weakness, pain, snapping, and loss of rotation.

Contraindications include acute dorsal DRUJ instability, malalignment of either of the forearm bones, advanced degenerative changes in the DRUJ, ulnar-plus variance with evidence of ulnocarpal impingement (3), rheumatoid disease, and Ehlers-Danlos-like laxity. A relative contraindication is obvious disruption of the TFC or the base of the ulnar styloid, as this may be amenable to direct repair without augmentation.

Acute subluxations usually respond to reduction in supination and 6 weeks' immobilization in a long-arm cast. Osseous deformities require osteotomies, realignment, length adjustment, and internal fixation. Rheumatoid deformity often can be improved by radiolunate arthrodesis, whereas ulnar head resection may accelerate instability. Collagen deficiency problems are unlikely to respond to augmentation procedures.

## PREOPERATIVE PLANNING

Examination confirms prominence of the ulnar head as compared with the opposite wrist, particularly while the forearm is pronated (Fig. 2A, B). There

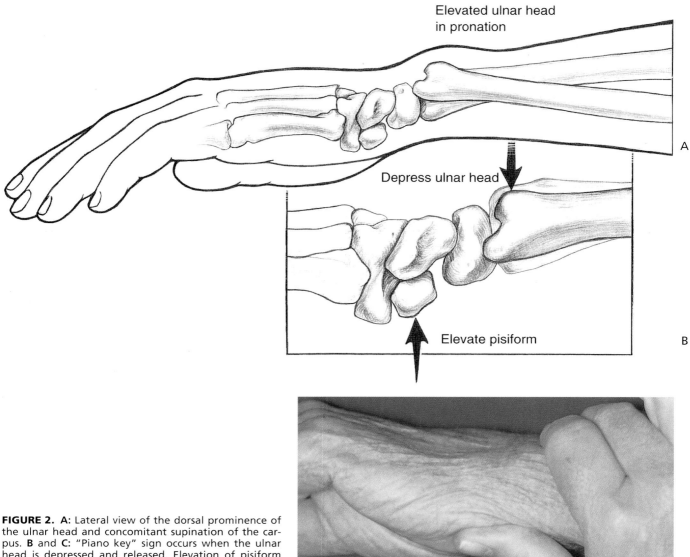

**FIGURE 2. A:** Lateral view of the dorsal prominence of the ulnar head and concomitant supination of the carpus. **B** and **C:** "Piano key" sign occurs when the ulnar head is depressed and released. Elevation of pisiform and ulnar head depression restores normal alignment.

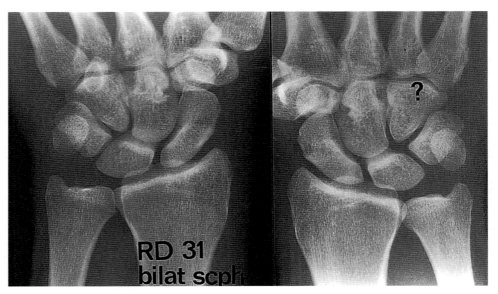

**FIGURE 3.** Standard radiographs are often nondiagnostic.

may be an obvious, painful jerk during rotation. A positive "piano key" test is noted if the ulnar head is depressed and released. An even more dramatic test is to depress the ulnar head with the thumb while elevating the pisiform with the fingers (Fig. 2C). A crepitant relocation with a sense of relief may be experienced by the patient.

Standard radiographs may not be helpful as the deformity is not readily obvious on anteroposterior films. Sagittal films are notoriously difficult to interpret for radioulnar deformity for two reasons: They are seldom truly lateral, thus often portraying apparently displaced superimposed silhouettes; and the radiograph usually is taken in neutral rather than pronation (Fig. 3). Cross-sectional computed tomography scans through the DRUJ are diagnostic, but carpal supination is not always appreciated (2). Surgery is indicated when the above conditions interfere with the ability to work or the enjoyment of normal activities.

## SURGERY

The patient is positioned supine on the operating table with the arm abducted on a hand table and a pneumatic tourniquet applied below the axilla after an axillary block or before induction of general anesthesia. A standard antiseptic preparation is followed with draping to just below the cuff. The joint is manipulated and surface anatomic features marked with a surgical pen.

### Technique

With the forearm pronated, a straight incision is made over the subcutaneous border of the forearm. The flexor carpi ulnaris is exposed from the pisiform well into the musculotendinous junction, as the tendon is relatively short. The tendon is split in a natural groove (Fig. 4). The ulnar half is cut proximally, left attached distally to the pisiform, and wrapped in a saline-soaked sponge. The pisotriquetral capsule is perforated proximally for later introduction of the tendon end.

The incision is curved dorsally over the distal hamate. The dorsoulnar sensory nerve is exposed and protected. The dorsal retinaculum is split over the extensor

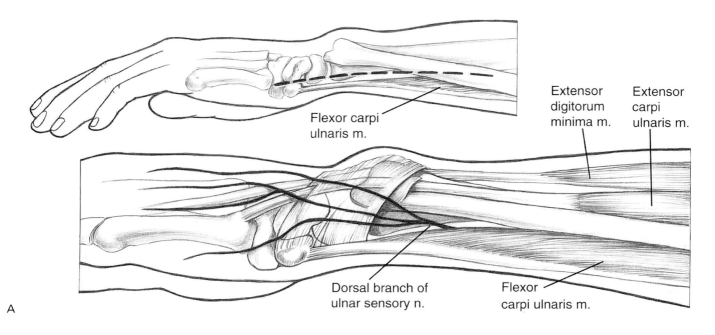

Flexor carpi
ulnaris m.

Extensor
digitorum
minima m.

Extensor
carpi
ulnaris m.

Dorsal branch of
ulnar sensory n.

Flexor
carpi ulnaris m.

A

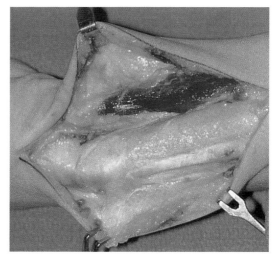

**FIGURE 4. A** and **B:** The surgical approach is made over the ulnar aspect of the wrist and forearm with the arm exsanguinated, and a pneumatic tourniquet is applied about the upper arm. The superficial dorsal sensory branches of the ulnar nerve are protected. The extensor retinaculum is split over the extensor carpi ulnaris and reflected in either direction. The deep component of the retinaculum, which holds the extensor carpi ulnaris in position in its groove in the ulnar neck, is retained.

B

digiti minimi (EDM) and the ulnar leaf reflected from over the deep ligament, forming the roof of the sixth dorsal compartment (Fig. 5).

The dorsal capsule of the DRUJ is opened longitudinally, taking care not to injure the dorsal radioulnar ligament. The capsule of the ulnotriquetral and triquetrohamate joint is opened so that the TFC may be inspected from either side. The triquetrohamate joint also may be exposed by incising the capsule distally. The TFC origins from the styloid process and fovea are inspected. If disrupted, secondary preparation for reattachment is made. At this point, a 2.0-mm bit in a power drill is used to drill obliquely from the ulnar neck into or adjacent to the fovea. When satisfied with the position, a 4.0-mm or 5.0-mm bit is used to enlarge the hole sufficiently to allow tendon passage (Fig. 6). A curved tendon passer is inserted dorsally ulnar to the triquetrum and pushed through the previous pisotriquetral capsular window. The tendon end is grasped and extracted dorsally (Fig. 7). Next, the tendon is brought through the TFC if a central defect exists or over the dorsal limb of the TFC if intact. The former technique helps to reestablish an insertion at the fovea if TFC integrity is compromised and the latter exerts a depression effect on the ulna when the TFC is intact.

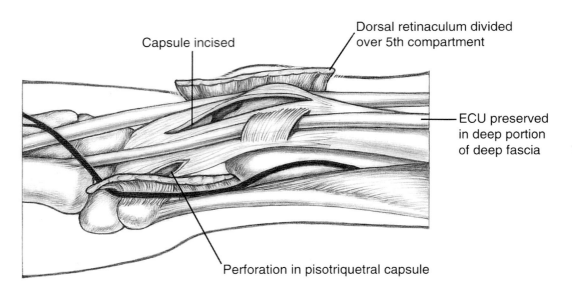

Capsule incised

Dorsal retinaculum divided
over 5th compartment

ECU preserved
in deep portion
of deep fascia

Perforation in pisotriquetral capsule

**FIGURE 5.** The dorsal capsule of the distal radioulnar joint is incised. This incision is continued longitudinally into the lunotriquetral capsule, which is freed up so that it may be imbricated during closure. A perforation is made in the pisotriquetral capsule for passage of one-half the flexor carpi ulnaris. ECU, extensor carpi ulnaris.

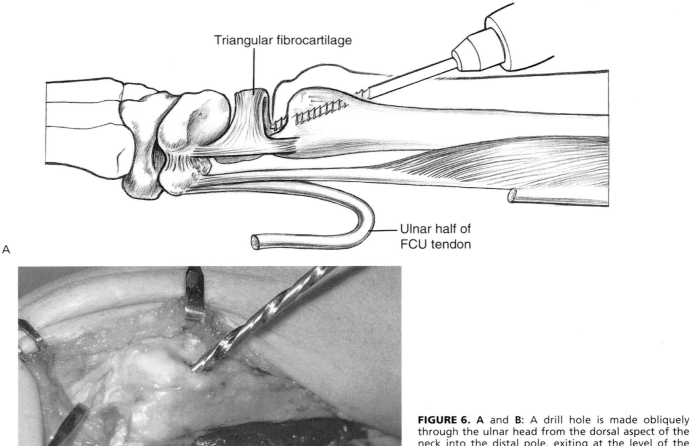

Triangular fibrocartilage

Ulnar half of
FCU tendon

A

B

**FIGURE 6. A** and **B:** A drill hole is made obliquely through the ulnar head from the dorsal aspect of the neck into the distal pole, exiting at the level of the fovea. The medial aspect of the flexor carpi ulnaris (FCU) has been freed at the level of the musculotendinous junction and stripped distally to the pisiform.

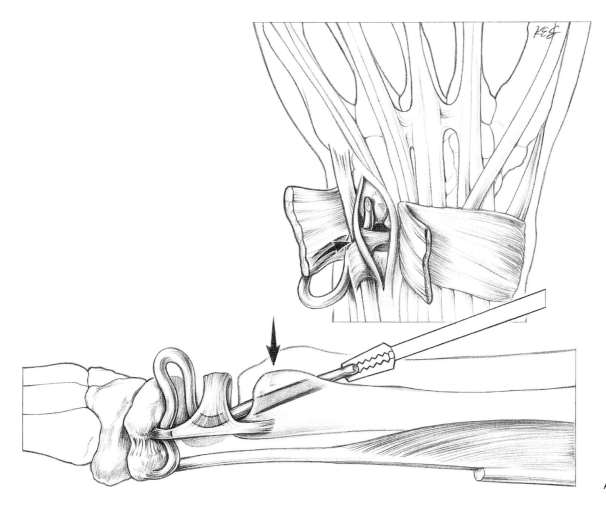

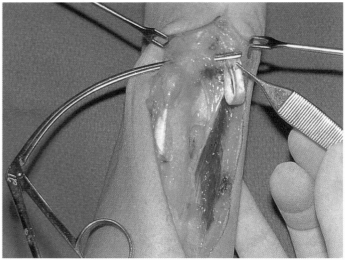

**FIGURE 7. A:** The flexor carpi ulnaris is brought into the ulno-carpal joint through a small defect in the proximal aspect of the pisotriquetral joint. A tendon passer is then inserted through the ulnar head, through the triangular fibrocartilage or dorsal to it, and used to extract the tendon. **B:** An anteroposterior view during extraction of the flexor carpi ulnaris into the ulno-triquetral joint.

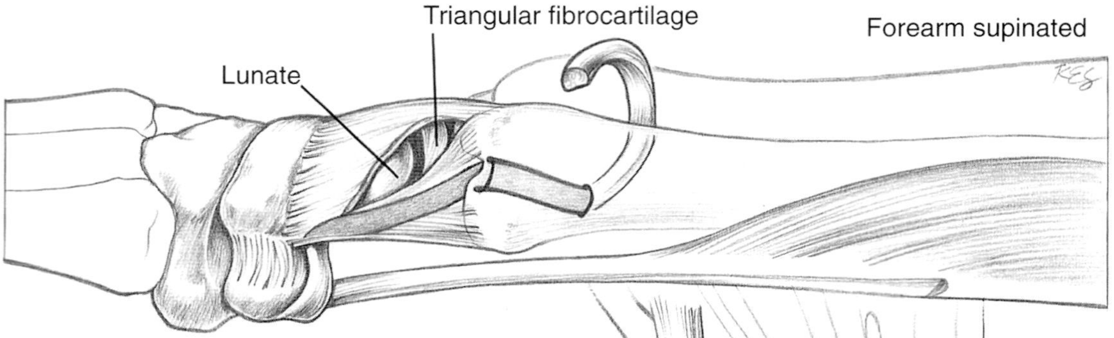

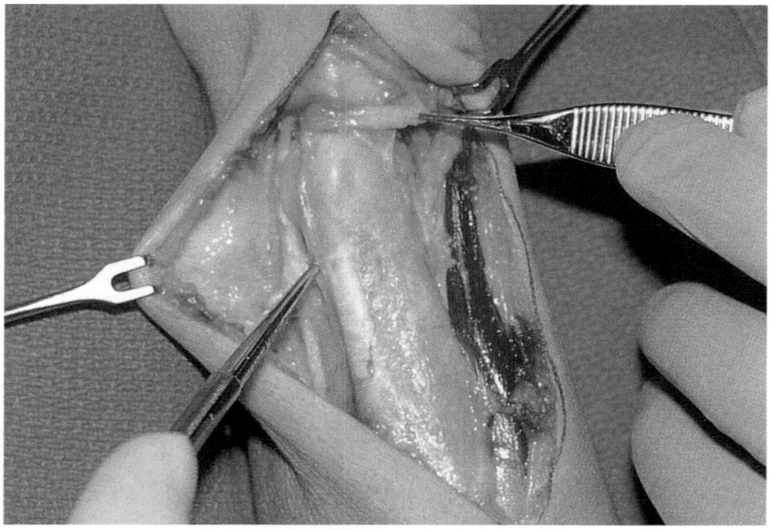

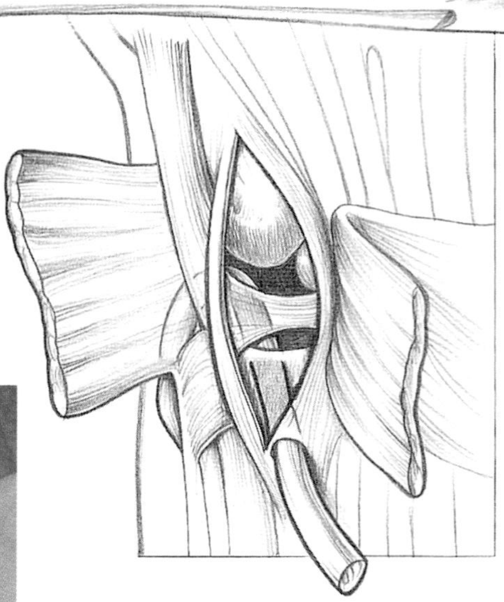

**FIGURE 8. A** and **B:** The forearm is turned into supination, which helps to reduce the dorsal subluxation. A 0.062-in. K-wire may be drilled from the ulna into the radius at this point to hold the reduced position, or an oblique wire may be drilled through the ulna into the triquetrum distally to maintain reduction of the ulnocarpal aspect of the subluxation. The tendon is pulled taut and sutured to the periosteum or fascia at the ulnar neck with several nonabsorbable sutures. **C:** Anteroposterior view. The tendon is extracted proximally from the hole in the ulnar neck.

The tendon is grasped with a straight tendon passer inserted into the drill hole in the ulnar head and extracted proximally at the ulnar neck, where it is pulled taut while the carpus is elevated by support under the pisiform. The tendon is snugly sutured with nonabsorbable 3–0 suture to the bone, periosteum, or capsule. The free end is reversed and sutured distally. The forearm is supinated and a K-wire drilled through the ulna and into the radius to hold the reduced position (Fig. 8).

The dorsal capsular incisions over both the carpus and DRUJ are imbricated closed to assist in constraining the carpal supination (Figs. 9, 10). The dorsal retinaculum then is overlapped and closed (Fig. 11). Skin incisions are closed with subcuticular absorbable sutures and a plaster-reinforced long-arm compressive dressing is applied.

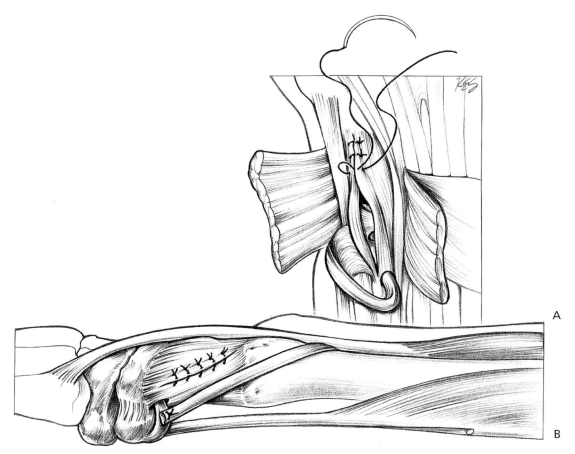

**FIGURE 9. A:** The tendon is pulled taut, sutured first proximally and then distally. Imbrication of the dorsal capsule is begun. **B:** The ulnocarpal capsule is imbricated tight in the repair. The flexor carpi ulnaris strip is pulled distally and sutured into its insertion on the pisiform.

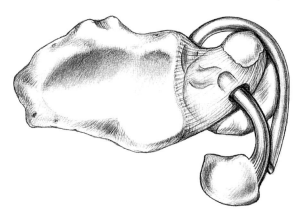

**FIGURE 10.** Schematic cross-sectional view of the path of the tendon strip. This helps to elevate the ulnar carpus and depress the ulnar head.

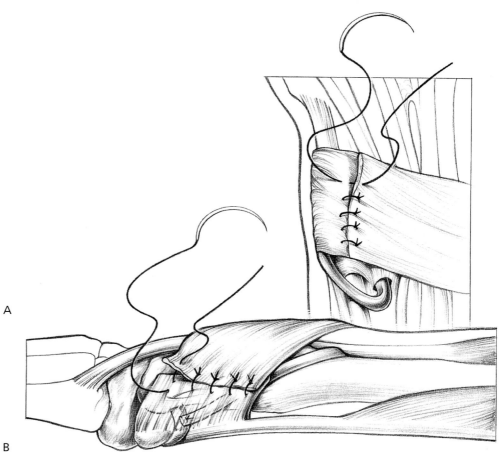

**FIGURE 11. A:** Anteroposterior view showing repair of the dorsal retinaculum by imbrication in pants-over-vest fashion. **B:** The sagittal view is the same.

## POSTOPERATIVE MANAGEMENT

The initial dressings are removed after a few days, and if postoperative swelling is minimal, a long-arm cast is applied. This is left in place for 4 weeks and then removed, as is the K-wire. An orthoplast ulnar gutter splint is fabricated, and gentle motions are encouraged several times a day out of the splint. Pronation usually is limited at this point but improves slowly over the next 6 weeks. Active assisted rotation exercises are undertaken with the aid of a hand therapist. The use of a long-handled broom or staff gripped firmly is helpful in increasing the torque during rotatory exercises, which are carried out with the elbows locked against the sides. The handle is extended slowly above the hand to increase the rotatory torque the handle imparts as it swings downward. It is occasionally necessary to apply a dynamic pronation splint if progress is slow. This is worn for 2- to 3-hour intervals as tolerated between exercises. Maximum improvement is expected to occur in 3 months.

## COMPLICATIONS

Complications include recurrence of dorsal instability, loss of pronation, and progressive degenerative changes. Recurrent instability may be due to inadequate initial reduction or stretching of the repair over time. Instability produces a shear stress on the articular cartilage of the ulnar head as it subluxes over the dorsal rim of the sigmoid notch. The protracted erosions produce increasing degenerative arthritis. Failure to regain pronation is due most likely to capsular contracture or to articular irregularity.

## ILLUSTRATIVE CASE FOR TECHNIQUE

A 29-year-old gymnastics teacher injured her left wrist in a fall 1 year previously. She had weakness and pain, particularly while twisting her wrist, and supination was limited to 20°. The ulnar head was dorsally prominent, and the piano key sign was positive. The carpus was supinated on the forearm. Reduction could be obtained by depressing the ulnar head and elevating the pisiform simultaneously. The patient was offered a ligamentous augmentation.

The procedure described in the sections Surgery and Technique was performed. Cast immobilization was discontinued at 6 weeks and pronosupinatory exercises were begun. Initially pronation was limited to 10° and wrist motion was limited to 50% of the opposite arm. Motion and strength were regained slowly. At 1 year pronation was 60°, supination was 70°, and wrist motion was slightly less than the contralateral side. Grip strength was 80% of the opposite hand. The previous pain, snapping, and ulnar head subluxation were no longer troublesome.

## RECOMMENDED READING

1. Bowers, W. H.: The distal radioulnar joint. In: *Operative Hand Surgery*, vol 2, edited by D. P. Green, Churchill Livingstone, New York, pp. 939–989, 1988.
2. Darrow, J. C., Linscheid, R. L., Dobyns, J. H., Mann, J. M., Wood, M. B., Beckenbaugh, R. D.: Distal ulna recession for disorders of the distal radioulnar joint. *J. Hand Surg.*, 10A: 482–491, 1985.
3. Hui, F. C., Linscheid, R. L.: Ulnotriquetral augmentation tenodesis: a reconstructive procedure for dorsal subluxation of the distal radioulnar joint. *J. Hand Surg.*, 7: 230–236, 1982.
4. Linscheid, R. L.: Biomechanics of the distal radioulnar joint. *Clin. Orthop.*, 275: 46–55, 1992.
5. Mino, D. E., Palmer, A. K., Levinsohn, E. M.: The role of radiography and computerized tomography in the diagnosis of subluxation and dislocation of the distal radioulnar joint. *J. Hand Surg.*, 8: 23–31, 1983.

# 22

# Partial Excision of the Triangular Fibrocartilage Complex

Erich E. Hornbach and A. Lee Osterman

## INTRODUCTION/INDICATIONS

Tears of the triangular fibrocartilage complex (TFCC) are caused by a fall on an outstretched hand that results in a combination of extension, pronation, and axial loading to the wrist. The TFCC is a complex anatomic structure with multiple functions. It provides a surface for axial load bearing, and its peripheral ligaments play a key role in stability of the distal radial ulnar joint (DRUJ) and ulnar carpus. Its central portion is horizontal and avascular, and its thickness is variable (3,4,7). The peripheral portion of the triangular fibrocartilage (TFC) is highly vascular (4) and blends with the ulnocarpal ligaments. It has attachments to the radius, ulna, lunate, triquetrum, and other carpal bones. In 1989, Palmer developed a classification system of injuries to the TFCC (6) (Table 1). Acute traumatic injuries were defined as *class I injuries,* and degenerative injuries were defined as *class II injuries*. Treatment of class I injuries depends on many factors, but in general peripheral lesions with the capacity to heal are treated with repair, and central lesions with poor healing capacity are treated with débridement. Class II, degenerative lesions represent an ulnar impingement or impaction process. As noted by the classification, TFC wear deteriorates to an attritional tear, followed by increasing chondral changes on the lunate and distal ulna, eventually resulting in lunatotriquetral ligament perforation. Besides TFC débridement, surgical procedures used to treat class II lesions should address the mechanical overload by wafer resection or ulnar shortening osteotomy.

Primary indications for partial excision of the TFC are class IA or IIC TFCC perforations. The patient with a class IA tear often presents with a traumatic twisting or rotation injury to the wrist that results in ulnar-sided wrist pain. Swelling is present, but not dramatic, and the patient notes pain on forceful grasp and rota-

**TABLE 1. CLASSIFICATION OF TRIANGULAR FIBROCARTILAGE COMPLEX (TFCC) INJURIES**

Class I: Acute–traumatic injuries
  A. Central—just medial to the radial attachment, volar-dorsal orientation, unstable flap.
  B. Ulnar/medial—tear along the ulnar border of the TFCC at the base of the styloid or with fracture of the ulnar styloid. This portion of the TFCC is associated anatomically with the sheath of the extensor carpi ulnaris.
  C. Distal—detachment from the lunate or triquetrum with injury to the ulnolunate or ulnotriquetral ligaments. This may result in a supination deformity of the carpus on the ulna.
  D. Radial—avulsion of the TFCC from the sigmoid notch of the radius, linear in nature and oriented in a volar-dorsal nature.
Class II: Degenerative (ulnocarpal impaction syndrome)
  Chronic–degenerative injuries
  A. Degeneration of the horizontal portion of the TFCC without perforation
  B. Degeneration of the horizontal portion of the TFCC without perforation
      + Lunate and/or ulnar chondromalacia
  C. Full thickness perforation of the horizontal portion of the TFCC
      + Lunate and/or ulnar chondromalacia
  D. TFCC perforation
      + Lunate and/or ulnar chondromalacia
      + Lunotriquetral ligament perforation
  E. TFCC perforation
      + Lunate and/or ulnar chondromalacia
      + Lunotriquetral ligament perforation
      + Ulnocarpal arthritis

tion. In the subacute phase, audible crepitation may develop with forearm rotation; intermittent swelling may be present as well. Patients with degenerative lesions may have symptoms brought on by an acute traumatic episode, or may report a more insidious onset of pain and symptoms. Often a history of repetitive motion or previous wrist injury is present. Symptoms and findings are similar to class I tears.

Initially, wrists with suspected tears of the TFC that have normal radiographs and no evidence of DRUJ instability are treated with relative rest, with or without immobilization, nonsteroidal antiinflammatory agents, and therapy. With resolution of symptoms, patients are returned to their previous level of activity gradually. If this is ineffective after 3 to 4 months and the symptoms are sufficiently disabling, operative treatment is indicated.

## CONTRAINDICATIONS

Contraindications to arthroscopic treatment include uncontrolled medical problems, open wounds or concomitant infections, lymphedema, and previous open wrist surgery. Treatment of the central TFCC tear alone in an ulnar-positive patient may fail because it does not address the biomechanical cause of the tear.

## PREOPERATIVE ASSESSMENT

The diagnosis of a TFCC lesion is based primarily on the history and physical examination. Usually, patients report a twisting injury or traumatic event that leads to persistent ulnar-sided wrist pain. Complaints such as recurrent pain with activity, swelling, limitation of range of motion, and audible crepitation suggest TFC complex injury. A differential diagnosis of ulnar-sided wrist pain is listed in Table 2 (2). In addition to a comprehensive evaluation of the upper extremity, we routinely include the following findings and provocative tests when assessing

## TABLE 2. DIFFERENTIAL DIAGNOSIS OF ULNAR-SIDED WRIST PAIN

Extensor carpi ulnaris subluxation
Lunotriquetral interosseous ligament injury
Chondral lesions of the ulnar lunate or midcarpal joint
Triquetral avulsion fracture
Pisotriquetral arthrosis
Ulnar artery thrombosis
Dorsoulnar sensory nerve neuritis
Ulnar neuropathy at Guyon's canal
Triangular fibrocartilage complex injury

ulnar-sided wrist pain: (a) point of maximal tenderness; (b) TFCC grind, performed by deviating the wrist ulnarly and applying axial load and rotation (a positive test being painful clicking that reproduces the patient's symptoms); (c) shuck and lunotriquetral (LT) ballottement for LT injury; and (d) shear test for pisotriquetral arthrosis. Tests are done to confirm DRUJ (tested in supination) and extensor carpi ulnaris (ECU) stability as well. Grip strength and forearm circumference are recorded.

Plain radiographs should include a zero-rotation posteroanterior view to determine ulnar variance (Fig. 1). Also included is a clenched fist, ulnar deviation view to rule out dynamic ulnar impingement. Like arthrography, magnetic resonance imaging (MRI) is accurate for radial and central TFC tears (Fig. 2), particularly if a dedicated wrist coil is used. It provides no information on the size, configuration, or reactive joint synovitis, and poor information on the LT ligament. Unlike arthrography, MRI is noninvasive, and can offer information on ulnar impaction such as marrow changes in the lunate, ulnar head, or triquetrum (Fig. 3). Wrist arthrography, while accurate for radial and central TFC perforations, is rarely used at this time because it provides no information on the size of the tear or the joint reaction to the tear (synovitis). A midcarpal arthrogram may be considered if LT ligament integrity is a concern. MRI remains our choice for advanced imaging in the workup of suspected TFCC disorders.

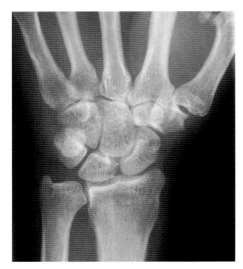

**FIGURE 1.** Zero-rotation posteroanterior view.

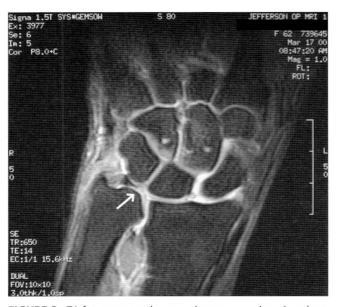

**FIGURE 2.** T1 fat-suppressed magnetic resonance imaging demonstrating central triangular fibrocartilage tear (*arrow*).

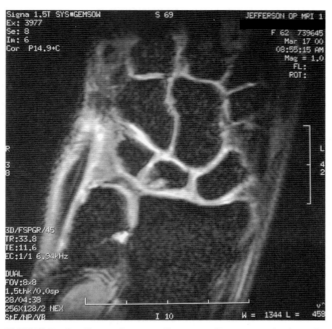

**FIGURE 3.** Gradient echo revealing a small amount of edema in the dorsal lunate.

## TABLE 3. RADIOCARPAL ARTICULATION

Articular surfaces
  Radius
    Scaphoid facet
    Lunate facet
  Lunate
Extrinsic ligaments
  Radioscaphocapitate
  Long radiolunate
  Radioscapholunate
Intrinsic ligaments
  Scapholunate interosseous ligament

## TABLE 4.  ULNOCARPAL ARTICULATION

Articular surfaces
  Lunate
  Triquetrum
  Ulnar head (if visible through perforation)
Extrinsic ligaments
  Ulnolunate
  Ulnotriquetral
Intrinsic ligament
  Lunatotriquetral ligament
Triangular fibrocartilage complex (TFCC)
  Radial attachment
  Peripheral attachments
  Tension

## OPERATIVE MANAGEMENT

Operative management can be performed openly or arthroscopically. Presently, we perform a diagnostic and therapeutic arthroscopy of the wrist for treatment of the TFCC and associated pathology. Open treatment of these lesions may be performed, and is easily combined with a shortening osteotomy or wafer procedure. A list of anatomic structures evaluated is presented in Tables 3 and 4. We generally evaluate all these structures in sequence, prior to treatment of the TFCC lesion. Photographic documentation of the diagnostic arthroscopy is an integral part of the procedure. We routinely document the pathology with arthroscopic photographs and videotape.

## TECHNIQUE

The procedure is performed under general or axillary block anesthesia. Wrist arthroscopy requires distraction, which can be obtained by the use of a vertical

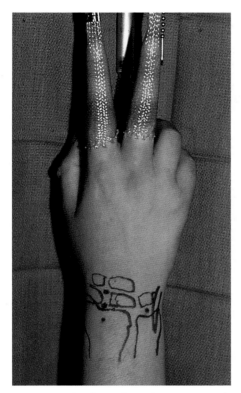

**FIGURE 4.** Outline of pertinent anatomic structures and preliminary portal sites before arthroscopy.

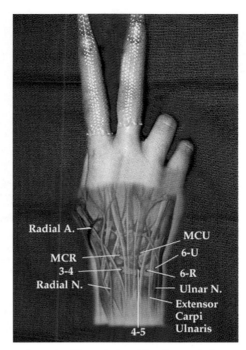

**FIGURE 5.** The relationship of portal site to underlying anatomic structures. MCR, midcarpal radial; MCU, midcarpal ulnar.

distraction arthroscopy tower (preferred) or by horizontal traction over the hand table. A tourniquet is applied in all cases, but not inflated unless the arthroscopic field is obscured by bleeding. The arm is prepped and draped. The patient's fingers are placed in the finger traps. When using the arthroscopy tower, a towel is placed between tower and elbow, as well as the tower and volar forearm. This helps protect the olecranon and ulnar nerve. Velcro straps are used to secure the arm and forearm to the arthroscopy tower. Next, the wrist is flexed 15° to 20° and distraction is applied to 15 pounds, anatomic landmarks are drawn, and preliminary portal sites are identified. Because of the change in surface anatomy with the distraction of the joint, it is important to have the traction applied prior to drawing any landmarks (Figs. 4, 5).

The landmarks used include the following: Lister's tubercle, the ECU, extensor pollicis longus, common extensors, and extensor digiti quinti. The 3–4 portal is marked 1 cm distal to Lister's tubercle. The midcarpal radial portal is marked 1 cm distal to the 3–4 portal in line with the radial border of the long finger metacarpal. The ECU tendon is identified, and the 6R portal (which is the portal primarily used) is marked in the soft spot just distal to the ulnar head at the level of the ulnar styloid. The 6U portal may be marked, but is rarely used. Landmarks are reassessed, and an 18-gauge needle is introduced into the 3–4 portal along the slope of the articular surface of the radius. With the needle in the radiocarpal joint, 10 to 15 cc of saline is injected. The pattern of distension is noted, and filling of the midcarpal joint is assessed. An 11-blade scalpel is then used to longitudinally incise the skin only. Using a hemostat, blunt dissection down to the level of the capsule is performed. Next, a blunt trochar is introduced into the radiocarpal joint along the slope of the articular surface. Firm pressure with a gentle twisting motion is used to penetrate the capsule. Any difficulty with insertion of the trochar should prompt immediate reevaluation of the anatomic placement of the

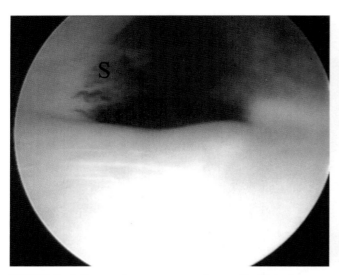

**FIGURE 6.** Arthroscopic appearance of synovitis (S) in the prestyloid recess.

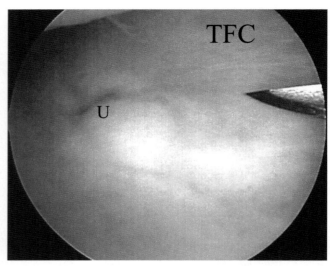

**FIGURE 7.** Visualization of a class IIC triangular fibrocartilage (TFC) tear through the 3–4 portal in a right wrist. Note 18-gauge needle distal to the triangular fibrocartilage serving as an outflow portal. U, ulnar head.

portal. Excessive force or difficulty with joint entry that causes plunging into the radiocarpal joint can result in devastating injuries to the articular surfaces or scapholunate interosseous ligament.

A 2.9-mm small joint arthroscope is used in most instances, with the inflow system attached to an arthroscopy pump. After the 3–4 portal is established, the arthroscope is directed ulnarly, and the dorsoulnar portion of the TFCC and capsule are visualized. After palpation over the previously marked 6R portal, adjustments in the placement of the outflow portal are performed as needed. Carefully, a preliminary outflow portal is made by introducing an 18-gauge needle into the ulnocarpal joint distal to the TFC. After the joint has been lavaged and a preliminary assessment has been performed, a probe is introduced through the 6R portal. Preliminary débridement of synovitis or redundant capsular tissue improves visualization and is performed as needed.

The radial side of the wrist is evaluated first. Table 3 lists the structures to evaluate. Assessment of the articular surfaces, as well as intrinsic and extrinsic ligaments, is completed and documented. Moving to the ulnar side of the wrist, a detailed evaluation of the ulnocarpal articulation and TFCC is performed. The presence of any synovitis should also be documented (Fig. 6). Next, the ulnar extrinsic ligaments should be palpated, using a probe to evaluate their integrity. The assessment of the TFC begins with an evaluation of its general appearance (Fig. 7). The ulnar side of the lunate should be assessed for any chondromalacia, suggestive of an ulnocarpal impaction syndrome (Fig. 8). If there is no obvious tear of the TFC, it is palpated with the probe to check for tension. Any loss of tension is suggestive of a significant peripheral tear. When assessing a central or chronic tear, the tear will have unstable flaps. Manipulation of the torn portion of the TFC can be done with the probe (Figs. 9, 10). When the anatomy of the tear has been defined, the unstable portion of the tear is débrided back to a stable rim. To complete the radiocarpal evaluation, the arthroscope should be placed in the 6R portal to evaluate the LT interosseous ligament. Injecting fluid or air into the midcarpal joint further defines the presence of any abnormal midcarpal to radiocarpal communication.

Many arthroscopic instruments, including small joint Shutts, banana blade, full-radius oscillating shaver, radiofrequency ablation probes, suction punch, and laser, exist to assist with débridement of the TFC. We routinely use the suction punch and a 2.0- to 3.0-mm arthroscopic shaver to remove the unstable portions

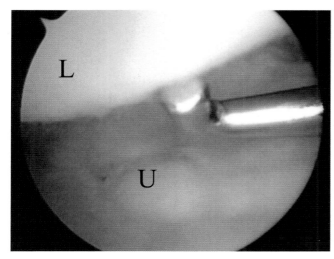

**FIGURE 8.** Probe on the lunate (L) demonstrating early chondromalacia. U, ulnar head.

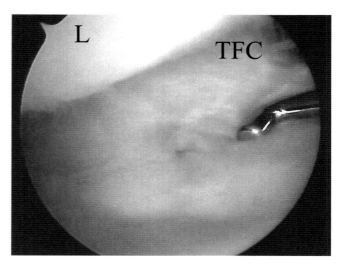

**FIGURE 9.** Chronic, degenerative central triangular fibrocartilage (TFC) tear with ulnar head visible through the tear. Note chondromalacia on ulnar head. L, lunate.

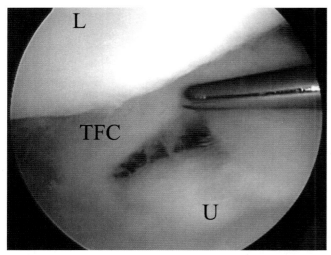

**FIGURE 10.** The same tear with the triangular fibrocartilage (TFC) lifted using the probe, further exposing the ulnar head (U). L, lunate.

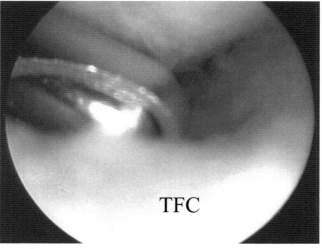

**FIGURE 11.** Full radius shaver in the 3–4 portal débriding the dorsal border of the central triangular fibrocartilage (TFC) tear.

of the TFC (Fig. 11). Our working portal for a majority of the débridement is the 6R portal (Fig. 12). The 4–5 portal is used on occasion. Use of any of the above instruments through the 6R portal allows access to the volar, central, and radial aspects of the TFC. Switching the arthroscope to the 6R portal and bringing the instrument through the 3–4 portal allows access to the dorsal and ulnar margins of the TFC. The resection of the TFC should be limited to the loose or damaged parts within the central region. To prevent significant biomechanical changes resulting in instability, the resection should always be less than two-thirds of the disk, and should preserve the peripheral 2 mm of the disk (1,8). After the resection of all loose tissue has been completed, we routinely use the arthroscopic shaver or radiofrequency ablation probe to contour and smooth the remainder of the central TFC (Figs. 13–15). Arthroscopic evaluation of the midcarpal joint is performed on a routine basis using both midcarpal radial and midcarpal ulnar portals. This allows for a further assessment of LT interface congruity and helps rule out any hamate chondral lesion.

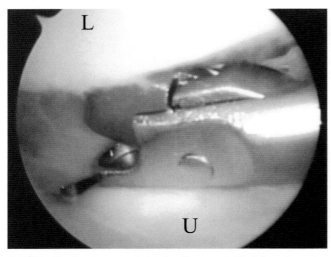

**FIGURE 12.** Suction punch in the 6R portal débriding the volar border of the triangular fibrocartilage back to a stable rim. L, lunate; U, ulnar head.

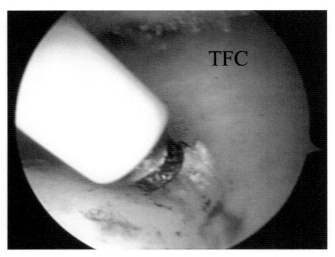

**FIGURE 13.** Radiofrequency ablation probe in the 3–4 portal contouring the triangular fibrocartilage (TFC).

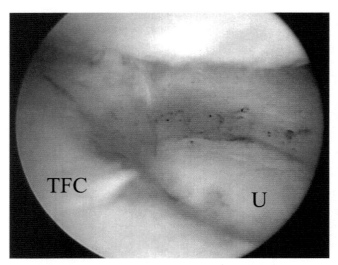

**FIGURE 14.** Appearance of triangular fibrocartilage (TFC) after débridement with arthroscope in the 3–4 portal. U, ulnar head.

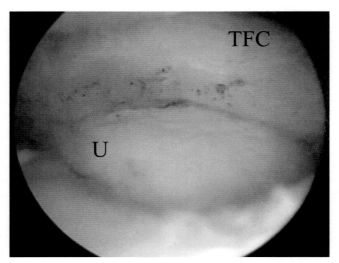

**FIGURE 15.** Appearance of the triangular fibrocartilage (TFC) after débridement with the arthroscope in the 6R portal. U, ulnar head.

Following the débridement, the distal ulna is evaluated for any chondral changes by gently supinating and pronating the wrist. If significant chondromalacia is present, ulnar variance is neutral or positive, and no LT instability is present, an arthroscopic wafer resection of the distal ulna may be performed. Alternatively, in the same situation, an open ulnar shortening osteotomy may be performed. Class II D or E lesions are the end stages of the ulnar impaction syndrome and represent a wide spectrum of pathology including LT ligament disruption, varying degrees of LT instability, and ulnocarpal arthrosis. A full discussion of treatment for these lesions is beyond the scope of this chapter, but a brief discussion of arthroscopic evaluation and treatment is presented. Following débridement of the TFC as in a class IIC lesion, the frayed portions of the LT ligament are débrided. If the LT ligament is frayed or perforated, midcarpal evaluation of the LT joint reveals no articular step-off (no instability), and there are no chondral changes on the hamate, an arthroscopic wafer procedure (particularly useful in an older patient) or an ulnar shortening osteotomy is performed. If evidence of instability, such as fraying of the ulnocarpal extrinsic ligaments, LT joint incongruity from the midcarpal evaluation, and chondral changes on the hamate exist, an ulnar shortening osteotomy is performed to tighten the extrinsic ligaments. This can be combined with an arthroscopic reduction and pinning of the LT joint.

## POSTOPERATIVE MANAGEMENT

Postoperative management depends on the abnormalities treated. If only a simple TFC débridement has been performed, the patient is given a removable wrist splint to be used for comfort, and range-of-motion exercises for the hand and wrist are begun. At 4 weeks progressive strengthening is started. Approximately one-half of the patients enroll in a supervised therapy program. Return to sport or vigorous activity is restricted for 10 to 12 weeks. Following an osteotomy, a short-arm cast is worn for 4 to 8 weeks. At that time, a graduated therapy program is begun and a protective splint is worn for 4 more weeks. Return to vigorous activity is restricted until the osteotomy is healed completely and range of motion and strength have returned to preoperative levels.

## COMPLICATIONS

The incidence of complications in arthroscopy has been estimated at 2% (5). Complications have been categorized by Warhold and Ruth (9). They include complications related to traction and arm positioning, complications related to establishment of portals, procedure-specific complications, and general arthroscopic complications. To avoid complications associated with portal placement such as nerve or tendon laceration, meticulous palpation of surface anatomy and identification of portal sites are mandatory. Following skin incision, a small hemostat is used to spread down to the wrist capsule gently. This helps move important structures away from the portal site. As previously mentioned, introduction of the trochar and cannula is performed with gentle pressure and a twisting motion. Any difficulty with entry should prompt an immediate reevaluation of anatomy and a possible change in portal placement. Plunging with the trochar in the cannula can cause significant chondral or ligament damage. An iatrogenic cartilage lesion is equivalent to carving one's name on a tree. The damage is lifelong and irreparable.

## ILLUSTRATIVE CASE FOR TECHNIQUE

A 40-year-old, right-hand dominant surgical technician presented for evaluation of pain and clicking about the ulnar aspect of his left wrist. He reported no specific history of injury, only occasional ulnar-sided wrist pain in the past year. Three weeks previously, the pain increased, and he developed clicking with wrist movement, as well as occasional episodes of locking. Examination at that time revealed a positive TFCC stress test and pain with forearm rotation. There was no DRUJ instability. Radiographs from the initial office visit are shown (Figs. 16–18). He was initially treated with a short-arm splint, but this did not relieve his symptoms. Four weeks later, at the next office visit, this was converted to a long-arm removable splint. Over the following 6 weeks, the patient noted significant reduction in pain while using the splint, but a return of crepitation and pain while out of the splint.

Because of continued symptoms and the inability to perform tasks required at his job, surgical treatment was undertaken. An MRI was ordered that confirmed the diagnosis of a central TFC tear, while revealing no LT ligament tear. Surgical

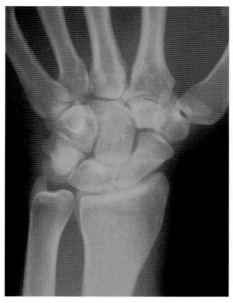

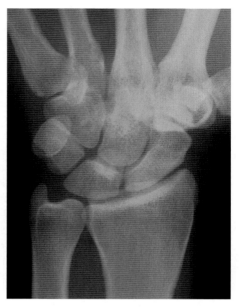

**FIGURE 16.** Preoperative posteroanterior radiograph (in ulnar deviation).

**FIGURE 17.** Preoperative posteroanterior radiograph (with grip loading).

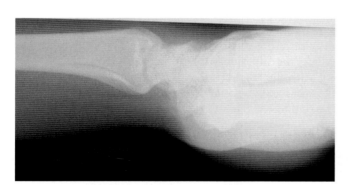

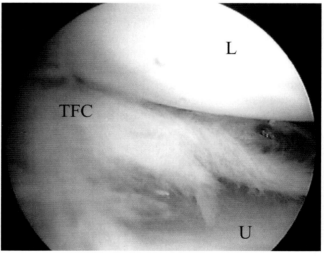

**FIGURE 18.** Preoperative lateral radiograph.

**FIGURE 19.** Initial arthroscopic view through 3–4 portal. L, lunate; TFC, triangular fibrocartilage; U, ulnar head.

treatment consisted of a wrist arthroscopy, which demonstrated a degenerative central flap tear of the TFC (Fig. 19), chondromalacia of the lunate and ulnar head (Figs. 20, 21), and a large, complete perforation of the LT ligament. Minimal step-off of the LT joint was seen on midcarpal arthroscopy. An oblique, 4-mm shortening osteotomy was performed using the stacked blade technique, and a five-hole LC-DCP plate was applied (Figs. 22, 23).

Postoperatively, he was placed in a cast for 4 weeks and then converted to an orthoplast splint. At this time, he began range-of-motion exercises. At 10 weeks postoperatively, with uneventful healing of the osteotomy, he was weaned from his splint, and began strengthening in a formal therapy program. At 14 weeks postoperatively, he reported minimal pain and no crepitation with wrist motion. He was returned to his job without restrictions.

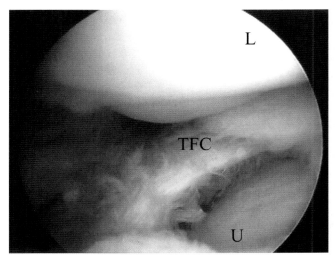

**FIGURE 20.** Arthroscopic view through 3–4 portal after preliminary débridement. L, lunate; TFC, triangular fibrocartilage; U, ulnar head.

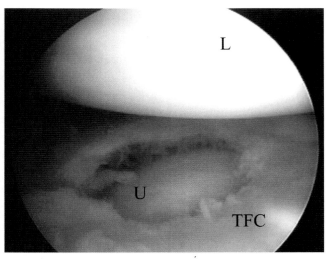

**FIGURE 21.** Arthroscopic débridement through 3–4 portal just prior to final contouring. Note chondromalacia of ulnar head (U). L, lunate; TFC, triangular fibrocartilage.

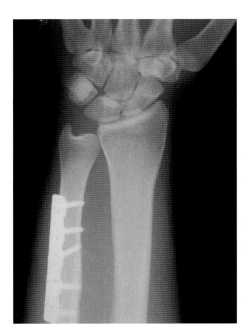

**FIGURE 22.** Posteroanterior radiograph 1 month postoperative.

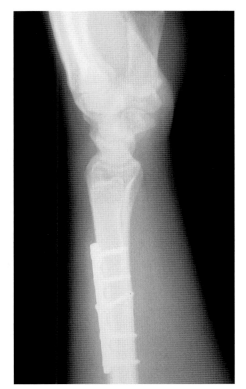

**FIGURE 23.** Lateral view 1 month postoperative.

## ACKNOWLEDGMENTS

The authors would like to thank Andrew K. Palmer, M. D. for his work on the initial chapter, which forms the basis of our chapter. We also would like to acknowledge the AV help of Michael Roth.

## RECOMMENDED READING

1. Adams, B. D.: Partial excision of the triangular fibrocartilage complex articular disk: a biomechanical study. *J. Hand Surg.*, 18A: 334–340, 1993.
2. Bednar, J. M., Osterman, A. L.: The role of arthroscopy in the treatment of traumatic triangular fibrocartilage injuries. *Hand Clin.*, 10(4): 605–614, 1994.
3. Bednar, M. S., Arnoczky, S. P., Weiland, A. J.: The microvasculature of the triangular fibrocartilage complex: its clinical significance. *J. Hand Surg.*, 16A: 1101–1105, 1991.
4. Chidgey, L. K.: Histologic anatomy of the triangular fibrocartilage. *Hand Clin.*, 7(2): 249–262, 1991.
5. Culp, R. W.: Complications of wrist arthroscopy. *Hand Clin.*, 15(3): 529–535, 1999.
6. Palmer, A. K.: Triangular fibrocartilage complex lesions: a classification. *J. Hand Surg.*, 14A: 594–606, 1989.
7. Palmer, A. K., Glisson, R. R., Wemer, F. W.: Relationship between ulnar variance and triangular fibrocartilage complex thickness. *J. Hand Surg.*, 9A: 681–683, 1984.
8. Palmer, A. K., Werner, F. W., Glisson, R. R., Murphy, D. J.: Partial excision of the triangular fibrocartilage complex. *J. Hand Surg.*, 13A: 403–406, 1988.
9. Warhold, L. G., Ruth, R. R.: Complications of wrist arthroscopy and how to prevent them. *Hand Clin.*, 11: 81–89, 1995.

# 23

# Arthroscopic Repair of the Triangular Fibrocartilage Complex

Gary G. Poehling and Rafael M. M. Williams

## INDICATIONS/CONTRAINDICATIONS

The peripheral attachments of the TFC are made up of thick, strong collagen bundles that are well vascularized. The thin central portion of the articular disk, however, is relatively avascular with short, randomly oriented collagen fiber bundles (Figs. 1, 2) (2,7,8). Because of this difference in blood supply, there is an improved healing capacity following injury to the peripheral portions of the TFC. It is therefore possible to treat injuries to the vascularized (peripheral) areas of the TFC with arthroscopic repair. Injuries to the avascular (central) portion of the TFC, however, are amenable only to arthroscopic débridement (1,10). Lesions of the TFCC can be placed into one of two broad categories based on arthroscopic appearance and location as either traumatic (type I) or degenerative (type II) (Table 1) (9).

Traumatic injuries to the TFCC usually occur following a hyperextension, twisting injury of the wrist with impaction of the ulnar-sided carpus on the distal ulna. The most common traumatic tear pattern courses from dorsal to palmar adjacent to the sigmoid notch of the distal radius in line with the orientation of the collagen fibrils (type IA) (Fig. 3A). Peripheral detachment or avulsion of the TFC insertion at the base of the ulnar styloid (type IB) may be associated with distal radius fractures or with other injuries to the upper extremity that are remote from the TFCC itself (Fig. 3B). Tears also may involve the ulnocarpal ligaments (ulnolunate and ulnotriquetral) (type IC) (Fig. 3C).

Complete detachment (usually an avulsion injury) of the radial origin of the TFCC from the sigmoid notch of the distal radius (type ID) is associated with instability of the DRUJ and is caused by a severe impact or twisting injury to the wrist and forearm (Fig. 3D). In general, traumatic injuries to the TFCC are rare in patients who have open physis or who are beyond the fifth decade of life. In con-

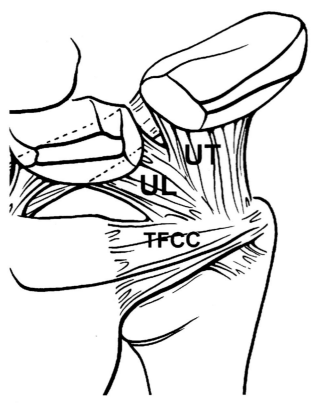

**FIGURE 1.** Components of the triangular fibrocartilage (TFCC) complex. UL, ulnolunate; UT, ulnotriquetral.

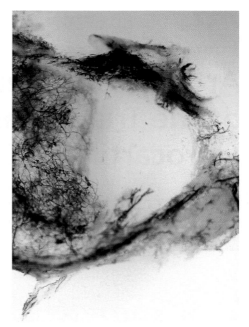

**FIGURE 2.** Blood supply of the triangular fibrocartilage. Well-perfused peripherally, avascular at central portion of disk. (From Chidgey, L. K.: Histological and vascular anatomy of the triangular fibrocartilage complex. In: *Operative Arthroscopy*, 2nd ed., edited by J. B. McGinty, R. W. Caspari, R. W. Jackson, and G. G. Poehling, Lippincott–Raven, Philadelphia, 1996, with permission.)

trast, the incidence of degenerative lesions to the TFCC increases with increasing age (7,9–12).

Degenerative lesions almost always occur in the centrum of the articular disk, are usually round with rough edges, and appear to result from impaction of the ulnar carpus on the ulnar head. Type IIA, the earliest stage of ulnocarpal abutment, is characterized by thinning of the articular disk without perforation. Type IIB lesions are associated with thinning of the articular disk as well as changes in the hyaline cartilage consistent with chondromalacia on the adjacent surfaces of the ulnar head and lunate. Perforation of the articular disk with chondromalacia on the ulnar head and lunate is seen in type IIC. With progression to type IID lesions, there is partial tearing of the lunotriquetral (LT) ligament, further destruction of articular cartilage, and subchondral bone changes.

These lesions immediately precede the more severe degeneration of the articular surfaces characteristic of type IIE lesions. In type IIE lesions, there is fibrillation and fissuring of the articular surfaces of the radioulnar joint, with disruption of the articular disk and the LT ligament as well as synovitis (12).

Arthroscopy of the wrist is indicated for the patient who, by history, physical examination, and x-ray, has a mechanical disruption of the TFCC with clinically significant symptoms. The average patient has a history of some trauma to the wrist, which, when treated by rest, becomes painless; with activity, however, the patient has pain, popping, and catching on the ulnar side. In addition, the injury presents as

**TABLE 1. LESIONS OF THE TRIANGULAR FIBROCARTILAGE COMPLEX (TFCC)**

**Class I—Traumatic**
  A. Central perforation
  B. Ulnar-sided avulsion with or without fracture
  C. Distal avulsion (ulnolunate and/or ulnotriquetral ligaments)
  D. Radial avulsion with or without sigmoid notch fracture
**Class II—Degenerative**
  A. TFCC wear (no perforation)
  B. TFCC wear (no perforation) with lunate or ulnar chondromalacia
  C. TFCC perforation with lunate or ulnar chondromalacia
  D. TFCC perforation with chondromalacia and lunotriquetral ligament perforation
  E. TFCC perforation with chondromalacia, lunotriquetral ligament perforation, and ulno-
     carpal arthritis

From Palmer, A. K.: Triangular fibrocartilage complex lesions: a classification. *J. Hand Surg.*, 14A: 594–606, 1989, with permission.

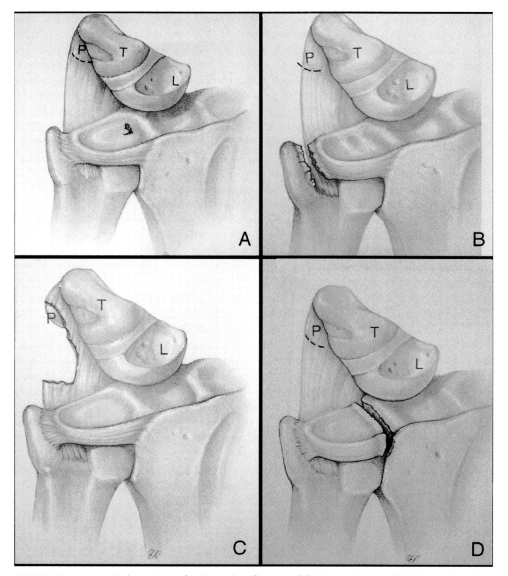

**FIGURE 3.** Anatomic depictions of Palmer classification: **(A)** Palmer IA tear; **(B)** Palmer IB peripheral tear; **(C)** Palmer IC tear of ulnolunate and ulnotriquetral ligament tears; **(D)** Palmer ID tear at radial margin. L, lunate; P, peripheral; T, triquetrum. (From illustrations by Elizabeth Roselius 1993. In: *Operative Hand Surgery*, 3rd ed., edited by D. P. Green, Churchill Livingstone, New York, 1993, with permission.)

a diagnostic dilemma or has failed to respond to conservative management consisting of splinting and a period of nonsteroidal antiinflammatory medication (4).

The general contraindications to TFCC repair are similar to those that would normally preclude wrist arthroscopy: poor medical status, open wounds at or near the surgical site, infection, and complex regional pain syndrome. The physician also must pay attention to the degree of ulnar variance when simple, partial débridement of the TFC is planned. A positive ulnar variance may be associated with ulnar-carpal abutment and require distal ulnar resection or shortening in addition to débridement of the TFC to achieve optimal long-term results.

## PREOPERATIVE PLANNING

Most patients with traumatic lesions of the TFCC describe pain on the ulnar side of the wrist, which is exacerbated by any activity that requires forearm rotation. Weakness, catching, and snapping also are noted. Although the pain may improve with rest, symptoms frequently return once activities are resumed.

Physical examination often demonstrates a pattern of tenderness and painful motion that can help identify the specific type of TFCC injury. Type IA lesions are associated with dorsal tenderness as well as pain with pronation and supination. Type IB lesions are also painful with forearm rotation and generally present with weakness, catching, and snapping; pain is localized to the ulnar side of the wrist. If there is a complete avulsion of the ulnar attachment of the TFC (with or without an ulnar styloid fracture), patients generally present with gross instability at the DRUJ; these injuries typically are associated with fractures of the distal radius. Tenderness over the palmar aspect of the TFCC (pisiform) associated with pain and catching that occurs during forearm rotation, extension, and radial deviation suggests a type IC lesion. Diffuse tenderness associated with an unstable DRUJ usually follows a more severe injury and may indicate a type ID tear/avulsion.

Examination is performed most efficiently with the patient seated and the elbow resting on the examination table. With the forearm initially stabilized, the wrist is brought into maximal dorsiflexion and ulnar deviation (ulnar impaction test), thus impacting the ulnar carpus against the distal ulna (Fig. 4); this maneuver commonly causes immediate pain in patients with tears of the TFCC. A similar maneuver can be performed throughout a range of pronation and supination as well as with the wrist palmar-flexed. The amount of dorsal-palmar translation of the ulnar carpus and the stability of the DRUJ should be assessed as well and compared with that of the normal wrist.

Radiographic examination should include plain and stress radiographs. In patients with type IA and ID lesions, triple-injection arthrograms demonstrate dye leaking from the radiocarpal joint to the DRUJ through the radial side of the TFC. Patients with type IB lesions demonstrate pooling of the dye at the base of the ulnar styloid process. Type IC lesions may be associated with instability of the distal ulna; radiocarpal arthrography may demonstrate communication between the radiocarpal and midcarpal joints. These findings may cause type IC lesions to be mistaken for tears of the LT ligament.

Magnetic resonance imaging (MRI) also has a role in the assessment of the TFCC (Fig. 5). With regard to the detection of a tear, when prospectively compared with arthroscopy, MRI was found to have a sensitivity of 100%, a specificity of 90%, and an accuracy of 97%. With regard to the location of a tear, MRI was 100% sensitive, 75% specific, and 92% accurate (13).

## SURGERY

Diagnostic arthroscopy is accomplished using standard traction apparatus (Fig. 6). The 3–4, 4–5, and 6R portals are used routinely for complete visualization and

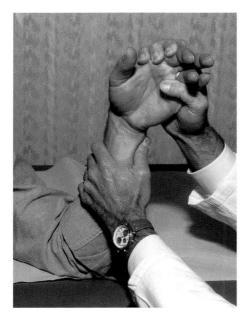

**FIGURE 4.** Ulnar abutment test. With the patient's elbow firmly supported, an axial load is placed on the wrist with ulnar deviation. This test should be performed throughout a range of pronation and supination as well.

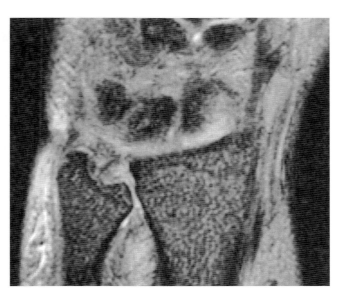

**FIGURE 5.** Magnetic resonance imaging of a triangular fibrocartilage complex tear. (Courtesy of Carol A. Boles, M. D., Winston-Salem, North Carolina.)

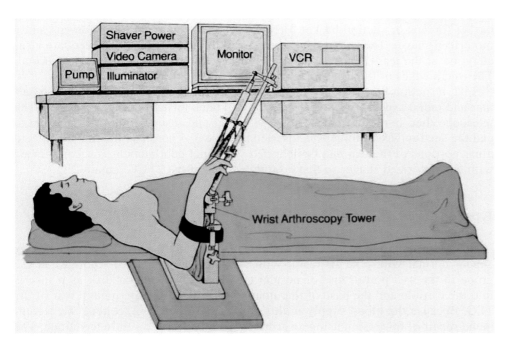

**FIGURE 6.** Standard wrist arthroscopy setup.

probing of the TFCC (Fig. 7) and the LT and scapholunate ligaments, as well as the articular surfaces of the scaphoid, lunate, triquetrum, and distal radius. The arthroscope (includes the outflow and pressure-monitoring system) is placed initially into the 3–4 portal; the 4–5 portal is then established. It usually is necessary to use a shaver (we prefer to use a 2.9-mm, full-radius, motorized suction shaving device) in the 4–5 portal to débride the extensive synovitis that is often present on the ulnar side of the wrist to visualize the joint fully.

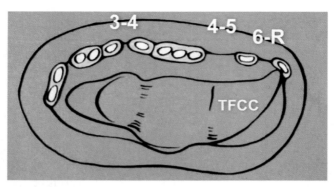

**FIGURE 7.** Anatomy of wrist arthroscopy portals. TFCC, triangular fibrocartilage complex.

Once the diagnosis and location of a TFCC tear is established by direct visualization, use a probe to assess the stability of the tear. Then perform arthroscopic treatment based on the location and type of lesion found; injuries to the vascularized (peripheral) areas of the TFCC can be repaired in most cases, but those involving the avascular (central) portion of the TFCC (traumatic or degenerative) are amenable only to arthroscopic débridement.

### Type IA Lesions

Débridement of the unstable portion of the TFCC is accomplished with 2.9-mm basket forceps or suction basket forceps, as well as with grasping forceps and a motorized shaver. The telescope is maintained in the 3–4 portal for adequate visualization of the tear (Fig. 8A), and a shaving device is placed into the 4–5 portal. The rough edges of the tear are débrided with the suction shaving device.

Next, a suction basket forceps is inserted into the 4–5 portal, and the loose palmar and radial aspects of the tear are trimmed back to stable tissue (Fig. 8B). The telescope then is removed from the 3–4 portal and inserted into the 4–5 portal, and the suction basket forceps is inserted into the 3–4 portal so that the dorsal and ulnar portions of the tear can be débrided. The final débridement is accomplished with the motorized shaver so that no rough edges of the TFCC remain (Fig. 8C).

### Type IB Lesions

The radial, central, dorsal, and palmar aspects of the articular disk usually appear normal with type IB tears. With the telescope in the 3–4 portal and the probe in the 4–5 portal, loss of normal tension in the articular disk as it inserts into the capsule and the base of the ulnar styloid suggests a peripheral tear of the TFC. Because the blood supply in this area of the TFCC is excellent, we recommend repair of this lesion using an arthroscopically assisted suture technique. The shaver is placed into the 6R portal and the margins of the articular disk are trimmed, as is the adjacent surface of the dorsal capsule.

Place the telescope in the 4–5 portal for better visualization of the tear (Fig. 9). Insert an empty Toughy 20-gauge needle (used by anesthesiologists for placement of epidural catheters—its inner edge is beveled and will not cut suture) into the 1–2 portal (Fig. 10). Push it through the periphery of the tear in the TFCC, then through the capsule and skin on the ulnar wrist.

Thread a 2–0 PDS suture through the needle (Fig. 11); the needle tip is withdrawn into the joint to be reinserted 5 to 10 mm away from the first needle puncture. Push the needle again through the articular disk, capsule, and skin (Fig. 12A). Pull the

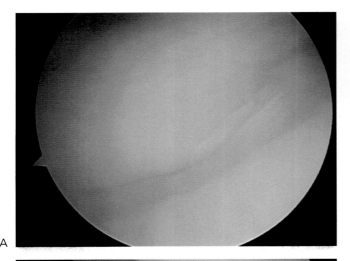

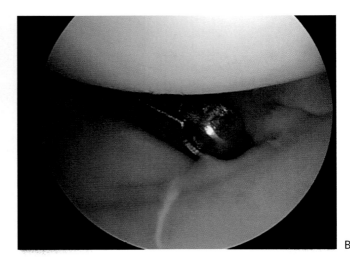

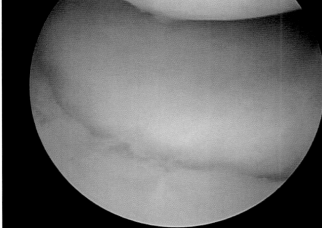

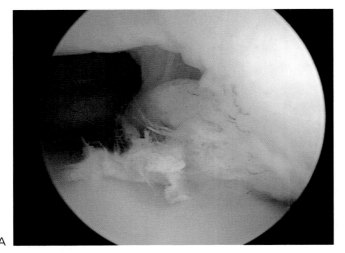

**FIGURE 8.** **A:** Arthroscopic picture of a Palmer IA tear prior to treatment. **B:** Débridement of a Palmer IA tear with a suction basket placed in the 4–5 portal. **C:** Débrided Palmer IA tear.

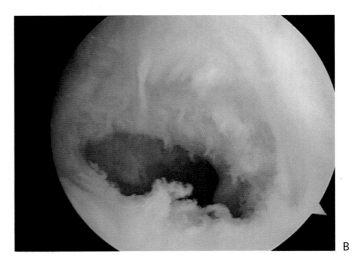

**FIGURE 9.** **A:** Arthroscopic image of a Palmer IB tear. **B:** Close-up.

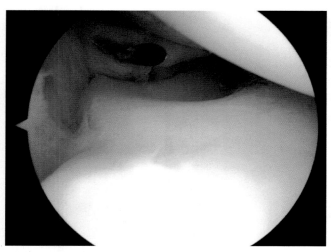

**FIGURE 10.** Arthroscopic view from 4–5 portal of Toughy needle entering from the 1–2 portal.

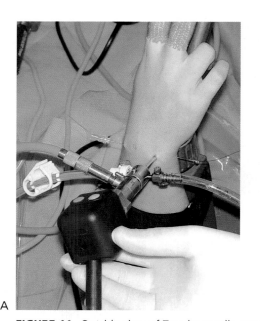

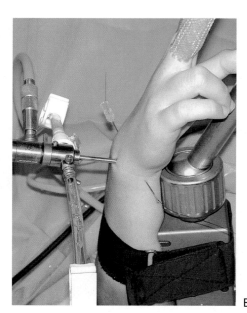

A                                                                                    B

**FIGURE 11.** Outside view of Toughy needle entering 1–2 portal and exiting at the ulnar side of the wrist. **A:** Anterior view. **B:** Lateral view.

suture out of the tip of the needle and withdraw the needle (Fig. 12B). This technique leaves a horizontal mattress suture through the torn TFCC (Fig. 13). Make a 1- to 2-cm longitudinal incision between the sutures so that the capsule can be visualized; bring the sutures into the wound and tie them over the capsule (Fig. 14). Take care not to entrap the ulnar sensory nerve (Fig. 15). This maneuver firmly approximates the ulnar border of the TFCC and the capsule (Fig. 16).

### Type IC Lesions

Type IC lesions are treated with débridement of the free ligamentous tissue to prevent impingement and interference in the normal gliding of the wrist joint. Most of these tears are partial, and they maintain sufficient stability such that sub-

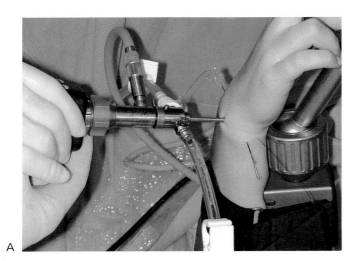
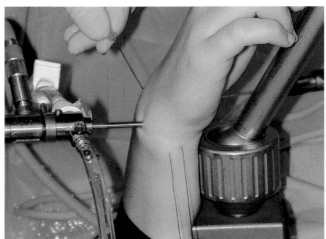

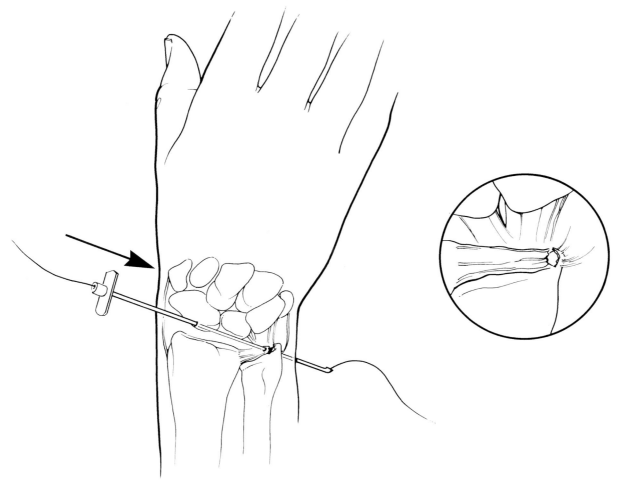

**FIGURE 12.** Second pass with Toughy needle through the triangular fibrocartilage complex with both ends of stitch exiting the ulnar side of the wrist. **A:** Needle pushed through for second pass. **B:** Needle withdrawn. **C:** Diagram of first pass with capture of the triangular fibrocartilage complex detachment. (*continued.*)

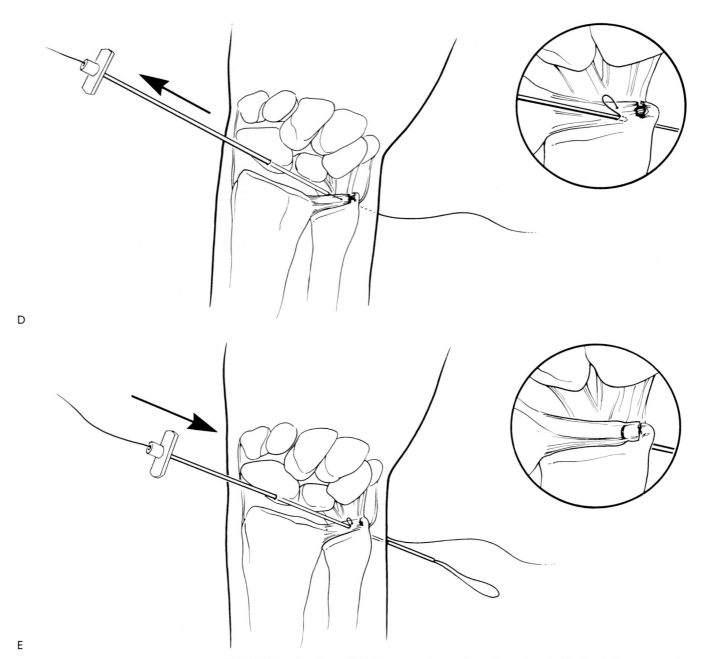

D

E

**FIGURE 12.** (*continued.*) **D:** Diagram of retraction of needle into the joint. **E:** Diagram of second pass followed by pulling the suture out the distal end of the needle.

sequent reconstruction is not necessary. We have found that most patients have excellent symptomatic relief with débridement alone if a TFCC tear is their only intraarticular problem.

### Type ID Lesions

Type ID lesions are seen most often in distal radius fractures and can be treated simply with reduction of the fracture in most cases. Arthroscopic treatment generally is not indicated because realignment of the bony avulsion fragment along the radial edge of the TFCC with the distal radius leads to satisfactory healing with a stable, painless DRUJ.

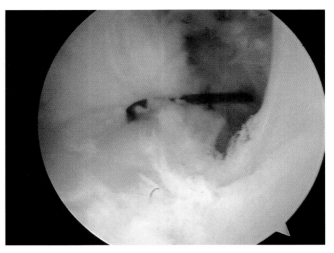

**FIGURE 13.** Arthroscopic view of horizontal mattress stitch through the detached triangular fibrocartilage complex prior to being tied down.

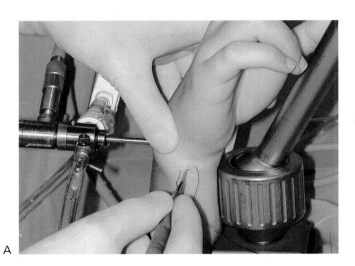

A

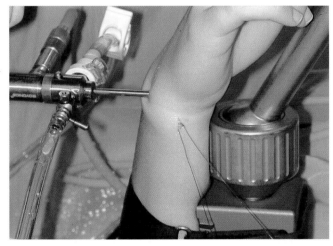

B

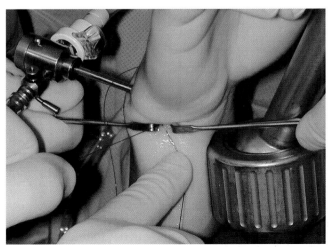

C

**FIGURE 14.** The triangular fibrocartilage complex is tied down with a 2–0 PDS suture. **A:** A 1-cm longitudinal incision is made between the two ends of the 2–0 PDS suture. **B:** Both ends of the PDS suture are pulled out through the incision. **C:** The PDS suture is tied down over the ulnar retinaculum. Take care to identify and protect the dorsal cutaneous branch of the ulnar nerve.

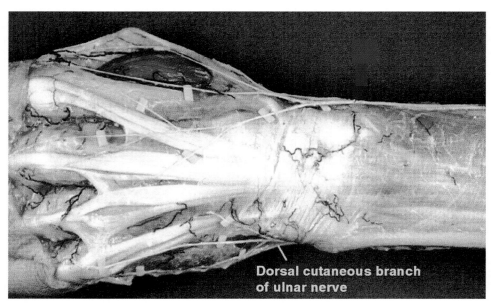

**FIGURE 15.** Anatomic dissection depicting vulnerability of the dorsal cutaneous branch of the ulnar nerve as it courses dorsally across the ulnar side of the wrist. (Courtesy of Pau Golano, PhD. Barcelona, Spain.)

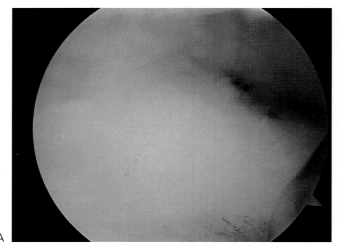

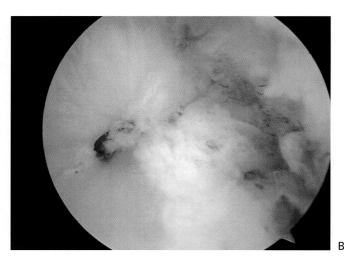

A

B

**FIGURE 16. A:** Arthroscopic view of the repaired ulnar detachment of the triangular fibrocartilage complex with the 2–0 PDS suture. **B:** Close-up.

### Degenerative Tears

Arthroscopic treatment includes débridement of the unstable portion of the degenerated articular disk with intraarticular resection of the ulnar head (the wafer procedure) and débridement of the unstable portion of the LT ligament tear. With the telescope in the 3–4 portal, the 2.9-mm shaver in the 4–5 portal, and the outflow and pressure-monitoring system in the 6R portal, débride the unstable portion of the TFCC in patients with stage IIA or IIB lesions. These lesions rarely are seen because most patients are asymptomatic until the TFC becomes perforated.

With stage IIC lesions, débridement of associated flap tears of the articular surface may be necessary as well. Carefully examine the adjacent articular surfaces of the lunate, the triquetrum, and the ulnar head; stress the wrist into ulnar deviation to assess any impingement of the ulnar carpus on the distal ulna. The information obtained during arthroscopy is correlated with the preoperative clinical evaluation to determine whether resection of the ulnar head is warranted.

Débridement of the articular disk is necessary for complete visualization before the ulnar head is resected. The ulnar head resection is accomplished with the telescope in the 3–4 portal and a 2.9-mm motorized abrader in the 4–5 portal. Remove the distal 2 to 3 mm of ulnar head, including the articular cartilage and subchondral bone, under direct visualization. It is necessary to rotate the forearm fully to expose the entire ulnar head through the TFC tear. Leave the articular cartilage of the DRUJ intact to preserve normal forearm rotation. Copious irrigation is necessary to ensure evacuation of all osseous and cartilaginous debris. (We also have found arthroscopy to be of benefit in assessing the adequacy of resection after the open wafer procedure or in assessing ulnocarpal impingement after diaphyseal ulnar shortening procedures.)

Frequently, type IID lesions are associated with instability of the LT joint. It is necessary to insert a probe into the 3–4 portal with the telescope in the 4–5 portal to assess the stability of this joint. Insert the probe into the articulation in an attempt to separate the two bones. Under direct visualization, manually stress the LT joint to assess dorsal palmar stability.

If the joint appears stable but there is a partial tear, carry out débridement with a power shaver in the 6R portal, with the telescope in the 4–5 portal. If instability is noted, however, débride all loose, unstable tissue back to the bleeding tissue. Then reduce the LT joint under direct visualization and pin it percutaneously, with radiographic guidance for placement of the pins. Arthroscopic visualization of the LT joint from both the radiocarpal and midcarpal joints is necessary to ensure anatomic alignment. Such patients also often require débridement of the articular disk and ulnar shortening, as previously described.

Patients with stage IIE lesions do not respond well to débridement procedures, because advanced arthritis currently is not amenable to arthroscopically assisted treatment.

## POSTOPERATIVE MANAGEMENT

At the completion of the wrist arthroscopy, infiltrate the joint with a mixture containing 5 cc of 0.25% sensorcaine, 0.1 cc epinephrine (1;1,000), and 1 cc morphine (4 mg). Inject all portal sites subcutaneously with 0.25% sensorcaine. Do not close these portal sites with suture, but close any ulnar incision that has been made (repair of IA tears) with a 4–0 nylon suture.

After débridement of the TFCC is performed (traumatic or degenerative), apply a wrist splint for 2 days and initiate active exercise thereafter. Symptomatic relief and restoration of motion can be expected within 6 to 12 weeks of surgery. Rarely have we found it necessary to reoperate on these wrists, although occasionally a second tear will develop in a previously débrided area. This tear responds well to repeat débridement.

If repair of the TFCC is performed, place the patient in a below-elbow splint for 1 month with the wrist in a neutral position, followed by 2 weeks in a cock-up wrist splint. Institute aggressive occupational therapy within 5 days to maintain range of motion at the metacarpophalangeal and interphalangeal joints as well as at the elbow. Forearm rotation and wrist motion are restricted for 1 month. Most patients, especially high-level athletes, report stiffness for up to 3 months. Determination of return to full athletic participation must be made on an individual basis, depending on the type of sport and level of competition.

## RESULTS

Our experience has been that arthroscopic débridement or repair of a torn TFCC provides significant patient satisfaction with regard to pain relief, range of

**TABLE 2. LITERATURE REVIEW OF ARTHROSCOPIC TRIANGULAR FIBROCARTILAGE COMPLEX (TFCC) REPAIR/DÉBRIDEMENT**

| Authors | Treatment | Number of patients | Average follow-up | Excellent/ good | Fair/ poor | Unique findings |
|---|---|---|---|---|---|---|
| Corso, Savoie, Geissler, et al (3) | Repair of peripheral detachment | 44 | 37 mo | 29/12 (Mayo wrist score) | 1/3 | Multicenter study<br>93% returned to work/sports<br>Grip strength = 75% |
| Haugstvedt, Husby (5) | Repair of peripheral detachment | 20 | 41 mo | 7/7 (Mayo) | 4/2 | Range of motion = 90%<br>Grip strength = 83%<br>100% returned to work |
| Minami, Kato (6) | Ulnar shortening with débridement of tears | 25 | 35 mo | 12/9 | 2/2 | Osteotomies healed at 7 wk<br>92% with complete relief or occasional mild pain |
| Terry, Waters (14) | Repair | 29 | 21 mo | 24/3 (Mayo) | N/A | Pediatric/adolescent patients<br>86% with coexisting pathology |
| Trumble, Gilbert, Vedder (15) | Repair before 4 mo | 24 | 34 mo | N/A | N/A | Range of motion = 89%<br>Grip strength = 85%<br>Pain relief ($p$ <.01)<br>75% returned to work/sports |
| Trumble, Gilbert, Vedder (16) | Repair after 6 mo with ulnar shortening | 21 | 29 mo | N/A | N/A | Range of motion = 81%<br>Grip strength = 83%<br>Pain relief ($p$ <.01)<br>12 of 14 remained intact at follow-up study |
| Westkaemper, Mitsionis, Giannakopoulos, Sotereanos (17) | Débridement of TFCC tear | 28 | 15.4 mo | 13/8 (Mayo) | 8/2 | Involvement with workers' compensation did not affect results |

N/A, not available.

motion, and grip strength. Our clinical results closely resemble those previously reported in the literature (Table 2) (3,5,14–17).

## COMPLICATIONS

In our experience, the most common postoperative complication is prolonged stiffness with limited pronation/supination. It can be avoided most effectively with an aggressive rehabilitation program. Tenderness can occur at the level/distribution of the dorsal cutaneous branch of the ulnar nerve if the surgeon does not take care to identify and protect this nerve as sutures are tied down to the ulnar retinaculum.

Although the exact incidence is not known, re-tear at the edge of the initial débridement or fixation site may occur and should be suspected if there is a recurrence of symptoms. Appropriate immobilization, rehabilitation, and activity modification are the only ways to limit re-tear.

Continued instability may occur if there is inadequate fixation or healing at the base of an associated ulnar styloid fracture or radial avulsion. It is important to recognize injuries that are not amenable to arthroscopic repair or closed treatment. Displaced, irreducible fractures at the base of the ulnar styloid generally require open fixation (pin fixation with tension banding) to maintain stability at the DRUJ. If the TFC is dorsally detached, it can be sutured to the dorsal retinaculum/extensor carpi ulnaris subsheath under direct visualization during this approach.

Failure to recognize and treat ulnar positive variance during treatment for a degenerative lesion can result in continued pain with perpetuation of the ulnar abutment. Finally, all problems associated with distal radius fractures, especially malreduction at the lunate facet and shortening (with subsequent ulnar positive variance), must be recognized as being potential causes for delayed or inadequate healing of the TFCC.

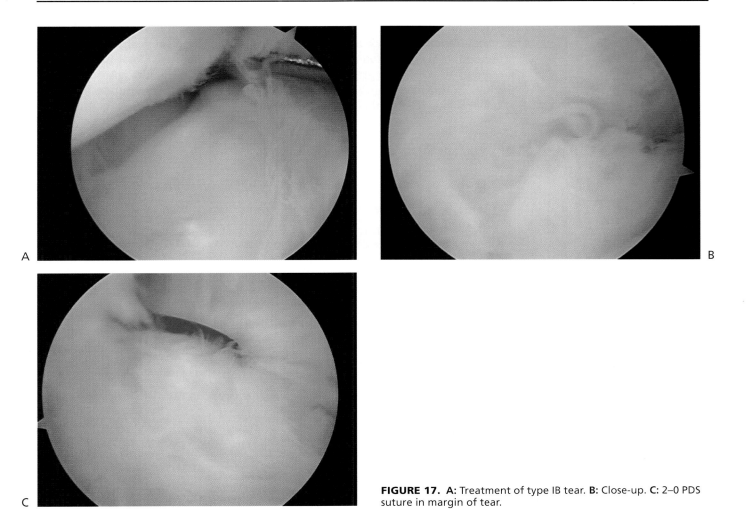

**FIGURE 17.** **A:** Treatment of type IB tear. **B:** Close-up. **C:** 2–0 PDS suture in margin of tear.

## ILLUSTRATIVE CASE FOR TECHNIQUE

A 28-year-old, right-hand dominant male presented with a 2-month history of right wrist pain that began after falling on his outstretched right arm while playing tennis. He denied any paraesthesias or paralysis to the hand and complained primarily of pain over the ulnar side of the wrist. The pain was only minimally alleviated with antiinflammatories and was exacerbated by playing tennis (especially forehand strokes).

Physical examination revealed intact skin with no ecchymosis. The hand was neurovascularly intact with no appreciable weakness. Tenderness was elicited over the ulnar side of the wrist (at the level of the 6U portal). He was nontender over the scaphoid as well as the radial side of the wrist. A palpable click was noted with palpation of the ulnar side of the wrist throughout pronation and supination. Plain radiographs of the wrist showed no evidence of fracture or intercarpal ligamentous damage.

Symptoms persisted despite conservative therapy with protected motion (wrist splint), activity modification (no tennis), and a long course of nonsteroidal antiinflammatories. Diagnostic arthroscopy was performed that demonstrated a traumatic type IB tear of the TFC. Using a Toughy needle, repair was performed with a single 2–0 PDS suture that was passed through the ulnar border of the TFC and tied over the ulnar retinaculum (Fig. 17). Postoperatively, the patient was placed in a below-elbow wrist splint for 4 weeks. Range of motion at the metacarpophalangeal and interphalangeal joints was maintained throughout this period. After 4 weeks, a removable cock-up wrist splint was applied, and gradual wrist and forearm motion was instituted. Once the patient had pain-free, normal range of motion at 10 weeks, he gradually returned to tennis. At 6 months postoperatively, the patient remained pain free and was able to play competitive (club level) tennis at his previous level without any symptoms.

## RECOMMENDED READING

1. Bednar, J. M.: Arthroscopic treatment of triangular fibrocartilage tears. *Hand Clin.*, 15: 479–488, 1999.
2. Chidgey, L. K.: Histologic anatomy of the triangular fibrocartilage. *Hand Clin.*, 7: 249–262, 1991.
3. Corso, S. J., Savoie, F. H., Geissler, W. B., Whipple, T. L., Jiminez, W., Jenkins, J.: Arthroscopic repair of peripheral avulsions of the triangular fibrocartilage complex of the wrist: a multicenter study. *Arthroscopy*, 1: 78–84, 1997.
4. Fulcher, S. M., Poehling, G. G.: The role of operative arthroscopy for the diagnosis and treatment of lesions about the distal ulna. *Hand Clin.*, 14: 285–296, 1998.
5. Haugstvedt, J. R., Husby, T.: Results of repair of peripheral tears in the triangular fibrocartilage complex using an arthroscopic suture technique. *Scand. J. Plast. Reconstr. Surg. Hand Surg.*, 33: 439–447, 1999.
6. Minami, A., Kato, H.: Ulnar shortening for triangular fibrocartilage complex tears associated with ulnar positive variance. *J. Hand Surg.*, 23A: 904–908, 1998.
7. Palmer, A. K.: The distal radioulnar joint. Anatomy, biomechanics and triangular fibrocartilage complex abnormalities. *Hand Clin.*, 3: 31–40, 1987.
8. Palmer, A. K., Werner, F. W.: Triangular fibrocartilage complex of the wrist—anatomy and function. *J. Hand Surg.*, 6: 153–162, 1981.
9. Palmer, A. K.: Triangular fibrocartilage complex lesions: a classification. *J. Hand Surg.*, 14A: 594–606, 1989.
10. Palmer, A. K.: Triangular fibrocartilage complex lesions: injury patterns and treatment. *Arthroscopy*, 6: 125–132, 1990.
11. Palmer, A. K.: Partial excision of the triangular fibrocartilage complex. In: *Master Techniques in Orthopaedic Surgery: The Wrist*, edited by R. H. Gelberman, Raven Press, New York, pp. 207–218, 1994.
12. Palmer, A. K., Harris, P. G.: Classification and arthroscopic treatment of triangular fibrocartilage complex lesions. In: *Operative Arthroscopy*, 2nd ed., edited by J. B. McGinty, R. W. Caspari, R. W. Jackson, and G. G. Poehling, Lippincott–Raven, Philadelphia, pp. 1015–1022, 1996.
13. Potter, H. G., Asnis-Ernberg, L., Weiland, A., Hotchkiss, R. N., Peterson, M. G., McCormack, R. R.: The utility of high-resolution magnetic resonance imaging in the evaluation of the triangular fibrocartilage complex of the wrist. *J. Bone Joint Surg.*, 79A: 1675–1684, 1997.
14. Terry, C. L., Waters, P. M.: Triangular fibrocartilage injuries in pediatric and adolescent patients. *J. Hand Surg.*, 23A: 626–634, 1998.
15. Trumble, T. E., Gilbert, M., Vedder, N.: Isolated tears of the triangular fibrocartilage: management by early arthroscopic repair. *J. Hand Surg.*, 22A: 57–65, 1997.
16. Trumble, T. E., Gilbert, M., Vedder, N.: Ulnar shortening combined with arthroscopic repairs in the delayed management of triangular fibrocartilage complex tears. *J. Hand Surg.*, 22A: 807–813, 1997.
17. Westkaemper, J. G., Mitsionis, G., Giannakopoulos, P. N., Sotereanos, D. G.: Wrist arthroscopy for the treatment of ligament and triangular fibrocartilage complex injuries. *Arthroscopy*, 14: 479–483, 1998.

# 24

# Ulnar Shortening Osteotomy

Tung B. Le and C. Vaughan A. Bowen

## INTRODUCTION

The term *ulnocarpal impingement* is used to describe a spectrum of ulnar-sided clinical problems in which pain occurs because of increased loading at the ulnocarpal joint. It is also known as *ulnocarpal abutment* or *ulnar impaction syndrome*.

Experimental studies by Palmer and Werner (10) demonstrated that load transmission across the ulnocarpal joint changes greatly with ulna variance. In ulna-neutral variance wrists, in which the distal radius and ulna are the same length on standardized radiographs, approximately 82% of the compressive load across the wrist joint is borne by the radiocarpal articulation, and the remaining 18% is transmitted across the ulnocarpal joint. Ulna-positive or ulna-plus variance, in which there is long ulnar length relative to the distal radius on standardized radiographs, significantly increases force transmission across the ulnocarpal joint.

Most cases of ulnocarpal impingement occur in ulna-plus or ulna-neutral wrists. Variation in ulnar length may be "normal" or result from abnormal development, trauma, or previous surgery. Distal radius malunion, posttraumatic premature closure of the distal radial physis, and proximal migration of the radius after radial head excision are among the most common causes of ulnocarpal impingement. Wrist fusion in the immature skeleton may lead to ulna-plus variance as well. Developmental causes of the syndrome usually are associated with deformity of the wrist and include Madelung's deformity (11) and multiple enchondromatosis. Ulnar-plus variance can be "normal" but may become symptomatic when associated with repetitive loading (1,9).

The abnormalities caused by ulnocarpal impingement are now well understood (7). The condition can be viewed as part of a wide spectrum of ulnar carpal derangements resulting from a local increase in load transmission (8,9).

Patients present with a variety of these degenerative problems, depending on the chronicity of impingement. As ulna variance changes with different degrees of forearm rotation (4), ulnocarpal impingement symptoms may occur intermittently and may be related only to certain specific activities. The onset or exacerbation of symptoms usually follows specific tasks in which the wrist is axially loaded, ulnar deviated, and supinated. This dynamic form of ulnocarpal impingement can occur in work, sports, and recreational activities. Many people with ulna-plus variance never load their wrists enough to develop symptoms. Others, however, use their arms in such a way that loads are transmitted repeatedly across the ulnocarpal joint, and this brings on symptoms. It is possible for people with neutral- or negative-ulna variance to develop the condition if they engage in sufficiently provocative activities. Because such a wide range of etiologic factors can be responsible for the development of this condition, it is not surprising that it can affect individuals of either sex and at any age.

## MANAGEMENT

Nonoperative treatment is carried out initially, with patient education, activity modification, physiotherapy, splinting, and nonsteroidal antiinflammatory medications. These measures may be effective for patients with small amounts of ulna-plus variance and no underlying anatomic malalignment.

Surgical options should be considered for patients who do not respond adequately to nonoperative treatments. The medical literature describes many different operations that have been used for ulnocarpal pain. None are suitable for all patients, thus individual clinical problems should be analyzed carefully and the appropriate operation recommended.

Ulnar shortening osteotomy is used primarily for patients with ulnar abutment syndromes associated with ulna-plus variance and/or triangular fibrocartilage complex (TFCC) tears, but without significant structural malalignment (1,3,7,8). The procedure also has been used to treat ulnar-sided wrist pain associated with isolated TFCC tears (1). The rationale is that ulnar shortening unloads the ulnocarpal joint without violating the articular surfaces of the distal ulna. Ulnar shortening osteotomy has been successfully used for treating distal radioulnar joint (DRUJ) malalignments as well, such as those seen in distal radius fracture malunions or in Madelung's deformity. Here the procedure improves DRUJ congruity as well as reducing ulnocarpal load transmission (6). Shortening the ulna also has the effect of tightening the ligamentous attachments of the TFCC at the distal end of the ulna. This effect can be used for managing patients with these ligamentous instabilities, although the results of using the operation for this purpose are not well documented.

## INVESTIGATION

### History

It is important to look for possible underlying causes of ulnocarpal impingement. Is the condition secondary to fracture in the distal radius (Fig. 1), or is it insidious in onset (Fig. 2)? The usual clinical feature is ulna wrist pain aggravated by grip, especially grip with rotation. As the history is taken, questions are asked to rule out other possible causes of ulnar wrist pain.

### Clinical Examination

Observation may reveal prominence of the distal ulna, although this usually is not marked (except in extreme cases). Range of motion is often fully maintained in cases associated with "normal" ulna-plus variance and patients with a TFCC tear. If the condition is secondary to fracture of the distal radius, there may be

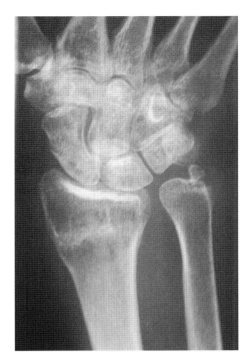

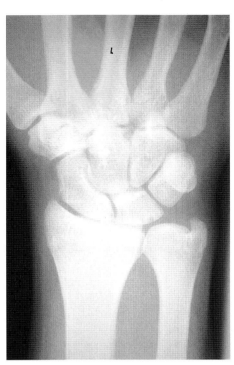

**FIGURE 1.** Neutral rotation posteroanterior radiograph of a wrist with a previous fracture of the distal radius. The fracture has united with shortening, leaving the patient with ulna-plus variance and ulnocarpal impingement.

**FIGURE 2.** Neutral rotation posteroanterior radiograph of a wrist that has developed with a small amount of "normal" ulna-plus variance. The patient presented with ulnar wrist pain and was clinically diagnosed as having ulnocarpal impingement. Note the cyst in the proximal surface of the lunate, where it impinges on the distal ulna. L, left.

limited flexion and extension, and supination may be blocked. Ulnar deviation of the wrist is often painful. On palpation there is localized tenderness over the ulnocarpal joint. Point tenderness on the proximal articular surface of the triquetrum is an almost pathognomonic feature. The distal ulna should be stable, and there should be no pain from the DRUJ on compression and forearm rotation. There should be no evidence of tendonitis in the extensor carpi ulnaris (ECU) and flexor carpi ulnaris tendons, and the ECU should be stable when the forearm is supinated forcibly with the ECU under tension. The pisotriquetral joint should glide smoothly without localized discomfort or crepitus. The hook of hamate should not be tender. Grip strength is often diminished by pain. The ulnocarpal grind test is usually painful. Tests for ligamentous stability, such as Lichtman's test and the Watson shift test, should be negative. Grip strength often is diminished because of associated pain.

## Imaging Techniques

**Plain Radiographs.** Supination and radial deviation increase ulna variance. This phenomenon explains some of the clinical features and are considered when measurements are taken from plain radiographs. Care must be taken when ulna variance is measured. Standardized radiographs are used so that assessments of variance are comparable in the same patient on different occasions and from one patient to another. The accepted convention is that neutral rotation posteroanterior (PA) wrist radiographs are used for the evaluation of ulna variance. Ulnar variance is expressed in millimeters and as plus or minus. Lateral radiographs of the

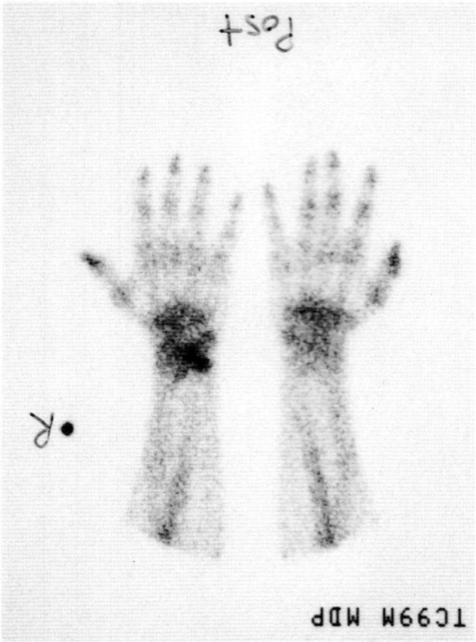

**FIGURE 3.** Tc99 MDP bone scan of a wrist with ulnar carpal impingement showing increased uptake in adjacent locations in the distal ulna and the proximal part of the lunate.

wrist also are obtained. Obliques usually are not necessary, unless they are required to rule out other conditions.

Most cases of ulnocarpal impingement have ulna-plus variance. Additionally, there may be cyst formation (Fig. 2) in adjacent surfaces of the distal ulna and in the proximal lunate, close to the LT joint. Associated conditions, such as malunion of the distal radius fracture, can be assessed on the plain radiographs as well.

**Tc99 MDP Bone Scan.** Sometimes a Tc99 MDP bone scan (Fig. 3) can be useful if there is doubt about the correct diagnosis. In cases in which degenerative changes are occurring at the ulnocarpal joint, there may be adjacent areas of increased uptake in the distal ulna and proximal lunate. In general, Tc99 MDP bone scans are not needed.

**Computed Tomography Scan.** A computed tomography scan is obtained to investigate or rule out other conditions, such as distal radius malunions or DRUJ incongruity; however, they do not provide much useful information in most cases of ulnocarpal impingement.

**Magnetic Resonance Imaging.** Magnetic resonance imaging is used frequently to aid in the diagnosis of wrist pain. It produces detailed images of both skeletal and soft tissue structures. Modern scanners have the ability to show tears in the TFCC, and it is possible to identify abnormalities in the intercarpal ligaments. It is important to realize, however, that care must be taken when images are interpreted. Findings should be correlated with clinical features. False positives should be identified; in particular, the finding of a TFCC tear should be considered very carefully, as this can reflect normal wear and tear that may not be the cause of a patient's symptoms.

**Arthrogram.** Wrist arthroscopy is replacing arthrography as the standard technique to investigate TFCC tears. If an arthrogram is used to seek defects in the TFCC, then a double injection technique is used: one injection into the ulnocarpal joint, and a second injection into the DRUJ.

**Arthroscopy.** Diagnostic arthroscopy is increasingly becoming an accepted method of assessing wrist abnormalities. In the majority of cases of ulnocarpal impingement, the diagnosis is made by history and physical examination, with radiographic studies to assess the degree of ulna variance. Wrist arthroscopy documents associated TFCC tears, assesses the extent of ulnocarpal chondromalacia, and documents the stability of the triquetrolunate joint. After the diagnosis is confirmed, arthroscopy is also useful for débriding or repairing TFCC tears and for carrying out a partial synovectomy and/or chondroplasty. When significant LT arthritis is seen along with tear of the LT ligament, we recommend LT arthrodesis in addition to ulnar shortening osteotomy. Arthroscopy is done immediately before the shortening osteotomy using the same anesthetic. Alternatively, it may precede the shortening osteotomy by 4 to 6 weeks if the effect of joint débridement alone is being assessed.

## PATIENT SELECTION

The ideal patient is one who presents with a history of ulnocarpal pain aggravated by grip and especially by grip with rotation. On physical examination the distal ulna is stable and has point tenderness over the TFCC and on the proximal articular surface of the triquetrum, but no features to suggest other pathology. Radiographs show ulna-plus variance. Other imaging techniques might be used occasionally, but usually are not needed. Arthroscopy is done to confirm the diagnosis, to rule out other diagnoses, and when indicated, to test the effect of TFCC débridement and/or repair. Ulnar shortening osteotomy is indicated primarily for ulnocarpal impingement and is also useful for the management of patients with TFCC tears. Consider the procedure for patients who are ulna-neutral and even, occasionally, in those with ulna-minus variance. The operation also can be helpful in the management of patients who have had a fracture of the distal radius with shortening, Madelung's deformity, and some cases of ligamentous laxity or instability on the ulna side of the carpus.

## PREOPERATIVE PLANNING

Preoperative planning initially involves discussing the proposed anesthetic and operation with the patient. Information is given about the regional anesthetic technique and details of the operation are described, specifically the surgical technique, perioperative risks and complications, the rehabilitation program, and the expected outcome. It is important to point out that the procedure works by unloading the ulnocarpal joint rather than by directly fixing any degeneration that may be present. It therefore may still be possible for patients to experience symptoms postoperatively if their activities are such that excess loading is applied to the region.

Technical planning for the procedure involves determining how much bone is to be removed. It is essential that good quality neutral posteroanterior radiographs are used for measurements. The amount of bone removed is calculated as follows:

*The amount of bone to be removed in millimeters equals the number of millimeters of ulna-plus variance measured on the preoperative radiograph plus the number of millimeters of ulna-minus variance that the surgeon wants to produce.*

In the operating room it must be remembered that the saw blade, used to make the osteotomies, has a certain thickness. This varies from blade to blade. The surgeon should know how much bone his particular blades remove and take this into consideration when the osteotomies are done. At operation it should be found that the disk of cortical bone taken out of the ulna is less than the measured amount of shortening by the thickness of two saw cuts.

## TECHNIQUE

Regional or general anesthetic is induced with the patient supine on the operating table. The operation is done with the surgeons seated at a hand table. A pneu-

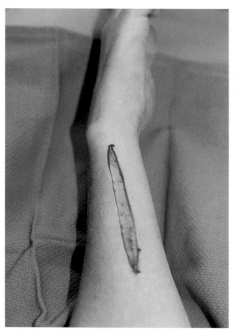

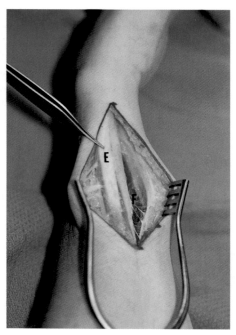

**FIGURE 4.** The skin incision is over the subcutaneous border of the ulna. The length of the incision is the length of an AO 6-hole dynamic compression plate with an extra 3 cm proximally for the application of the AO tension device.

**FIGURE 5.** The dissection is taken to bone between the extensor carpi ulnaris and flexor carpi ulnaris tendons. The forceps are pointing to the extensor carpi ulnaris tendon (E).

matic tourniquet is placed around the arm above the elbow. The whole limb is prepped with iodine from the tourniquet to the fingertips. The arm is draped free.

An incision is drawn out on the skin along the subcutaneous border of the ulna. The distal end of the incision is 2 cm proximal to the tip of the ulna styloid. The incision should be long enough to apply an AO small fragment six-hole dynamic compression (DC) plate and external tension device.

The arm is exsanguinated using an Esmarch bandage, and the tourniquet is inflated.

The skin incision (Fig. 4) is made using a #15 blade. As it is deepened into the subcutaneous tissue, small vessels are cauterized, while larger ones are ligated and divided. The approach extends into the plane between the ECU and flexor carpi ulnaris tendons (Fig. 5), and progresses till it reaches the periosteum covering the subcutaneous border of the ulna. A single knife cut is used to divide the periosteum of the ulna for the length of the incision.

The six-hole AO DC plate is temporarily positioned (Fig. 6) over the cut periosteum with its distal end placed at the flair of the distal metaphysis, approximately 2 cm proximal to the tip of the ulna styloid. A marking pen is used to color the tissue at the center of the plate (Fig. 7). This will be the location of the osteotomy. The plate is handed back to the scrub nurse.

Subperiosteal dissection (Fig. 8) is done to expose the bone circumferentially for approximately 2 cm on each side of the marked osteotomy site. The fixation plate is realigned with the ulna and the osteotomy site is marked on the exposed bone itself, again using the marking pen. The surgeon now determines if the plate will be placed on the dorsal or volar aspect of the ulna. Whenever possible the plate should be placed volarly, but occasionally it will sit better on the dorsal surface. Subperiosteal dissection is done on the chosen surface for the length of the plate and 3 cm proximal.

Once the osteotomy has been made the distal fragment is very mobile, and it is difficult to screw the plate to it. For this reason the plate is screwed to the distal fragment before the osteotomy is made (Fig. 9).

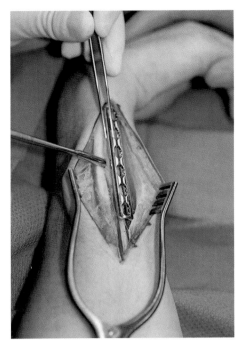

**FIGURE 6.** The fixation plate initially is positioned temporarily with its distal end against the flair of the distal ulna metaphysis to determine the osteotomy site that will be at the center of the plate.

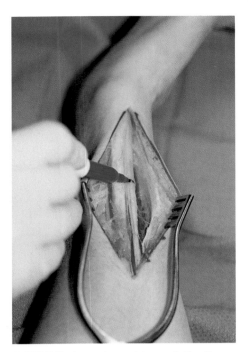

**FIGURE 7.** A pen is used to mark the tissues at the osteotomy site.

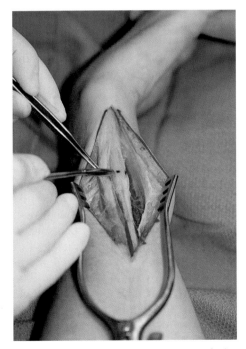

**FIGURE 8.** Subperiosteal dissection of the ulna is circumferential at the osteotomy site, but further along the bone is only done on the surface where the plate will lie.

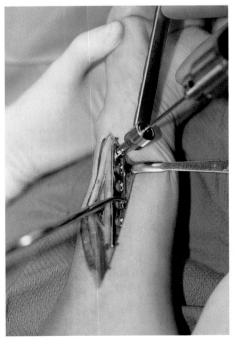

**FIGURE 9.** The plate is repositioned and clamped to the ulna. It is screwed to what will become the distal ulna fragment.

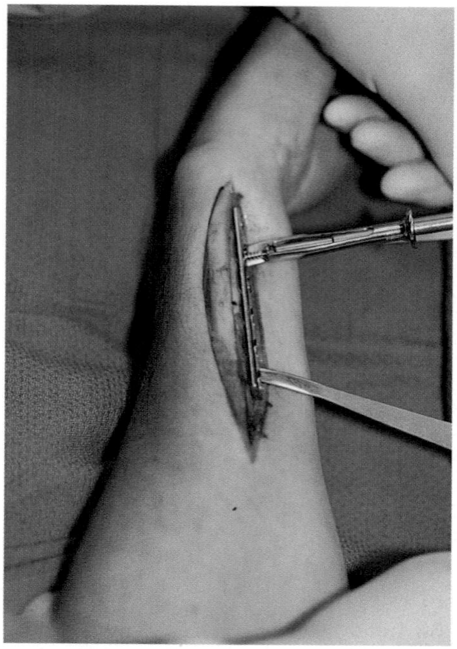

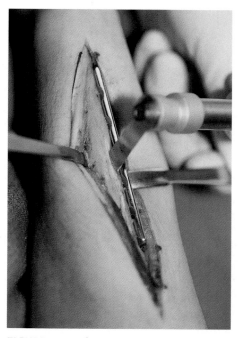

**FIGURE 10.** At this stage, only the distal three screws are inserted. The three proximal screws will not be placed until after the osteotomy had been made.

**FIGURE 11.** Before the plate is removed, a longitudinal groove is cut into the ulna so that rotational alignment can be assessed accurately when the shortened ulna is reduced. The groove should be long enough so that it remains clearly visible, both proximally and distally, after the ulna segment has been removed.

Place the plate against the chosen surface of the ulna as distally as possible. Use a reduction forceps with serrated jaws to hold it against the bone. Ensure that the plate is parallel to the bone for its whole length. Insert AO 3.5-mm screws into the distal three holes (Fig. 10) using the neutral drill guide and standard AO technique. Next, check to see that the bone is still satisfactorily marked at the central portion of the plate. Additionally, cut a longitudinal groove into the ulna at the site of the osteotomy (Fig. 11). This allows rotation to be gauged correctly after the bone is divided. The longitudinal groove must be long enough proximally so that a portion still remains after the bony segment is removed. When this has been done, take out the screws, remove the plate, and return them to the scrub nurse for careful storage.

The patient is ready for the osteotomy at this point. We use a Stryker Command saw (Stryker, Paoli, PA) with a 25.0 mm × 9.0 mm blade, but any small oscillating saw will suffice. Make sure that you know the thickness of bone your blade will remove. Next, a ruler is used to mark the location of the two osteotomy cuts accurately (Fig. 12). The measurement should take into consideration the thickness of the saw blade. The amount of shortening is calculated from good-quality preoperative neutral rotation posteroanterior radiographs. The two osteotomy cuts should be marked so that the thickness of bone removed plus two times the thickness of bone removed by a single saw cut equals the total amount of shortening needed. Two parallel transverse cuts are then made in the bone at the marked locations (Fig. 13). Both cuts are made simultaneously, with the saw moving from one to the other as each 1 mm to 2 mm is cut. Care is taken to ensure that each osteotomy is at right angles to the bone in every plane. Normal saline is squirted over the bone as it is being cut to prevent overheating and osteocyte death. The distal osteotomy should be the first to go completely through the bone, as this leaves more bony stability for completing the second cut, which will be in the proximal fragment. Once the two cuts are completed, the resected bone segment is removed (Fig. 14).

The plate is reapplied to reduce and stabilize the distal ulna fragment in its shortened position (Fig. 15). First the plate is reattached to the distal fragment,

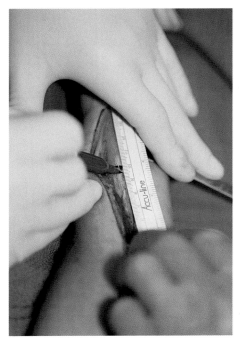

**FIGURE 12.** The amount of bone to be removed is determined from preoperative neutral rotation posteroanterior radiographs. Using a ruler, ink marks are placed where the proximal and distal saw cuts will be made.

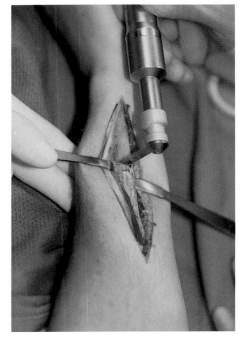

**FIGURE 13.** The proximal and distal osteotomies are made simultaneously, moving the saw from one to the other. Care must be taken to keep the saw perpendicular to the bone in every plane to keep the two saw cuts parallel.

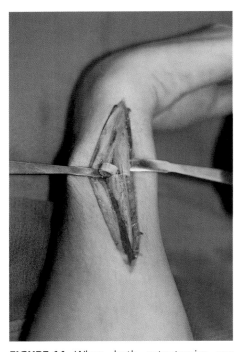

**FIGURE 14.** When both osteotomies are complete, the resected bone segment is removed. The bone segment will measure less than the predetermined shortening. The difference will be the amount of bone removed by the saw blade.

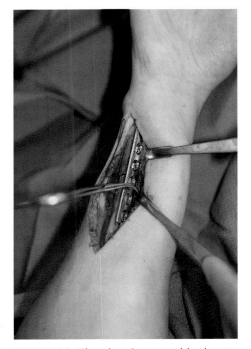

**FIGURE 15.** The plate is screwed back onto the distal fragment, which can be very mobile and difficult to handle after the osteotomy is complete. The predrilled screw holes greatly facilitate this stage of the procedure. The osteotomy is reduced, and the plate is clamped to the proximal fragment with as much ulna shortening as can be obtained easily.

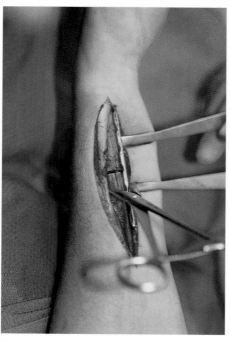

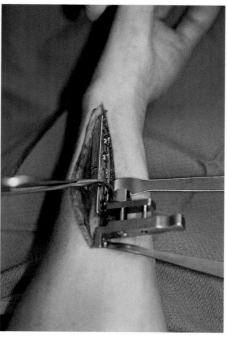

**FIGURE 16.** It is not essential to achieve complete closure of the osteotomy at this stage. It is important, however, to ensure that correct rotational alignment is restored. This illustration shows the longitudinal groove being used to judge rotational alignment.

**FIGURE 17.** The AO tension device is hooked into the most proximal hole in the fixation plate and attached to the ulna with a single screw. The tension device should be opened as wide as possible before application, and care should be taken to position it in line with the plate. Once secured in place, the longitudinal screw on the AO tension device is tightened to close and compress the osteotomy.

then the hand and wrist are realigned rotationally, using the previously made longitudinal groove (Fig. 16). A reduction forceps with serrated jaws is used to hold the plate temporarily to the proximal fragment. Now take the AO tension device, hook it into the proximal screw hole, and screw to the ulna at the proximal end of the plate (Fig. 17). Ensure that the AO tension device is parallel to the plate. Tighten the AO tension device by turning its longitudinal nut with a wrench. Tighten until the osteotomy is closed and compressed.

The amount of shortening obtained at the wrist is checked radiographically. Correct positioning is not as easy as in the x-ray department, but care should be taken to obtain an image as close to a neutral rotation posteroanterior radiograph as possible (Fig. 18). If insufficient shortening has been obtained, loosen the AO tension device, release the plate from the proximal fragment, and make a further saw cut, removing bone from the distal end of the proximal fragment. Once this is done, again clamp the plate to the proximal fragment, reapply the AO tension device, tighten it, and obtain a new radiograph. If necessary, this process can be repeated until the correct degree of shortening is obtained. Once you are satisfied, insert screws into the proximal three screw holes in the plate. If more compression is desired, the off-center drill guide can be used. Once the plate is attached securely to the bone, remove the reduction forceps with serrated jaws and the AO tension device. The ulna is now accurately shortened, aligned, and rigidly plated with compression (Fig. 19).

The tourniquet is released at this point. Hemostasis is secured with cautery. The wound is washed and closed in layers (Fig. 20). 3–0 Dexon is used for the subcutaneous layer, and intracuticular 4–0 Dexon is used for skin. A dry dressing is applied, and a volar plaster slab is added for immobilization.

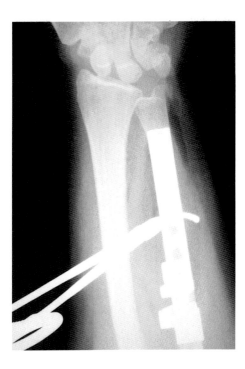

**FIGURE 18.** The AO tension device rigidly holds the reduction while a neutral rotation posteroanterior radiograph is taken. This image is used to measure the post-osteotomy ulna variance. If insufficient bone has been removed, additional shortening can be achieved by releasing the AO tension device, removing the reduction forceps with serrated jaws, and cutting more bone from the proximal fragment. It is not necessary to unscrew the plate from the distal fragment to do this.

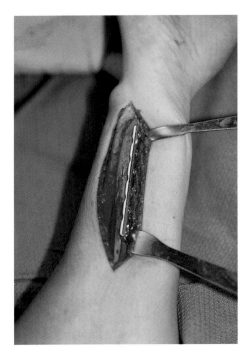

**FIGURE 19.** Once satisfactory shortening has been achieved, the plate is screwed to the proximal fragment. If additional compression is desired, the offset (gold) drill guide can be used. The reduction forceps with serrated jaws should not be removed until at least one of the proximal screws has been inserted and tightened. This prevents the plate, which is under tension, from springing off the bone. If there has been a lot of shortening, the longitudinal screw on the AO tension device may interfere with drill guide positioning at the most proximal hole. If this occurs, remove the AO tension device prior to inserting the last (most proximal) screw. After all six screws have been inserted and the AO tension device has been removed, the ulna is shorter by the predetermined measurement, and the osteotomy is accurately reduced and rigidly fixed with compression.

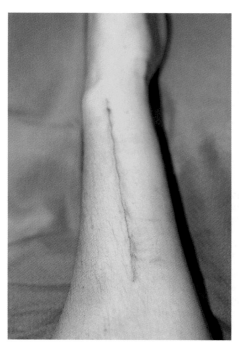

**FIGURE 20.** After the tourniquet has been deflated and hemostasis is secured, the wound is closed in layers. An intracuticular suture is used for skin closure.

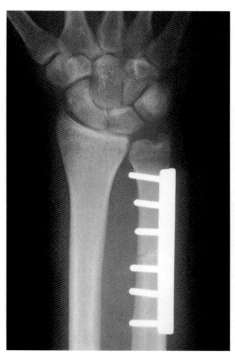

**FIGURE 21.** A neutral rotation posteroanterior radiograph at 6 weeks shows accurate shortening and rigid skeletal fixation. There is almost no callus formation at the osteotomy site. Union is achieved by primary bone healing.

## POSTOPERATIVE MANAGEMENT

The operation is done as an outpatient procedure. The patient returns home once fully recovered from the anesthetic. Instructions are given to keep the arm elevated and the operative site iced for the first 24 to 48 hours. The patient is encouraged to move the fingers and thumb as much as possible.

The patient is seen at the follow-up clinic 1 week after the operation. The plaster slab and dressings are removed, and wound healing is checked. A light dressing is applied, and the patient is referred to hand therapy.

The hand therapist supplies the patient with a removable static volar wrist splint and starts a rehabilitation program. The splint is used only for protection and should be removed frequently for exercise. Initial therapy concentrates on restoring range of motion. The therapist emphasizes the importance of regaining supination and pronation as well as working on flexion and extension. If there is any swelling or stiffness in the hand, this is treated as well.

When necessary, physical modalities are used. Our preferred initial method is to use contrast baths. In the early postoperative period, before wounds are healed, dry contrast is applied using hot and cold packs. Once wounds are healed, hot and cold water baths are used. From time to time, ultrasound may be needed to help with adhesion breakdown and range-of-motion improvement.

Once pain and swelling are controlled and range of motion is returning, the hand therapist moves the patient on to a strengthening program. At 6 weeks, a neutral rotation posteroanterior radiograph is obtained (Fig. 21). It can be difficult to know when bony union occurs because very little callus is seen. Union results from primary bone healing. Once union is achieved, the splint is no longer needed. Follow-up is maintained until full range of motion and strength have been regained and the patient has returned to normal activity.

## COMPLICATIONS

The operation of ulnar shortening osteotomy is generally very safe. The literature only contains one report in which substantial complications were encountered (14). Our own experience and those of other investigators (3) have reported that complications are not encountered often, although the usual early, late, local, regional, and general problems common to all surgical procedures are possible and may be seen on occasion.

The surgical approach is close to ideal. Entering the forearm at the subcutaneous border of the ulna between the territories of the ulna and radial nerves exposes peripheral nerves, major vascular structures, and muscle tendon units to almost no risk. The skeletal component of the operation is away from joints, and access involves almost no muscle dissection and very little soft tissue retraction. Postoperative swelling is minimal.

Potentially, the dorsal sensory branch of the ulna nerve can be damaged. This nerve lies in the volar flap and crosses to the dorsal aspect of the hand approximately 1 cm distal to the tip of the ulna styloid. Normally it is not seen in the surgical approach, but surgeons should be aware of its proximity. Damage can be prevented by meticulous dissection and careful placement of retractors.

Chun and Palmer (3) reported neither infections nor nonunions in their series of 30 ulnar shortening osteotomies. Nonunions, however, have been a cause for concern. The incidence has been related particularly to transverse osteotomies. A number of techniques, such as the oblique osteotomy with interfragmental lag screw fixation (12), have been developed to minimize their incidence. Our patients *(unpublished data),* treated with transverse osteotomies fixed with six-hole AO DC plates and compression, have experienced no nonunions. We believe that the nonunions associated with transverse osteotomies in the literature were related to inadequate internal fixation.

The most common late problem with the operation is plate pain. This is more likely to occur if the plate is placed dorsally, under the ECU tendon, rather than if it is put onto the volar surface. Affected patients complain of localized pain over the plate, especially after repetitive activity. On examination, there may be localized swelling and tenderness. The condition responds well to plate removal, but this should not be done during the first postoperative year. Use of reconstructive plates has produced less plate pain than our earlier cases, which used standard AO small fragment plates.

## DISCUSSION

A variety of surgical options have been recommended for the treatment of ulnocarpal impingement. There has been much debate about which is the best, and there is still no consensus of opinion.

The Darrach procedure has been widely used for many years. Although it can be a good solution for patients with ulnocarpal pain, results can be unpredictable and less than satisfactory. A particular concern is the potential for the distal end of the remaining ulna to become unstable after a Darrach procedure, a problem for which there is no satisfactory solution. The Darrach technique is now more or less restricted to patients with very low physical demand, such as the elderly or those with rheumatoid arthritis.

Concern about results from Darrach procedures has led to the development of mode variations. The most commonly done are the Bowers distal ulnar hemiresection and interposition technique, and the Watson distal ulnar matched resection. Indications for these procedures vary according to the training and experience of individual surgeons. These techniques are indicated for patients whose primary complaint is distal radioulnar joint pain from distal radioulnar joint arthritis or incongruity (2,15).

The Sauve-Kapandji technique is a popular alternative, as it has a wide spectrum of application and good results have been reported. It can be used to provide shortening as well as to obliterate DRUJ problems. The operation makes radical changes in the distal ulna region. Frequently, a lesser procedure is all that is necessary. In our practice we reserve its use for severe or advanced problems at the distal end of the ulna.

Feldon described a procedure known as the *wafer distal ulna resection* for the management of TFCC tears and/or ulnocarpal impingement syndrome (5). This approach eliminates the need for an ulna internal fixation plate and reduces the size of the surgical approach. It has the advantages of avoiding two problems that have been associated with the ulnar shortening osteotomy technique: ulnar nonunion and late fixation plate pain. The disadvantages of the wafer technique are that it cannot be used with patients with more than 4-mm ulnar-plus variance and it does not have the added effect of stabilizing the distal ulna.

The technique of ulnar shortening osteotomy that we use has a number of advantages: It is technically straightforward, shortening can be measured accurately, and skeletal fixation is rigid enough for early motion postoperatively. Its main disadvantage is that the incision is long. Use of a six-hole AO DC plate with the AO tension device produces good compression at the osteotomy site. There have been no nonunions with our compression plate technique. Late plate pain is uncommon and, when it does occur, responds well to plate removal. Plates are not taken out for at least 1 year after the osteotomy.

The amount of shortening needed is calculated based on the experimental studies of Palmer and Werner (10). In neutral-ulna variance the radiocarpal joint bears approximately 82% of compressive load, with the remaining 18% being transmitted through the ulnocarpal joint. In Palmer and Werner's study, shortening the ulna to 2.5-mm ulna-minus variance reduced ulnocarpal force transmission to 4%. At operation we shorten the ulna to between 2.0-mm and 2.5-mm ulna-minus variance. It is important to obtain accurate intraoperative neutral posteroanterior radiographs to assess the amount of shortening being achieved. The use of the fluoroscan imager has helped greatly as it allows multiple images to be obtained quickly. Radiographs need to be taken with the osteotomy closed but without definitively attaching the plate, in case adjustments are needed. We previously used a mandibular reduction clamp to hold the osteotomy temporarily while the radiograph was made (13). The AO tension device is more efficient, especially if a lot of shortening is needed.

In the early stages of transverse osteotomy use, nonunions were common. A variety of osteotomy techniques have been described to try to minimize this and other problems. The chevron osteotomy cuts the bone in a V-shaped manner. This increases surface contact area for bone healing, prevents rotation, and reduces the risk of angulation. The step-cut osteotomy allows for accurate measurement of shortening, prevents rotational malalignment, and can be fixed with interfragmental screws. The oblique osteotomy enables fixation to be achieved with a lag screw and neutralization plating. In the past, interosseous wires, compression screws, and metal plates have been used for internal fixation. Modern fixation techniques have led to much more predictable outcomes.

## RECOMMENDED READING

1. Boulas, H. J., Milek, M. A.: Ulnar shortening for tears of the triangular fibrocartilaginous complex. *J. Hand Surg.*, 15A: 415–420, 1990.
2. Bowers, W. H.: Distal radioulnar joint arthroplasty: the hemiresection-interposition technique. *J. Hand Surg.*, 10A: 169–178, 1985.
3. Chun, S., Palmer, A. K.: The ulnar impaction syndrome: follow-up of ulnar shortening osteotomy. *J. Hand Surg.*, 18A: 46–53, 1993.
4. Epner, R. A., Bowers, W. H., Guilford, W. B.: Ulnar variance: the effect of wrist postioning and roentgen filming technique. *J. Hand Surg.*, 7: 298–305, 1982.

5. Feldon, P., Terrono, A. L., Belsky, M. R.: Wafer distal ulna resection for triangular fibrocartilage tears and/or ulna impaction syndrome. *J. Hand Surg.*, 17A: 731–737, 1992.
6. Fernandez, D. L., Jupiter, J. B.: Malunion of the distal end of the radius. In: *Fractures of the Distal Radius*, edited by D. L. Fernandez, J. B. Jupiter, Springer-Verlag, New York, pp. 263–315, 1996.
7. Friedman, S. L., Palmer, A. K.: The ulna impaction syndrome. *Hand Clin.*, 7: 295–310, 1991.
8. Linscheid, R. L.: Ulnar lengthening and shortening. *Hand Clin.*, 3: 69–79, 1987.
9. Moy, O. J., Palmer, A. K.: Ulnocarpal abutment. In: *The Wrist: Diagnosis and Treatment*, vol 11, edited by W. P. Cooney, R. L. Linscheid, J. M. Dobyns, Mosby, St. Louis, pp. 773–787, 1998.
10. Palmer, A. K., Werner, F. W.: Biomechanics of the distal radioulnar joint. *Clin. Orthop.*, 187: 26–35, 1984.
11. Ranawat, C. S., DeFiore, J., Straub, L. R.: Madelung's deformity and end result study of surgical treatment. *J. Bone Joint Surg.*, 53A: 772–775, 1975.
12. Rayhack, J. M., Gasser, S. I., Latta, L. L., Ouellette, E. A., Milne, E. L.: Precision oblique osteotomy for shortening of the ulna. *J. Hand Surg.*, 18A: 908–918, 1993.
13. Richards, R. S., Bowen, C. V. A.: Recessional ulna osteotomy: use of reduction forceps for intra-operative radiography and plate application. *J. Hand Surg.*, 18: 56–57, 1993.
14. Segalman, K. A., Yahiro, J., DaSilva, M.: Complications of ulnar shortening osteotomies. Presented at the 54th meeting of the American Society for Surgery of the Hand, Boston, 1999.
15. Watson, H. K., Ryn, J., Burgess, R. C.: Matched distal ulnar resection. *J. Hand Surg.*, 11: 812–817, 1986.

# 25

# Darrach Procedure

Leonard K. Ruby and Charles Cassidy

## INDICATIONS/CONTRAINDICATIONS

Although early reports emphasized the sequelae of acute trauma, particularly dislocation (4), as the primary reason for ulnar head resection, present indications are somewhat different. Indications include the patient with rheumatoid arthritis who has intractable pain at the distal radioulnar joint (DRUJ); the rheumatoid or nonrheumatoid patient with uncorrectable deformity due to subluxation of the DRUJ with or without extensor tendon ruptures (1), and the nonrheumatoid patient who has painful arthritis of the DRUJ. More controversial indications include limited forearm rotation, DRUJ instability, and ulnar carpal impingement. In some patients, decreased forearm rotation may not be symptomatic or may be treated more effectively with forearm osteotomy. Instability usually is not improved by ulnar head excision and may be worsened. Therefore, in our opinion, radioulnar instability is a relative contraindication to ulnar head resection. Ulnar carpal abutment may be treated more effectively by ulnar shortening osteotomy.

Over the last few years, emphasis has shifted to preserving as much ulnar shaft length as possible to minimize radioulnar impingement (5) (Fig. 1). Some authors have felt that the ulnar head is important in maintaining the ulnar carpal ligaments, as it acts as a buttress, preventing carpal migration ulnarly and palmarly. These authors would consider total ulnar head resection to be contraindicated in situations in which ulnar translocation is likely to occur, such as in rheumatoid arthritis (Fig. 2). This point remains controversial. A recent long-term retrospective study (11) of patients with rheumatoid arthritis following distal ulna resection suggests that ulnar translocation is due more likely to progression of the rheumatoid disease, whereas ulnar stump impingement is due to excessive resection.

Because persistent pain after ulnar head resection (which may be secondary to instability of the ulnar remnant) is a common problem, many authors have described various procedures to stabilize the ulnar remnant. To date, none has demonstrated consistently successful long-term results. To prevent this problem, Bowers (3) has described his modification of ulnar head resection in which only a

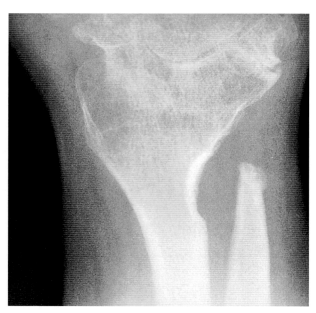

**FIGURE 1.** Patient with symptomatic ulnar stump impingement on radius status post-ulnar head resection and radiocarpal fusion.

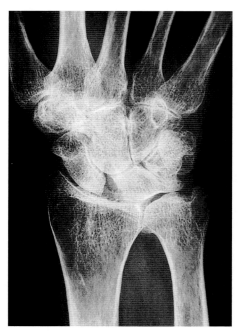

**FIGURE 2.** Ulnocarpal impaction in a patient with rheumatoid arthritis. Ulnar translocation is evident and may be exacerbated by distal ulna resection. In such an instance, radiolunate or total wrist arthrodesis should be performed in conjunction with the distal ulna resection.

portion of the distal ulna is removed, leaving intact the radioulnar and ulnar carpal ligaments as well as the triangular fibrocartilage attachment to the ulnar styloid base in an effort to preserve stability of the remaining ulna. He also described interposing tendon, muscle, or dorsal capsule in the resected area. He labeled this procedure the *hemiresection interposition arthroplasty* (see Chapter 27).

Watson (12) described a further modification of distal ulnar resection in 1985 and 1992, for which he coined the phrase *matched distal ulnar resection*. In his procedure, although the ulnar styloid and most of the head of the ulna are removed, an attempt is made to preserve ulnar length to the level of the radial articular surface and to taper the ulnar shaft for a distance of 5 to 6 cm into the shape of a pencil tip. This shape presents no bony surface for impingement on the radius or the ulnar carpus and exposes maximum cancellous bone so that the ulnar carpal ligaments can reattach to the ulnar remnant. Both techniques are reasonable alternatives to the method of distal ulna resection described in this chapter.

In 1990, the senior author (Ruby) reported on the results of an extensor carpi ulnaris (ECU) tenodesis to stabilize the ulnar stump (9). The early results were encouraging. However, the observation that the tenodesis eventually attenuated in some of the patients led him to develop the pronator quadratus interposition arthroplasty. This is our currently preferred technique for stabilizing the distal ulna (10). The rationale for the interposition of the pronator quadratus is three-fold: Interposition material is placed between the ulnar stump and the radius; the direction of pull of the pronator is such that it will tend to depress the ulna or elevate the radius to keep the two bones in more physiologic alignment; and the repair tends to stabilize the ECU over the distal ulna. Of interest, Kapandji, in his original paper, described placing the pronator quadratus between the resected ulna stump and the distal end of the ulna in an effort to prevent regrowth of the resected ulna (8).

## PREOPERATIVE PLANNING

Symptoms referable to the DRUJ include dorsoulnar wrist pain, weakness, and loss of forearm rotation (primarily supination). On examination, the distal ulna may be prominent dorsally. Tenderness is present at the dorsal aspect of the DRUJ. Pain may be elicited by compression of the radius against the ulna or with palmar displacement of the ulnar head. Increased translation of the ulnar head with respect to the radius may be noted. Patients with arthritis or incongruity of the DRUJ may present with crepitance or a click on active or passive rotation of the forearm.

Plain radiographs of the wrist are performed after the method of Epner et al (7); posteroanterior and lateral views are obtained with the shoulder at 90° abduction, the elbow at 90° flexion, and the forearm and wrist at neutral. In subtle cases, computed tomography may be helpful to demonstrate radioulnar subluxation or arthritis. These scans should include several cross-sectional views at the level of the DRUJ of both wrists in full pronation, neutral forearm rotation, and full supination. The symptomatic side must be compared to the normal side.

Once the surgeon has decided to perform a distal ulna resection arthroplasty of the DRUJ, it should be determined whether to do this as an isolated or combined procedure. In the case of the nonrheumatoid patient, an isolated procedure is often done so that the skin incision can be placed over the distal ulna. In the case of the rheumatoid patient, an isolated procedure is seldom done; a more extensive exposure is usually desirable. This means placing the skin incision obliquely over the radiocarpal joint with extension to the DRUJ (12).

## SURGERY

Position the patient with the arm outstretched on the standard hand table; internally rotate the shoulder and pronate the forearm as necessary to present a dorsal surface to the surgeon (Fig. 3). In common with most procedures on the dorsum of

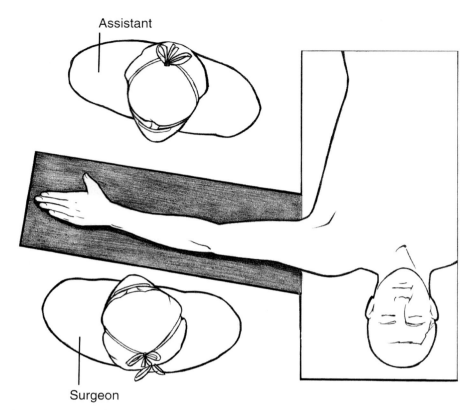

**FIGURE 3.** Position the patient supine with the arm outstretched on the standard hand table. The surgeon is toward the head of the patient, with the assistant on the axillary side.

the hand and wrist, the surgeon is near the head of the patient with the assistant on the axillary side. Prep and drape the upper extremity in standard sterile fashion with a pneumatic tourniquet about the proximal arm. If ulnar head resection is the sole procedure being performed, make a longitudinal incision over the distal ulna between the ECU tendon sheath and the extensor digiti quinti (EDQ) tendon sheath (Fig. 4). Elevate the skin flaps, being careful to identify and protect the dorsal sensory branch of the ulnar nerve, which is one finger-breadth distal to the ulnar head (Fig. 5). Continue the incision through the extensor retinaculum and the dorsal capsule of the DRUJ to the level of the bone. Expose the ulnar head subperiosteally beginning at the flare and proceeding proximally for a distance of 4 to 5 cm of the ulnar shaft (Fig. 6).

Perform the osteotomy at the metaphyseal flare using an oscillating saw, beveling the osteotomy toward the radius and dorsally. Trim the edges of the bone with a rongeur such that when the radius is brought from full pronation to full supination there is no prominence of the ulna that is likely to impinge on the radius.

Next, detach the pronator quadratus insertion on the palmar aspect of the ulna for its full distance of 4.5 to 7.0 cm (Fig. 7). This maneuver is facilitated by using a #64 Beaver blade followed by 1/2-in. and 3/8-in. curved osteotomes. It is important when performing this maneuver to include as much of the tendon (for insertion) and the periosteum at the edge of the pronator quadratus as possible for later reattachment. Pass the muscle flap between the radius and ulnar shafts through the interosseous space and suture dorsally over the ulnar shaft to the radial aspect of the ECU tendon sheath. Attempt to suture this edge as tightly as possible and imbricate it in an effort to prevent dorsal subluxation of the ulna remnant. Use 2–0 absorbable suture material in figure-of-eight or horizontal mattress fashion.

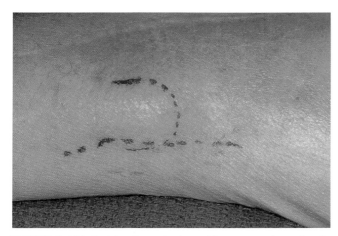

**FIGURE 4.** Skin incision is marked out. Ulnar stump is outlined.

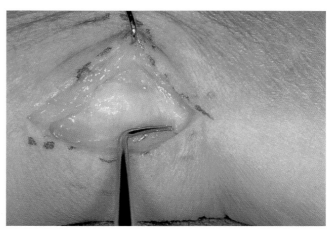

**FIGURE 5.** Skin incision is made. Dorsal sensory branch ulna nerve is identified and protected.

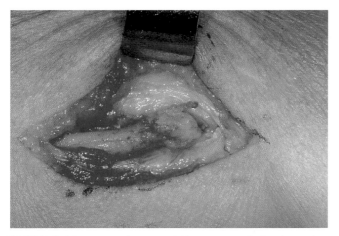

**FIGURE 6.** Ulna stump is exposed. Extensor carpi ulnaris tendon sheath is seen palmar; ulnar and pronator quadratus are not mobilized yet.

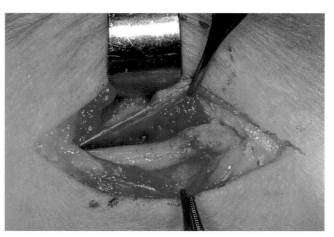

**FIGURE 7.** Ulna stump is trimmed. Pronator quadratus is mobilized and brought up between the radius and ulna.

There are three techniques that facilitate this maneuver (Fig. 8): The surgeon can place the sutures with the forearm in pronation, tying them with the forearm in supination; an assistant can depress on the ulna shaft while the surgeon sutures and ties; or the surgeon can work with the forearm in supination. We prefer the first approach, which is the easiest of the three techniques.

Use any available DRUJ capsule or extensor retinaculum to reinforce the repair. Skin closure is routine. A dressing is applied and the limb is placed in a U-shaped, above-elbow plaster splint with the forearm in 45° of supination and the wrist in neutral. The digits are free from the metacarpophalangeal joints distally.

## POSTOPERATIVE MANAGEMENT

Elevate the arm for 2 to 4 days, and encourage finger and shoulder motion. Remove sutures at 2 weeks postoperatively; care must be taken to keep the forearm in the 45° supinated position to prevent the pronator flap from separating from the ECU tendon sheath. A long-arm cast is placed with the forearm supinated 45° for an additional 2 to 4 weeks. After the above-elbow cast is removed, the limb is placed in a short-arm splint and the patient is encouraged to actively

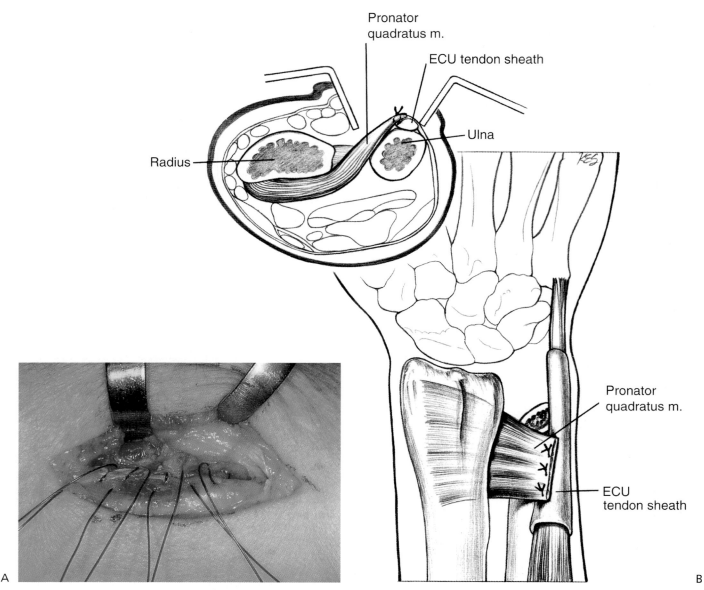

**FIGURE 8.** **A** and **B:** Pronator quadratus is sutured to the edge of the extensor carpi ulnaris tendon sheath. ECU, extensor carpi ulnaris.

supinate, pronate, and perform elbow extension exercises. Begin light strengthening exercises at the same time. Our therapy program usually includes the patient visiting the hand therapist three times per week. By 3 months, the patient should have nearly full forearm rotation without significant pain. Although there are no published studies that definitively answer the question of what one can expect in ultimate grip strength, we consider 70% to 75% of the normal side to be a good and achievable result.

## COMPLICATIONS

The most important problem is ulna stump instability and associated symptomatic impingement on the radius (2). As previously noted, this complication can be minimized by limiting the resection to the metaphyseal flare (6), careful tapering of the ulna resection margin, and adequate pronator quadratus bulk interposition. Rupture of the digital extensors over the ulnar stump is infrequent, and should be prevented by ensuring that the dorsal edge of the stump is smooth throughout the full arc of forearm rotation. Another potential complication is damage to the dorsal sensory branch of the ulnar nerve, although this has not occurred in our practice.

## ILLUSTRATIVE CASE FOR TECHNIQUE

A 41-year-old, left-hand–dominant engineer presented with pain and instability in the left wrist. He initially injured his left wrist 4 years earlier when a log fell and he attempted to catch it, sustaining a twisting injury to his left wrist. He recovered from this incident but reinjured the wrist 2 years later when pushing a large boulder. He then developed intermittent numbness in the little ring finger and ulnar-sided wrist pain.

He underwent ulnar head resection but his symptoms (ache, weakness, and a grating sensation) became worse after activity. He was able to work as an engineer but had more difficulty writing, and was very limited in participating in strenuous activities, as well as his hobbies, carpentry and shooting.

On examination he had full flexion, extension, supination, and pronation but there was an audible and palpable grating sensation in the left wrist with rotary movement. He had pain in all positions of the hand and wrist, but especially at the extremes of supination and pronation and upon compression of the forearm bones radius to ulna. Grip strength was 110 lb on the right and 85 lb on the left. Radiographs at that time showed a resection of the ulnar head without obvious erosions of the radius.

We elected to perform a revision of the ulna head resection with a pronator quadratus interposition. After general anesthesia, the left upper extremity was prepped and draped in standard sterile fashion with a tourniquet about the proximal arm. Skin incision was made through the old incision, which was on the dorsal ulnar aspect of the wrist, and extended proximally and distally between the fifth and sixth extensor compartments to provide adequate exposure of the ulnar remnant.

Intraoperatively there was a moderate amount of scar tissue over the ulnar remnant. The remnant itself was irregular in shape and had osteophytes where it had been impinging on the ulnar aspect of the radius. At this point the ulnar remnant was tailored for a distance of 2 cm into a point so as to present no prominence to the radius in pronation, neutral, or supination. The pronator quadratus insertion on the palmar aspect of the ulnar remnant was mobilized and brought between the ulna and radius through the interosseous space and sutured to the sheath of the ECU tendon using 2–0 polyglycolic suture. The wound was irrigated thoroughly, closed in layers, dry sterile dressing was applied, and a sugar-tong splint applied in the neutral position.

The patient's dressing and cast were changed, and sutures removed at 2.5 weeks. At 4 weeks a removable short-arm splint was applied, and he began supination and flexion/extension exercises—pronation was not allowed. At 6 weeks mobilization was discontinued, and he began strengthening exercises as well as pronation. At 3 months he had no pain. He had full motion and grip strength that was the same as on his normal side. He was able to play golf and perform all of the activities that he had been able to do before surgery.

## RECOMMENDED READING

1. Backdahl, M.: The caput ulnae syndrome in rheumatoid arthritis: a study of the morphology, abnormal anatomy and clinical picture. *Acta Rheumatol. Scand.*, 5: 1–75, 1963.
2. Bell, M. J., Hill, R. J., McMurtry, R. Y.: Ulnar impingement syndrome. *J. Bone Joint Surg.*, 67: 126–129, 1985.

3. Bowers, W. H.: Distal radioulnar joint arthroplasty: the hemiresection interposition technique. *J. Hand Surg.*, 10A: 169–178, 1985.
4. Darrach, W.: Anterior dislocation of the ulna. *Ann. Surg.*, 56: 802–803, 1912.
5. DiBenedetto, M. R., Lubbers, L. M., Coleman, C. R.: Long term results of the minimal resection Darrach procedure. *J. Hand Surg.*, 16A: 445–450, 1991.
6. Dingman, P. V. C.: Resection of the distal end of the ulna ("Darrach operation"); an end result of thirty-four cases. *J. Bone Joint Surg.*, 34A: 893–900, 1952.
7. Epner, R. A., Bowers, W. H., Guiltard, W. B.: Ulna variance: the effect of wrist positioning and roentgen filming technique. *J. Hand Surg.*, 7: 298–305, 1982.
8. Kapandji, I. A.: The Kapandji-Sauve operation. Its techniques and indications in non-rheumatoid diseases. *Ann. Chir. Main*, 5: 181–193, 1986.
9. Leslie, B. M., Carlson, G., Ruby, L. K.: Results of extensor carpi ulnaris tenodesis in the rheumatoid wrist undergoing a distal ulna excision. *J. Hand Surg.*, 15A: 547–551, 1990.
10. Ruby, L. K., Ferenz, C. C., Dell, P. C.: The pronator quadratus interposition transfer: an adjunct to resection arthroplasty of the distal radioulnar joint. *J. Hand Surg.*, 21A: 60–65, 1996.
11. Van Gemert, A. M. L., Spauwen, P. H. M.: Radiological evaluation of the long term effects of resection of the distal ulna in rheumatoid arthritis. *J. Hand Surg.*, 19B: 330–333, 1995.
12. Watson, H. K., Gabuzda, G. M.: Matched distal ulna resection for posttraumatic disorders of the distal radioulnar joint. *J. Hand Surg.*, 17A: 724–730, 1992.
13. Weil, C., Ruby, L. K.: The dorsal approach to the wrist revisited. *J. Hand Surg.*, 11: 911–912, 1986.

# 26

# Salvage of the Failed Darrach Procedure

Jeffrey A. Greenberg and William B. Kleinman

Excision of the entire distal ulna (seat, pole, and distal metaphysis) is a procedure used to decompress the painful ulnocarpal and distal radioulnar joints. By definition, the Darrach procedure (4) sacrifices the load-bearing seat of the ulna. Load transfer from the hand to the forearm passes through the seat, which also serves as the fulcrum for forearm rotation (7,11). Whereas many patients who have lower demands on their upper extremities do well functionally after Darrach resection, patients with higher demand can experience debilitating mechanical symptoms after removal of the distal ulna. Appropriate patient selection and meticulous intraoperative and postoperative care minimize the number of patients with poor clinical outcomes. Symptomatic radioulnar mechanical impingement (manifested by locking, catching, and erosion of the medial radial cortex) or excessive dorsal translational instability ("winging") can occur nevertheless (1) (Fig.1).

Salvage of the failed symptomatic Darrach resection is difficult. In addition to ulna-sided wrist pain and impaired hand function, secondary occupational and psychosocial hardships may develop (1,5). Many soft tissue reconstructive procedures have been designed to overcome instability or impingement following resection of the distal ulna, but employment of any of these procedures is difficult, particularly with respect to the availability of soft tissue for reconstruction.

If a Darrach resection of the distal ulna has been performed and fails, failure may be due to a variety of causes, including excessive bony resection; insufficient soft tissue structures remaining to tether the distal ulna stump; and postsurgical scarring or absence of usable bone and soft tissue. A variety of soft tissue and bony procedures have been described in recent years, each directed at management of these complications (2,3,6,8,13,15–17).

After distal ulna resection, anatomic bony alignment of the two bones of the forearm through a full arc of pronosupination cannot be maintained. Impingement of the radiocarpal unit against the ulna may occur as the interosseous space is allowed to progressively narrow. Muscle forces crossing the interosseous

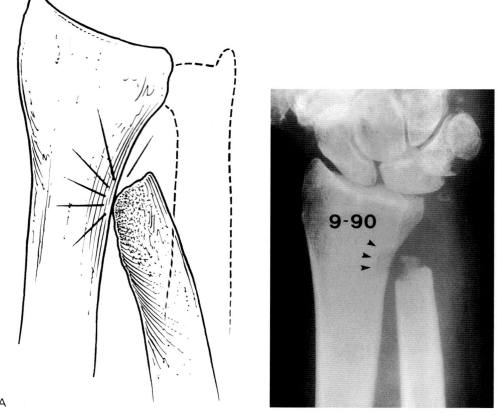

**FIGURE 1. A:** This figure illustrates radioulnar collapse, narrowing, and impingement of the resected ulna against the medial radius. **B:** Radiography of a wrist with symptomatic radioulnar impingement following distal ulna resection reveals that reactive bone at the distal ulna stump has developed. Scalloping of the medial cortex of the radius (*arrowheads*) is demonstrated.

space tend to accentuate convergence of the two forearm bones. After distal ulna resection, the pronator quadratus (PQ), normally a dynamic stabilizer of the distal radioulnar joint (DRUJ), actually becomes a strong deforming force, propagating impingement. In addition, normal elasticity and the contractile force of the two first dorsal compartment tendons (which obliquely span the interosseous space from medial to lateral) contribute to radioulnar impingement in the absence of DRUJ bony stability. Finally, loss of the stabilizing effect of the triangular fibrocartilage complex and associated ulnocarpal soft tissue stabilizers allows translation of the distal ulna with forearm rotation, promoting accentuated instability.

Clearly, symptomatic impingement following Darrach resection is a multifactorial problem caused by static loss of bone as well as soft tissue elements, accentuated by dynamic muscular forces. In an effort to avoid the creation of a functionally devastating one-bone forearm, many creative reconstructive procedures have been devised in an attempt to alleviate symptoms. These options utilize tendon transfers (alone or in combination), osteotomies, capsuloplasties, and combinations of these procedures.

Our approach to the problem uses a two-tendon, three-component reconstruction developed by the senior author (12), and is successfully used to salvage that small percentage of patients seen in clinical practice who have post-Darrach symptomatic impingement or winging. The approach is specifically designed to address post-Darrach winging (dorsopalmar translational instability), as well as painful mechanical radioulnar impingement.

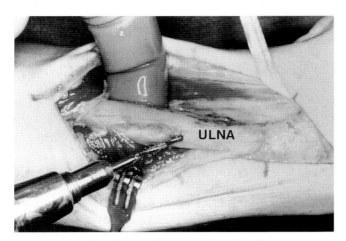

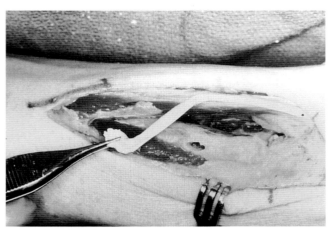

**FIGURE 2.** In this photograph, the patient's hand is to the right, left is proximal, and dorsal is toward the top. The previously prepared distal ulna is prepared for acceptance of the tendon transfer by reaming the medullary canal and creating a dorsal exit hole 1.5 cm proximal to the revised distal ulna osteotomy.

**FIGURE 3.** The harvested extensor carpi ulnaris tendon (held in forceps) has been left attached distally. Proximally, it has been divided with enough length maintained to allow passage through the medullary canal, exiting dorsally to be sewn to itself, and to the intact 50% extensor carpi ulnaris.

## SURGERY

Approach the long, remaining proximal stump of the resected distal ulna through the interval between the extensor carpi ulnaris (ECU) and flexor carpi ulnaris (FCU) tendons, along the line of the linea jugata. Take care to preserve the periosteal sleeve along the medial border of the distal ulna. Revise any irregularity or bony overgrowth of the end of the stump; remove any bony prominence that has developed while the ulna was impinging along the medial cortex of the radius. Maximum length, however, should be preserved. Remove as well any new bone that may have developed; it is essential to make certain that the entire DRUJ is decompressed. Prepare the distal ulna stump for intramedullary reception of the split-ECU tendon transfer by reaming the medullary canal with a side-cutting burr. Create an exit hole at the dorsomedial border, 1.5 cm proximal to the revised distal osteotomy (Fig. 2). Harvest half of the ECU from proximal to distal, and leave it attached within the still-intact sixth dorsal compartment fibroosseous tunnel. Harvest enough proximal length to allow the tendon to be passed into the medullary canal, out the exit hole, and back on itself in woven fashion (Fig. 3). It is critical to avoid destabilizing the fibroosseous canal of the deep sixth dorsal compartment. Tensioning and anchoring of the ECU are delayed until later in the procedure.

Attention is turned next toward harvesting the PQ. Flex the patient's elbow to 90°. Have an assistant support the forearm so that the fingers are towards the ceiling, with the arm on the hand table. Isolate the ulna insertion of the PQ and strip it from the volar surface of the distal ulna. It is essential to harvest as much tendon of insertion as possible; this usually is accomplished best with a small strip of periosteum. This material provides excellent additional soft tissue for anchoring the PQ to the *dorsum* of the ulna, directly into the preserved medial periosteum. Next, cut the interosseous membrane with Metzenbaum scissors, sufficiently proximal to allow transfer of the PQ easily through the interosseous space to the dorsum of the distal ulna (Fig. 4).

Use a laminar spreader to reestablish and maintain anatomic separation between the radius and ulna; confirm separation by fluoroscopy. With neutral forearm rotation maintained and a normal interosseous space radiographically confirmed, stabilize the radioulnar relationship with two divergent (or convergent) 0.062-in. K-wires. Place them proximal to the proximal border of the PQ so

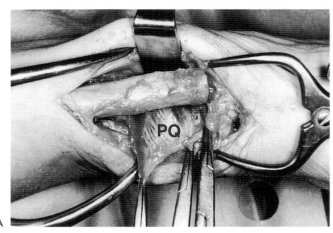
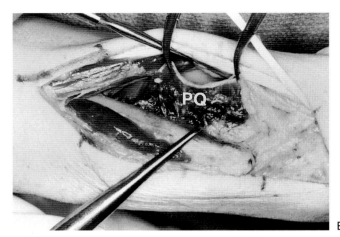

**FIGURE 4.** Harvesting of the pronator quadratus (PQ). **A:** The PQ has been detached from its insertion and is held by hemostats volar to the distal ulna. **B:** The PQ has been brought through the interosseous space and is now resting dorsal to the distal ulna.

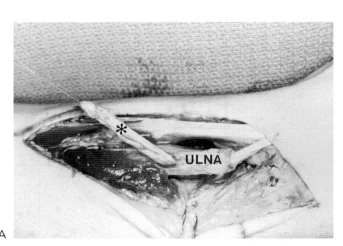
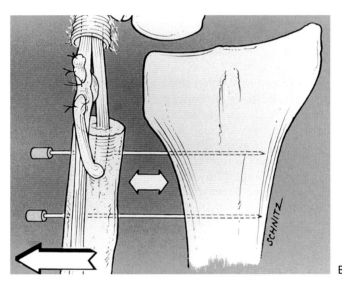

**FIGURE 5. A:** The extensor carpi ulnaris tendon (*asterisk*) has been passed through the distal medullary canal and out through the dorsal exit hole. **B:** The distal end of the tendon then is sutured to itself under the appropriate tension with multiple nonabsorbable sutures.

that they will not impede interosseous transfer of this muscle. Support the hand-fore-arm unit in 5° to 10° of ulnar deviation, and tension the ECU transfer. Pass the tendon through the distal end of the ulna, bring it out through the dorsal exit hole, and weave it in antegrade fashion into the intact remaining 50% of ECU. Suture it to itself with multiple nonabsorbable sutures (Fig. 5). Then transfer the PQ through the interosseous space, carry it dorsally over the distal ulna, and suture it to the residual medial periosteum of the ulna (Fig. 6). In those cases in which the soft tissue peri-osteal sleeve is deficient, secure the PQ to the distal ulna with suture anchors (Fig. 7).

After routine wound closure apply a long-arm, plaster-reinforced, bulky com-pressive dressing. Maintain the initial postoperative dressing for 2 weeks. At that time, remove the skin sutures and apply a long-arm cast. Remove the cast and K-wires at the end of the sixth postoperative week. Begin therapy exercises, consisting of active, active-assisted, and passive wrist, forearm, and elbow range-of-motion exercises at 6 weeks; use with interval short-arm splinting for comfort.

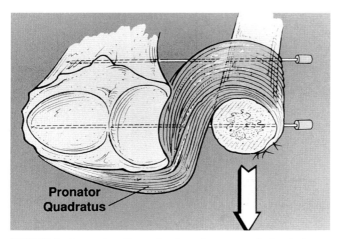

**FIGURE 6.** Reconstruction prior to extensor carpi ulnaris transfer. The distal radioulnar relationship has been stabilized by two divergent K-wires; the pronator quadratus has been transferred to the dorsal ulna through the interosseous space.

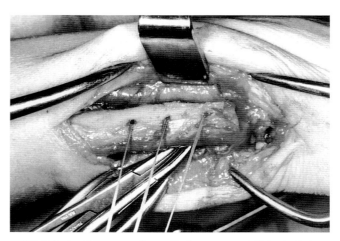

**FIGURE 7.** In this example, soft tissue was deficient. Suture anchors were required in the distal ulna to facilitate attachment of the transferred pronator quadratus.

## DISCUSSION

Although a variety of reconstructive procedures have been advocated to treat the symptomatic failed Darrach distal ulna resection, in general there is a paucity of literature regarding salvage of the failed Darrach; comparison among the many small series of clinical cases is difficult. Each published series contains a limited number of clinical cases and advocates a different approach to the painful, unstable distal ulna stump following Darrach resection.

Goldner and Hayes (6) described treatment of 50 patients for post-Darrach instability using a partial ECU tenodesis. Incorporation of a tenodesis with a distal ulna resection was reported by Tsai (15), who used 50% of the ECU; Hui and Linscheid (8) incorporated 50% of the FCU as an ulnotriquetral ligament augmentation for DRUJ instability. Neither group of authors used tenodesis for salvage of a failed Darrach resection. Breen and Jupiter (3) combined a partial ECU and FCU tenodesis to stabilize the unstable distal ulna in their series of eight patients; three were used as salvage for a failed Darrach. Good results were achieved in two of five patients in Tsai and Stillwell's report (16), in which a partial FCU tenodesis was utilized. Palmaris longus was the tendon of choice for stabilization in Noble and Arafa's report (13). Blatt's palmar capsulodesis (2) uses the volar DRUJ capsule, incorporated at the time of initial distal ulna resection. A variety of uses of the PQ have been advocated as well (10,12,14). Review of the literature on salvage of the failed Darrach reveals that many options exist, utilizing a variety of soft tissues (e.g., extensors, flexors, or ulnocarpal capsule) and even bone (17) for salvage reconstruction.

The success of our technique relies on the use of three components that separately address each facet of instability and impingement (Figs. 8, 9):

1. The PQ origin is detached from the palmarmedial ulna and transferred through the interosseous space to the dorsomedial aspect of the ulna. This substantial modification of Johnson's technique (9,10) serves multiple purposes. First, PQ tenotomy eliminates a strong deforming force; second, transferring the origin of the PQ from palmarmedial to dorsomedial provides a secure palmar-oriented dynamic tenodesis. Passing it through the interosseous space reduces the tendency of the distal ulna stump to wing. The transfer changes the "angle of attack" of the PQ, tethering the ulna palmarly and retarding the propensity for dorsal

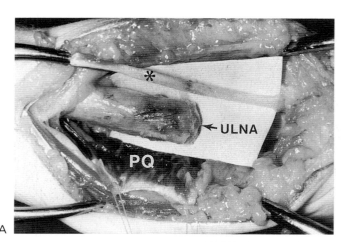

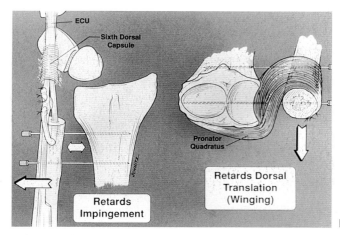

**FIGURE 8. A:** An intraoperative photograph demonstrating the soft tissue components of the reconstruction. Dorsally, the extensor carpi ulnaris (ECU) tendon is held by the forceps (*asterisk*); the released pronator quadratus (PQ) tendon remains volar to the distal ulna, tagged with sutures prior to dorsal intramedullary transfer. **B:** A diagrammatic representation of the reconstruction; each element of the reconstruction addresses an individual component of symptomatic distal ulna impingement and winging seen with failed Darrach resections.

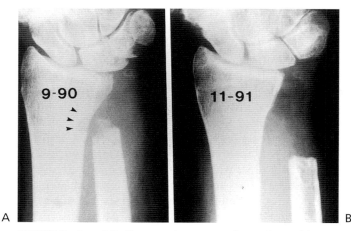

**FIGURE 9. A and B:** Comparative x-rays of a patient with symptomatic impingement demonstrating maintenance of a corrected radioulnar relationship 14 months following the combined reconstruction.

ulnar instability. Finally, the transferred muscle-tendon unit serves as interpositional material, further helping to prevent impingement of the resected distal ulna against the medial border of the radius.

2. Longitudinal ECU tenodesis to a point just proximal to the fibroosseous canal of the sixth dorsal compartment gives additional support to the unstable distal ulna stump and retards its tendency to translate medially toward the radius. Only half of the ECU is used; its fibroosseous canal and the linea jugata are left intact. A longitudinal tenodesis therefore is established using the remaining intact partial tendon of the ECU, just proximal to the unviolated, semirigid fibrous tissue of the sixth dorsal compartment.

3. The appropriate relationship between the distal radius and ulna is maintained securely by two divergent (or convergent) percutaneously placed 0.062-in. K-wires until soft tissue healing has occurred. Stability then can be maintained independently of the hardware.

## RECOMMENDED READING

1. Bell, M., Hill, R., et al.: Ulnar impingement syndrome. *J. Bone Joint Surg.*, 67B: 126–129, 1985.
2. Blatt, G.: Capsulodesis in reconstructive hand surgery. *Hand Clin.*, 3: 81–102, 1987.
3. Breen, T., Jupiter, J.: Extensor carpi ulnaris and flexor carpi ulnaris tenodesis of the unstable distal ulna. *J. Hand Surg.*, 14A: 612–617, 1989.
4. Darrach, W.: Partial excision of the lower shaft of the ulna for deformity following Colles' fracture. *Ann. Surg.*, 57: 764–765, 1913.
5. Field, J., Majkowski, R., et al.: Poor results of Darrach's procedure after wrist injuries. *J. Bone Joint Surg.*, 75B: 53–57, 1993.
6. Goldner, J., Hayes, M.: Stabilization of the remaining ulna using one-half of the extensor carpi ulnaris tendon after resection of the distal ulna. *Orthop. Trans.*, 3: 330–331, 1979.
7. Hagert, C. G.: The distal radioulnar joint in relation to the whole forearm. *Clin. Orthop.*, 275: 56–64, 1992.
8. Hui, F., Linscheid, R.: Ulnotriquetral augmentation tenodesis: a reconstructive procedure for dorsal subluxation of the distal radioulnar joint. *J. Hand Surg.*, 7: 230–236, 1982.
9. Johnson, R.: Muscle-tendon transfer for stabilization of the distal radioulnar joint. *J. Hand Surg.*, 10A: 437, 1985.
10. Johnson, R.: Stabilization of the distal ulna by transfer of the pronator quadratus origin. *Clin. Orthop.*, 275: 124–129, 1992.
11. Kleinman, W., Graham, T.: Distal ulnar injury and dysfunction. In: *Surgery of the Hand and Upper Extremity*, edited by C. Peimer, McGraw-Hill, New York, pp. 667–709, 1996.
12. Kleinman, W., Greenberg, J.: Salvage of the failed Darrach procedure. *J. Hand Surg.*, 20A(6): 951–957, 1995.
13. Noble, J., Arafa, M.: Stabilization of the distal ulna after Darrach's procedure. *Hand*, 15: 70–72, 1983.
14. Ruby, L., Ferenz, C., et al.: The pronator quadratus interposition transfer: an adjunct to resection arthroplasty of the distal radioulnar joint. *J. Hand Surg.*, 21A: 60–65, 1996.
15. Tsai, T., Shimizu, H., et al.: A modified extensor carpi ulnaris tenodesis with the Darrach procedure. *J. Hand Surg.*, 18A: 697–702, 1993.
16. Tsai, T., Stillwell, J.: Repair of chronic subluxation of the distal radioulnar joint (ulnar dorsal) using flexor carpi ulnaris tendon. *J. Hand Surg.*, 9B: 289–294, 1984.
17. Watson, H., Brown, R.: Ulnar impingement syndrome after Darrach procedure: treatment by advancement lengthening osteotomy of the ulna. *J. Hand Surg.*, 14A: 302–306, 1989.

# Hemiresection Interposition Technique of Distal Radioulnar Joint Arthroplasty

## William H. Bowers

## INDICATIONS/CONTRAINDICATIONS

Any consideration of arthroplasty as a procedure of choice presumes that restorative approaches are not feasible or have been unsuccessful. The procedure cannot succeed if the triangular fibrocartilage complex (TFCC) is not a functional structure, which most often occurs in severe rheumatoid arthritis or in traumatic disruption of the TFCC that cannot be reconstructed.

The hemiresection interposition technique (HIT) is useful in the early-to-middle disease state of rheumatoid arthritis. A patient with a painful swollen distal radioulnar joint (DRUJ) with impending or early descent of the ulnar carpus is an ideal candidate. The TFCC must be structurally intact, or isolated deficiencies in its attachment to the radius, ulnar, or carpal bones must be reconstructible. An ulnocarpal synovectomy is an integral part of the procedure. Late rheumatoid problems are best approached by the technique of radiolunate arthrodesis coupled with a modified Darrach procedure as described by Chamay et al. (2).

The basic HIT excels in patients with osteoarthritic DRUJ. Care is given to resect all osteophytes and to avoid stylocarpal impingement.

For patients with the ulnocarpal impingement syndrome, consider first a Feldon wafer resection (5), if radioulnar disease is not present and the variance is less than 2-mm positive, or a Milch shortening osteotomy (4,8), if radioulnar disease is not severe and shortening will not produce radioulnar incongruity (e.g., the variance is not greater than 3 mm to 4 mm and a competent sigmoid notch is present). In cases with a distorted sigmoid notch, the Milch shortening osteotomy will probably fail. Evaluate by preoperative, narrow-cut computed tomography (CT). In cases where the variance is greater than 2 mm and radioulnar disease is present, or the sigmoid is incompetent, HIT, with appropriate modifications such as interposition or shortening, is an excellent procedure.

If instability is the major problem and pain is a less prominent feature, first consider the possibility of restoring stability by reattachment or reconstruction of the deficient ligamentous structure or by correcting an underlying translational malalignment of the radius and/or ulna by osteotomy of the shafts. On occasion, correcting proximal/distal length discrepancies is effective in correcting length and translational malunions. If the unstable articulation has produced significant articular damage, the reconstructive attempt is abandoned and replaced by an arthroplasty, using HIT. HIT excels if its basic precepts are followed. Again, the operation does not restore stability but substitutes less painful instability and thereby improves rotation and grip strength.

Rotational contractures with radioulnar disease at the center of the problem should not be underestimated. The contracture may have had its genesis in a radioulnar dislocation or eventuated from positions of immobilization after fractures or ligamentous injuries of the wrist. The articular surfaces may be incompetent in the range of motion that has been lost and the cartilage may be soft and poorly attached. Dystrophic changes may be present in soft and osseous tissue. A full preoperative evaluation includes (a) comparison roentgenographic views of both forearms and wrists in several positions of rotation; (b) comparison CT scans of the DRUJ and carpal area in pronation, neutral, and supination; (c) arthrogram; and (d) bone scan.

Preoperative hand therapy includes baseline grip and motion evaluation and at least 2 months of therapy to reach a preoperative plateau of improvement as well as to acquaint the patient and therapist with rehabilitation methods and techniques. The problem should not be approached operatively if therapy has not been tried.

The operative approach considers the information gained in the workup. The author uses a dorsal and palmar exposure with capsular contracture release as a primary goal before HIT is considered. If palmar capsular release and limited interosseous division in the distal one-third of the forearm coupled with lysis of dorsal and palmar ulnocarpal capsular adhesions is successful in achieving the rotation desired and the articulation is structurally competent, the forearm is immobilized in the desired range (usually 50° to 60° of supination) and therapy begun again at 2 weeks after surgery. If the articulation is deficient (chondromalacia, malformed, arthritic, unstable, markedly positive ulnar-plus variance), HIT with appropriate shortening is added. In some cases, the Darrach procedure may be required. Therapy may be prolonged. Pain control is essential, initially using patient-controlled analgesia followed by appropriate oral medications. Transcutaneous nerve stimulation may be helpful as therapy begins.

Unreconstructible fractures entirely within the articular dome provide an instance where radioulnar incongruity is likely. The hemiresection technique may provide an early return to a functional state.

The basis for the procedure is a functionally adequate or reconstructible TFCC. Otherwise, no advantage over a Darrach (3) or its modifications is realized. Only in cases of severe arthritis is a modified Darrach coupled with a radiolunate arthrodesis a good primary choice.

The hemiresection arthroplasty is not used in arthritic or traumatic ulnar carpal translation. The procedure cannot restore stability in an unstable painful radioulnar joint. It simply substitutes less painful instability.

A correctly planned and performed arthroplasty using HIT may not alone restore rotation in a long-standing contracture. Loss of flexibility in the ulnocarpal ligament complex as well as the interosseous membrane may preclude a good result even if the central arthritic obstruction is removed. This poor result can be anticipated in patients with a dystrophic forearm such as occasionally seen following trauma.

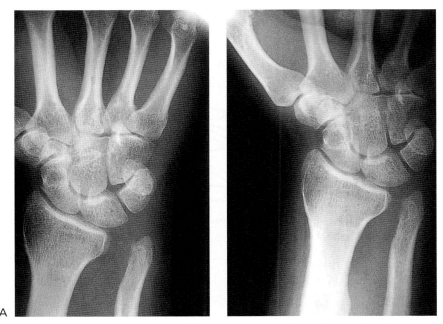

**FIGURE 1.** Relaxed **(A)** and grip **(B)** views after a hemiresection arthroplasty. Note the narrowing of space between radius and ulna with grip.

## PREOPERATIVE PLANNING

Range of motion is recorded, along with grip and pinch studies. Patients should be introduced to the hand therapists who will work with them postoperatively. It is also useful for patients to view the splints and therapy that might be used.

Radiographs include a posteroanterior series in 0° rotation (neutral) consisting of a relaxed, a fist-compressed, and an ulnar deviated view. In addition, a good 0° rotation lateral radiograph is required. CT scans are occasionally helpful but are most often used when reconstructive rather than arthroplasty alternatives are being considered. The radiographs are used to assess the likelihood of postoperative stylocarpal impingement. The usual maximum migration of radius and ulna toward each other after this procedure is 0.75 cm (i.e., in a grip view, the measured width from radial styloid to ulnar styloid is 0.75 cm less than before operation) (Fig. 1). If on a preoperative posteroanterior roentgenographic view in neutral rotation the amount of narrowing allows the styloid to come within 2 mm of the ulnar deviated carpus, one may anticipate impingement of the ulnar styloid on the carpus after the procedure. Some provision must be made for this postoperative biomechanical certainty to avoid the complication known as *stylocarpal impingement*. Reasonable modifications to consider are shortening of the ulnar shaft with subsequent compression osteosynthesis or interposition of bulk (anchovy) to the radioulnar joint void.

Arthrograms and arthroscopy are rarely indicated except when triangular fibrocartilage (TFC) function is suspect. If one is considering HIT following trauma, a DRUJ arthrogram will on occasion show a TFC detached from the ulna. While this must be addressed, it is usually obvious at surgery.

## SURGERY

The keys to exposure are the extensor carpi ulnaris (ECU) and extensor digiti minimi tendons (Fig. 2B). The ulnar head invariably can be made to present

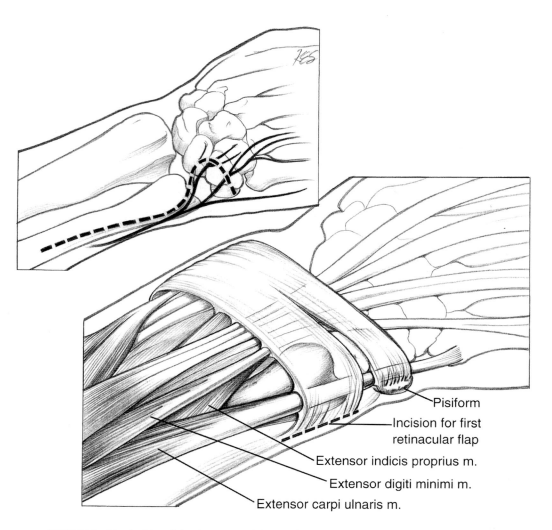

**FIGURE 2.** The incision **(A)** selection and design **(B)** of retinacular flaps. (Redrawn from Bowers, W. H.: The distal radioulnar joint. In: *Operative Hand Surgery*, edited by D. P. Green, Churchill Livingstone, New York, pp. 754–755, 1982, with permission.)

between these two tendons if the arm is pronated (Figs. 2B, 3). For exposure of the major portion of the ulnar articular surface, the procedure is begun in full pronation.

### Technique

The incision is begun laterally three finger-breadths proximal to the styloid along the ulnar shaft and curved gently around the distal side of the head of the ulna to end dorsally at midcarpus. For further distal exposure, the incision is curved back ulnarly.

The incision lies just dorsal to the dorsal sensory branch of the ulnar nerve, which is found and protected from vigorous retraction or pressure during the entire procedure (Fig. 2A). As the skin flaps are developed, dorsal veins are retracted rather than cut, if possible, and dissection is carried to the obliquely lying extensor retinacular fibers. Beneath the proximal border of the retinaculum the capsule of the ulnar head presents between the extensor digiti minimi and ECU (Fig. 3). A V-shaped portion of ulnar shaft disappears proximally between the deep-lying extensor indicis proprius muscle belly (Fig. 2B). The proximal and

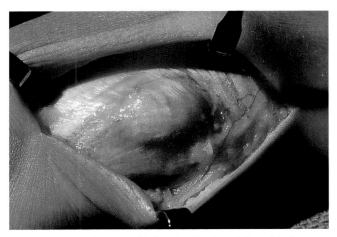

**FIGURE 3.** The rheumatoid distal radioulnar joint with forearm pronated prior to flap design.

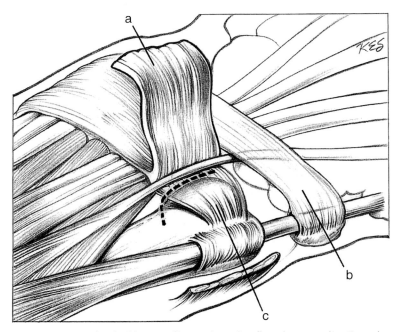

**FIGURE 4.** Capsular incision. a, first retinacular flap; b, second retinacular flap (if needed); c, capsular flap. (Redrawn from Bowers, W. H.: The distal radioulnar joint. In: *Operative Hand Surgery*, edited by D. P. Green, Churchill Livingstone, New York, pp. 754–755, 1982, with permission.)

ulnar half of the extensor retinaculum is reflected radially, uncovering the ECU and extensor digiti minimi tendons (Fig. 4). The base of this flap is the septum between the extensor digiti minimi and the extensor digitorum communis compartment. Take care not to enter the extensor digitorum communis compartment unnecessarily.

Retract the extensor digiti minimi, revealing the dorsal margin of the sigmoid notch of the radius and the TFC (Figs. 5, 6). Detach the capsule from the radius, leaving a 1-mm cuff for later repair. The capsule is then reflected toward the ulna, exposing the ulnar head for approximately 100° of its total convexity.

A small lamina spreader may be used to view the sigmoid notch. For better exposure of the underside of the TFC, the forearm should be brought to midrotation and a nerve hook or small right-angle retractor used to expose this area. Magnification is helpful in observing the pathologic changes in the TFC. To further

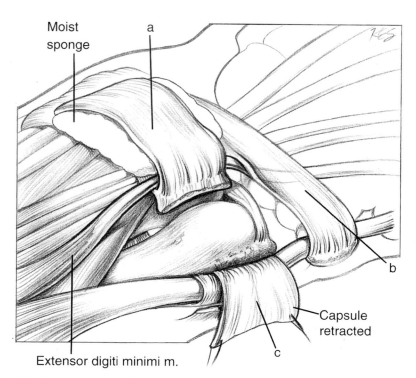

**FIGURE 5.** Exposure of joint. a, first retinacular flap; b, second retinacular flap (if needed); c, capsular flap. (Redrawn from Bowers, W. H.: The distal radioulnar joint. In: *Operative Hand Surgery*, edited by D. P. Green, Churchill Livingstone, New York, pp. 754–755, 1982, with permission.)

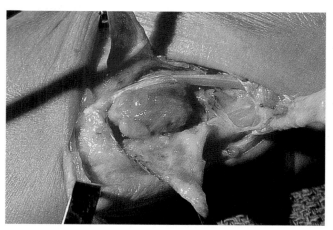

**FIGURE 6.** The proximal flap is radial, the distal flap ulnar, and the capsule is reflected, leaving the synovium of this rheumatoid joint exposed.

expose the TFC, both the extensor digiti minimi and ECU can be released from their retinacular compartments (Fig. 7). This is accomplished by reflecting the distal half of the extensor retinaculum toward the ulnar opposite to the first flap. The retinaculum is divided along the extensor digiti minimi septum; the base of the flap is the attachment of the ECU compartment nearest to the ulna. The ECU, where its groove is most pronounced, lies 1 to 2 mm ulnar to the attachment of the TFC. The ECU is fully released only if it is pathologically involved.

There is no need to enter the radiocarpal joint or expose the carpal surface of the TFC unless pathology is suspected therein. This is usually the case in rheumatoid

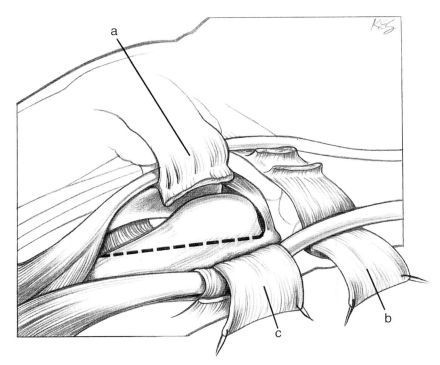

**FIGURE 7.** Entry into ulnar wrist. a, first retinacular flap; b, second retinacular flap; c, capsular flap. (Redrawn from Bowers, W. H.: The distal radioulnar joint. In: *Operative Hand Surgery*, edited by D. P. Green, Churchill Livingstone, New York, pp. 754–755, 1982, with permission.)

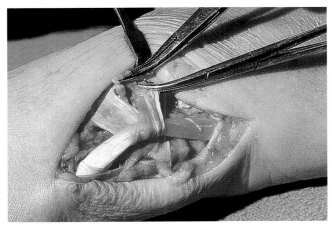

**FIGURE 8.** The extensor carpi ulnaris sling closure.

cases. The retinacular flaps are developed for exposure and to conserve tissue for dorsal stabilization of the ECU or augmentation of a deficient TFCC. If not needed for these purposes these flaps may be reattached, used for deep cover of the arthroplasty site, or excised. The ECU is *not* to be removed from its retinacular compartment if it is stable. Subperiosteal lateral reflection of the ECU compartment is possible and allows excellent exposure of the distal ulnar area with the assurance that when returned to its position it will reassume its stabilizing function. ECU stabilization is done only if it is displaced palmarly, as in rheumatoids, or if it is unstable in its compartment. In these instances, the ECU must be freed completely to its insertion on the fifth metacarpal. When the ECU is freed completely, the first proximal flap is used to create a sling to dorsally stabilize this tendon during closure (Fig.

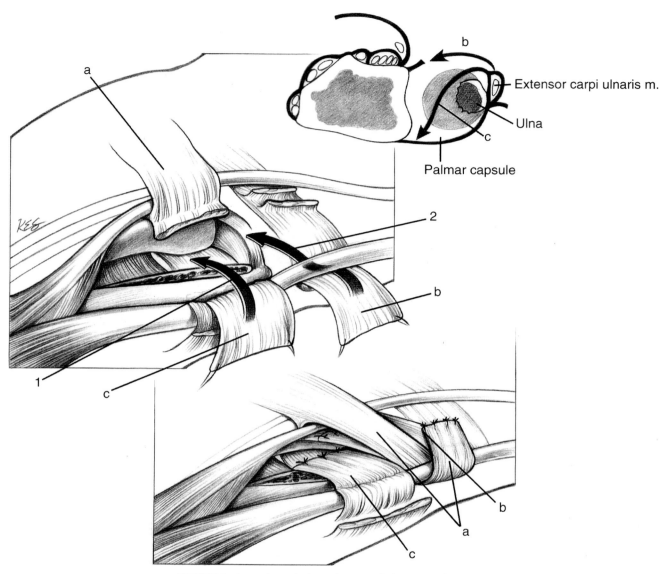

**FIGURE 9.** Resection of ulnar dome and closure. a, first retinacular flap; b, second retinacular flap; c, capsular flap. Arrows (1,2) show flap movement to final position. (Redrawn from Bowers, W. H.: The distal radioulnar joint. In: *Operative Hand Surgery*, edited by D. P. Green, Churchill Livingstone, New York, pp. 754–755, 1982, with permission.)

8). The flap is passed around the ECU and the distal end is sewn to the fourth compartment wall distal to its takeoff. This type of stabilization ensures a sling for the ECU rather than a noose, as would occur if the flap were sewn directly back to itself.

After development of the retinacular flaps, the capsule of the DRUJ is detached distally, radially, and proximally and turned to the ulnar side to expose the articular surface. A synovectomy is done and the ulnar articular surface and subchondral bone are removed with small osteotomes and rongeurs (Figs. 9–11). Inadequate bone removal is the likely technical error at this point. Large osteophytes around the sigmoid notch and all the bone of the ulnar head under the articular surface must be removed (Figs. 12, 13). The remaining shaft and styloid axis should be round in cross section and resemble a tapering 1-cm–diameter dowel (Fig. 14). A palmar portion of the head is particularly easy to miss in this resection.

The now-vacant DRUJ cavity is cleaned of the remaining synovium and the TFC is carefully inspected. Lesions of the TFCC will be readily apparent. If centrally

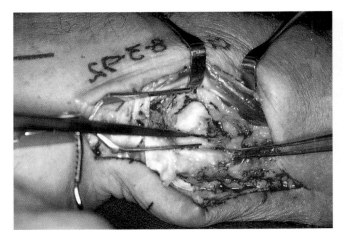

**FIGURE 10.** The osteotome is used to resect the ulnar head in a patient with traumatic arthritis. Arrow points to the wrist.

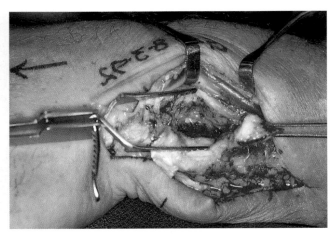

**FIGURE 11.** The forceps hold the resected head. Arrow points to the wrist.

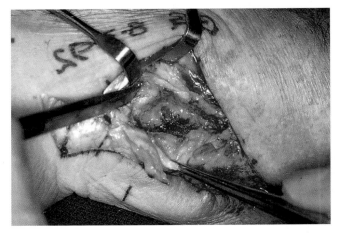

**FIGURE 12.** The osteotome is used to resect osteophytes about the sigmoid notch in the same cases shown in Figures 10 and 11.

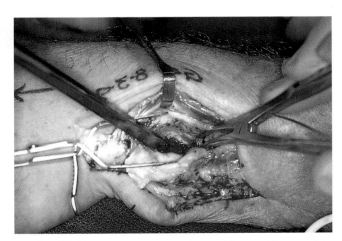

**FIGURE 13.** The osteotome is again used to provide complete resection of bone about the ulnar shaft after removal of the ulnar head. Arrow points to the wrist.

located, these perforations or tears are now functionally inconsequential, because resection of the ulnar head has accomplished full decompression. Repair of a central perforation is unnecessary. The lesions may be cleaned with minor débridement.

The decision about shortening, begun preoperatively with the radiographic impressions about possible stylocarpal impingement, is completed at this point. The radial and ulnar shafts are compressed and rotated with the wrist ulnarly deviated. A portable low-emission radiograph unit such as that shown in Figure 15 is helpful. If there is any question about impingement of the ulna on the carpus, the ulna is shortened. Shortening may be done through the metaphyseal base at the site of the previous ulnar head or by more proximal osteotomy with plating such as the Milch shortening (Fig. 16). If the former site is chosen, fixation is accomplished with a compression interosseous wire loop (Figs. 17, 18). If the preoperative assessment is equivocal (zero variant + or −1 mm) and the intraoperative assessment is equivocal, then the radioulnar space may be maintained by placing a carefully made ball of tendon or muscle about the size of the resected dome into the vacant DRUJ cavity (Figs. 19, 20), stabilizing it to the dorsal and palmar capsules with a few sturdy sutures. The tissue may be obtained from the palmaris longus (preferred), ECU, or flexor carpi ulnaris. This added interposition bulk seems

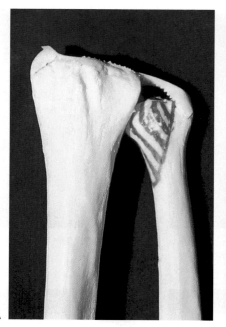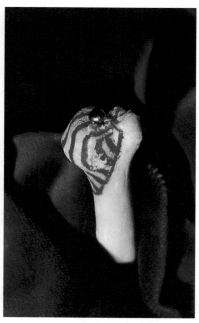

**FIGURE 14.** **A** and **B:** Graphic illustrations of the extent of resection required in the hemiresection interposition technique.

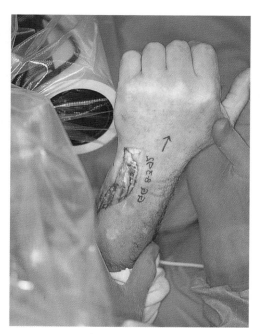

**FIGURE 15.** The wrist, after resection, is evaluated with a portable radiograph unit for stylocarpal impingement or for the need for additional bone resection.

to adequately counter radioulnar shaft approximation and therefore obviates stylocarpal impingement in the borderline cases (zero variant + or −1 mm). If no shortening is required, the capsule is the only material interposed (Figs. 9, 21).

The skin is closed without subcutaneous sutures. I use small silicone vessel loops in the incision as drains and do not release the tourniquet prior to dressing.

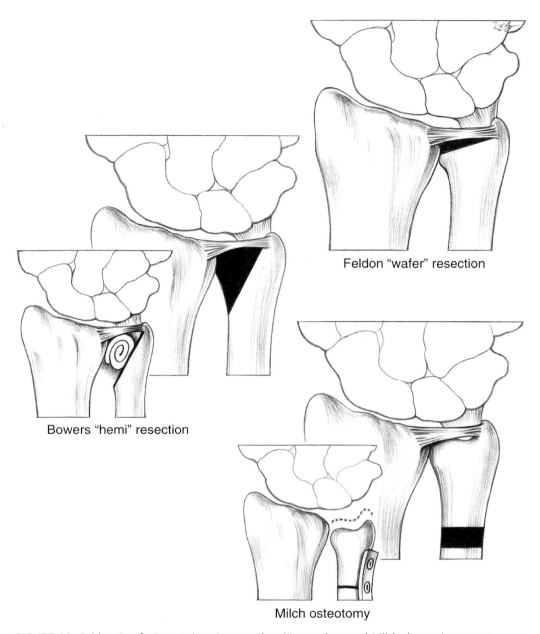

Feldon "wafer" resection

Bowers "hemi" resection

Milch osteotomy

**FIGURE 16.** Feldon "wafer" resection, Bowers "hemi" resection, and Milch shortening osteotomy. (Redrawn from Bowers, W. H.: Distal radioulnar joint arthroplasty. *Clin. Orthop. Rel. Res.*, 275: 104–109, 1992, with permission.)

## POSTOPERATIVE MANAGEMENT

If shortening is not done, the postoperative dressing is a short-arm bulky dressing with dorsopalmar plaster reinforcement. Finger motion is encouraged, whereas forearm rotation is neither encouraged nor discouraged. At 10 days, sutures are removed and a wrist splint is applied for 2 more weeks, allowing unrestricted rotation. If ulnar shortening is done in association with HIT, the initial plaster reinforcement splint goes above the elbow and, by supracondylar molding, limits forearm rotation to a few degrees. The postoperative dressing is converted to a short-arm cast with interosseous space molding at 2 weeks. This allows slightly more rotation and is removed 4 weeks later (at 6 weeks postoperatively).

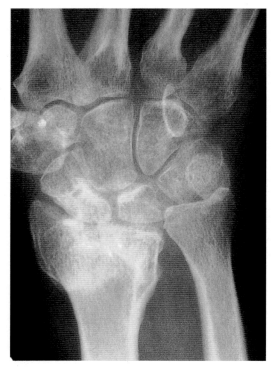

**FIGURE 17.** Severe settling of a radius fracture with ulnocarpal impingement. (See Case 2, text.)

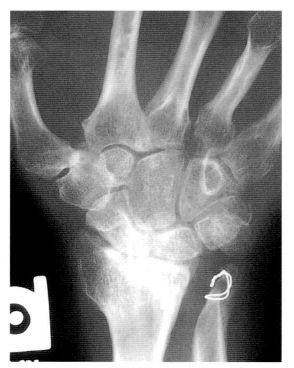

**FIGURE 18.** Radiograph following resection of head and adjacent shaft with osteosynthesis of the triangular fibrocartilage complex styloid to the shaft with a compression wire. (See Case 2, text.)

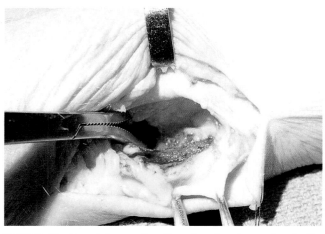

**FIGURE 19.** Remaining cavity after ulnar head resection in the rheumatoid patient shown in Figures 5–7.

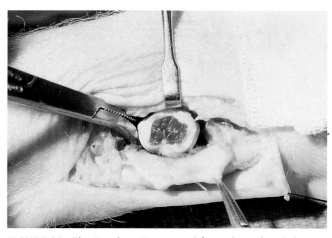

**FIGURE 20.** The "anchovy" prepared from the palmaris longus muscle tendon unit is inserted into the cavity as a means of preventing stylocarpal impingement in this rheumatoid patient.

A wrist splint is then used for the transition to full use over the next several weeks. The osteotomy, if done at the site of the ulnar head resection, usually heals in 6 weeks. If the resection is done at a shaft level and the forearm plate is used, this osteosynthesis must be protected until full healing. This is usually accomplished with an interosseous molded splint that allows wrist and elbow motion. This splint is shown in Figures 22 and 23.

I reported in 1985 (1) on 38 cases, 27 of which were rheumatoid. In its developmental stages, the procedure appeared very useful in this type of patient. In 1986, Watson et al. (10) reported on 44 cases (of which 34 were rheumatoid) treated by

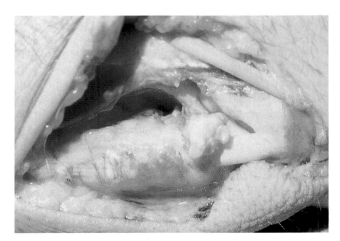

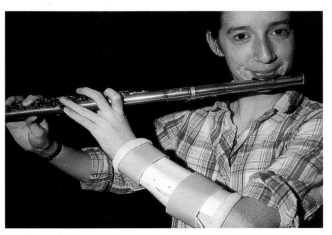

**FIGURE 21.** In this patient, no interposition bulk was required, and the capsule and retinaculum were both enfolded into the joint and sutured to the palmar capsule. This was the only interposition used.

**FIGURE 22.** The orthoplast forearm splint with interosseous molding. This allows wrist and elbow function but stabilizes the distal radioulnar joint after hemiresection interposition technique.

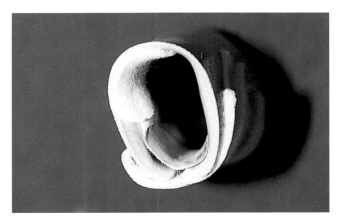

**FIGURE 23.** A cross section of the splint showing the pronounced interosseous molding required.

the "matched resection" technique—a procedure similar in technique and philosophy to HIT. Since these two initial reports, general awareness of DRUJ pathomechanics has increased dramatically and the procedure has found useful application in other types of patients. Minami et al. (9), Fernandez (6), and Imbriglia (7) have added their experience to the literature, and the combined series of 152 patients reflects the following diagnoses: 42% rheumatoid, 29% instability, 21% ulnocarpal impingement, 5% primary osteoarthrosis, and 3% a variety of other traumatic problems. Seventy-six percent were pain free and 24% had mild pain, better than preoperatively. Two percent of patients were treated with reoperation for stylocarpal impingement and were later classified as pain free. There were patients with poor results. There were none with instability; range of motion was reported variously as good to excellent.

My current expectations are similar. Patients normally require 3 to 4 months to achieve full range and comfort. Due to the mechanical alterations in joint structure, it is unlikely that the post-hemiresection DRUJ could hold up to maximum loaded rotational stress without problems. I do not advise or expect the patient treated with HIT to return to the "heavy use" vocation or avocation. For example, patients can play golf or tennis but can rarely return to structural carpentry or steel working.

## COMPLICATIONS

1. *Stylocarpal impingement*: The procedure will fail if stylocarpal impingement is not anticipated and interdicted. If the articular surfaces are removed with sufficient bone to unload an abnormally loaded ulnar carpal articulation and avoid contact with arthritic or unstable radial and ulnar shafts in rotation, a biomechanical fact becomes clear. The normal articular dome provides a stable seat for the radius to ride in its rotational arc. The absence of this seat allows the two shafts to come closer together (especially in power grip). Some provision is made for this predictable postoperative biomechanical certainty to avoid the complication known as *stylocarpal impingement*. Reasonable modifications to consider are shortening of the ulnar shaft with subsequent compression osteosynthesis or interposition of bulk tissue (anchovy) to fill the radioulnar joint void.

2. *Restricted rotation or pain with rotation*: In the absence of stylocarpal impingement, one considers an inadequate resection of bone from the margins of the shaft or the sigmoid notch. A CT scan in three positions of rotation is helpful. The problems and the solution will usually be obvious.

3. *Fracture of the shaft*: This usually occurs with the patient who has exceeded the biomechanical limitations of the arthroplasty. This is not usually a disaster and may be treated as any fracture. I prefer an interosseous mold splint as shown in Figures 22 and 23. A pseudarthrosis is not necessarily a bad outcome if it is not painful.

## ILLUSTRATIVE CASES FOR TECHNIQUE

### Case 1

This patient has osteoarthritis of the DRUJ with painful rotation. The radioulnar incongruity is well seen in Figure 24. The variance is negative and a straightforward hemiresection was successful in restoring pain-free motion. In Figure 25 the

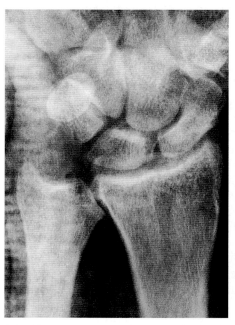

**FIGURE 24.** An osteoarthritic distal radioulnar joint with an ulnar gutter splint overlying the ulna.

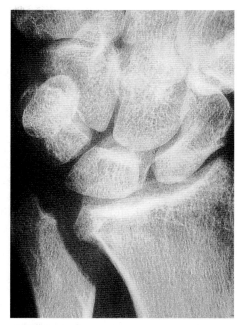

**FIGURE 25.** The patient has had a hemiresection interposition arthroplasty. A sigmoid osteophyte is noted.

postoperative appearance is shown. The sigmoid osteophytes should have been removed; however, in this case they did not interfere with the final good result.

### Case 2

In this patient, a severe distal radius fracture had healed with settling (Fig. 17). The major complaint was severe restriction of rotation and pain with grip loading. Although a wrist fusion was envisioned, HIT with shortening was planned in an attempt to restore better motion with decreased pain. The peripheral margins of the TFC were intact, although the central area was disrupted. This allowed a full resection of the head and the adjacent shaft with reattachment of the styloid to shaft preserving the function of the TFCC (Fig. 18). This provided stable and painless rotation. The patient was sufficiently satisfied after this initial procedure that no further operative procedure was required.

## RECOMMENDED READING

1. Bowers, W.: Distal radioulnar joint arthroplasty—the hemiresection interposition technique. *J. Hand Surg.*, 10A: 169, 1985.
2. Chamay, A., Santa, D. D., Vilaseca, A.: Radiolunate arthrodesis—factor of stability for the rheumatoid wrist. *Ann. Chir. Main*, 2: 5–17, 1983.
3. Darrach, W.: Partial excision of lower shaft of ulna for deformity following Colles' fracture. *Ann. Surg.*, 57: 764, 1913.
4. Darrow, J. C., Linsheid, R. L., Dobyns, J. H., Mann, J. M., Wood, M. B., Beckenbaugh, R. D.: Distal ulnar recession for disorders of the radioulnar joint. *J. Hand Surg.*, 10A: 482, 1985.
5. Feldon, P., Terrano, A. L., Belsky, M. R.: Wafer distal ulna resection for triangular fibrocartilage tears and/or ulna impaction syndrome. *J. Hand Surg.*, 17A: 731–737, 1992.
6. Fernandez, D. L.: Radial osteotomy and Bowers arthroplasty for malunited fractures of the distal end of the radius. *J. Bone Joint Surg.*, 10A: 1538, 1988.
7. Imbriglia, J.: The hemiresection interposition technique of distal radioulnar joint arthroplasty for the management of instability. Presented at the 43rd Annual Meeting of the American Society for Surgery of the Hand, Baltimore, Maryland, 1988.
8. Milch, H.: Cuff resection of the ulna for malunited Colles' fracture. *J. Bone Joint Surg.*, 23: 311, 1941.
9. Minami, A., Ogind, T., Minami, M.: Treatment of distal radioulnar disorders. *J. Hand Surg.*, 12A: 189, 1987.
10. Watson, A. K., Ryu, J., Burgess, R. C.: Matched distal ulnar resection. *J. Hand Surg.* 11A: 812, 1986.

# 28

# Matched Ulnar Resection Arthroplasty

Jeffrey Weinzweig and H. Kirk Watson

## INDICATIONS/CONTRAINDICATIONS

The distal radioulnar joint (DRUJ) is a complex structure that plays a significant role in permitting normal pronation and supination of the forearm, as well as facilitating normal function of the upper extremity. The articular surface of the ulna is a convex semicircle of 180° that opposes a concave radial sigmoid notch of 60° to 80°. Thus, at any position, 100° of ulnar articular surface is free from contact. Injury, destruction, dislocation, or subluxation of a portion of this articular surface is responsible for the clinical symptomatology seen with disorders of the DRUJ (Fig. 1) (1,2,4). A DRUJ affected by conditions such as degenerative arthritis, posttraumatic subluxation or dislocation, or rheumatoid arthritis, is often painful and causes loss of active rotation of the forearm (3,7). DRUJ subluxation or significant ulnar-positive variance may result in ulnar impaction syndrome as well, with substantial pain and diminished wrist function. The distal ulna with normal articular cartilage on both radius and ulna should be maintained if possible, employing lengthening, shortening, or stabilizing procedures in lieu of resection. The matched ulnar arthroplasty addresses the problematic DRUJ articular surface or untreatable malpositioned distal ulnar head and restores painless pronation and supination while preserving the triangular fibrocartilage complex and the ligamentous attachments of the distal ulna (Fig. 2) (5,6).

The success of the matched ulnar arthroplasty may be limited by concomitant carpal abnormalities, such as radiocarpal degenerative joint arthritis or carpal instability, but such an abnormality does not preclude the use of this technique for addressing disorders arising from the DRUJ or distal ulnar head. In addition, the matched ulnar arthroplasty is indicated in the patient with ulnar impingement on the radius following a Darrach resection. Salvage is possible by combining the matched ulnar resection with a step-cut ulnar lengthening (8).

The matched ulnar arthroplasty technique restores painless pronation and supination while preserving the full length of the ulna and structures crucial to stabil-

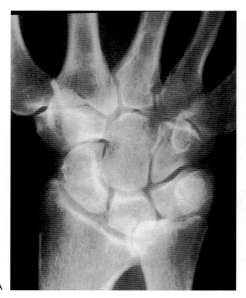
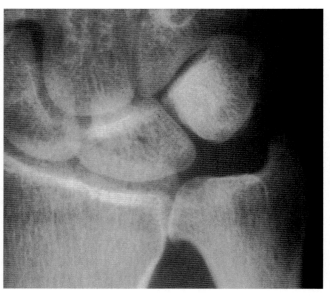

**FIGURE 1.** **A** and **B:** Complete destruction of the distal radioulnar joint is present, with no remnant cartilage and no potential for preserving the distal ulna. Matched ulnar arthroplasty is indicated.

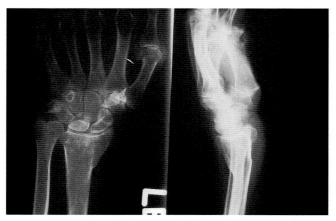

**FIGURE 2.** Dislocation or impaction and malalignment of this distal ulna most likely are managed best in this age group with a matched ulnar arthroplasty. The ulna is resected from the full pronation position to the full supination position of the radius. The resection is carried out such that the shape of the ulna matches the shape of the radius; it includes resection of the dorsal flare of the radius sulcus. It is not necessary to leave soft tissue attached, as the ulnar sling mechanism will reattach itself firmly to the broad cancellous ulnar surface. The sheath of the extensor carpi ulnaris can be left on the cortical portion of the ulna, but this is not necessary. It is important to leave the tip of the ulna at the level of the articular surface of the radius.

ity of the DRUJ without the need for soft tissue interposition (9,10). The resultant range of motion is nearly full and painless, and stability of the wrist and DRUJ is maintained. Impingement between the radius and ulna is rare, as the gap between them is equal and congruous throughout the full arc of pronation and supination. The matched ulnar arthroplasty is a reliable, predictable approach to the painful DRUJ. Patients with adequate cartilage on the distal half of the ulnar head may be treated with a modified DRUJ arthroplasty, without the need for a formal matched ulnar arthroplasty.

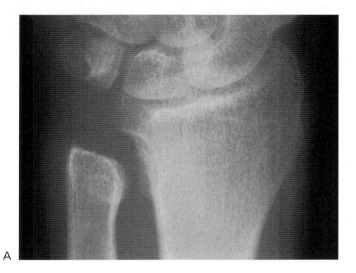

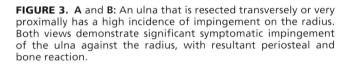

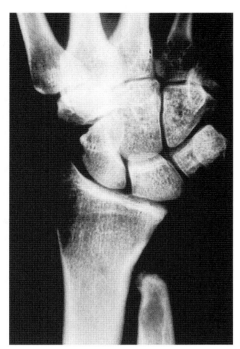

**FIGURE 3.  A** and **B:** An ulna that is resected transversely or very proximally has a high incidence of impingement on the radius. Both views demonstrate significant symptomatic impingement of the ulna against the radius, with resultant periosteal and bone reaction.

B

## PREOPERATIVE PLANNING

Preoperative evaluation of patients with abnormalities of the DRUJ and ulnar side of the wrist requires a focused physical examination and plain radiographic assessment. Patients usually present with complaints including generalized ulnar wrist pain (especially with attempted pronation and supination), loss of strength, and considerable restriction of motion. There may or may not be a specific history of previous wrist trauma.

Physical examination produces pain with radioulnar compression and demonstrates decreased pronation and supination. Clinical suspicion of an abnormality of the DRUJ or distal ulna is confirmed radiographically in many cases. Degenerative arthritis involving the DRUJ and abnormalities of the distal ulna, such as ulnar impaction and ulnar impingement, usually are detected on plain radiographs without the need for additional, or more invasive, radiologic studies (Fig. 3).

## SURGERY

To perform matched ulnar resection arthroplasty, position the patient supine and use standard positioning, prepping, and draping; use an upper-arm tourniquet. We generally do not administer perioperative antibiotics. The procedure is performed under general anesthesia in most cases, although regional block would be equally effective. With the arm fully abducted and pronated on the hand table, the surgeon can perform the procedure most comfortably seated on the cephalad side of the wrist.

### Technique

Approach the distal ulna through a longitudinal incision, approximately 4 cm in length, along the lateral aspect of the ulna, beginning at the level of the ulnar

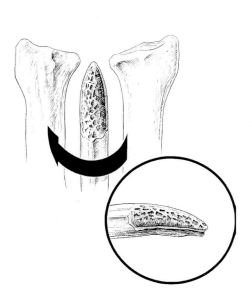

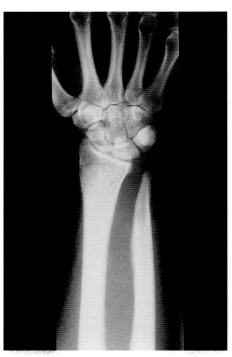

**FIGURE 4.** The alignment, position, and slope parallelism between the radius and the distal end of the ulna following matched ulnar arthroplasty are illustrated. This parallelism is maintained from full pronation to full supination.

**FIGURE 5.** After matched ulnar arthroplasty, the parallelism of surfaces between the radius and ulna is preserved throughout full pronation-supination. In addition, the tip of the ulna is maintained at the level of the articular surface of the radius. The preoperative radiograph for this patient is seen in Figure 1B.

head. Use spreading technique to preserve superficial veins as well as the dorsal branch of the ulnar nerve; continue the dissection down to the ulna.

The 180° arc of the ulna that is in contact with the radius from full pronation to full supination is resected in a long, sloping, convex curve, averaging 5 to 6 cm in length. This convex curve matches the contour of the opposing concave radius in three dimensions, thereby ensuring that there is no impingement during full pronation and supination of the forearm (Fig. 4). This resection is performed intraoperatively to verify the congruity of the opposing radial and ulnar surfaces. Once the head of the ulna has been resected, the ulna will shift toward the radius. This shift usually requires ulnar styloid resection, leaving the most distal tip of the resected ulna at or just proximal to the level of the articular surface of the radius (Fig. 5).

If the ulna impinges on the carpus in ulnar deviation, only the necessary minimal amount of distal ulna is resected to permit clearance. This resection is performed and periosteum and ligamentous attachments to the distal ulna may be maintained. However, it is not necessary to maintain attachments, as the ulnar sling mechanism will adhere to the cancellous ulna in any case. The 180° arc of posterior ulna cortex is maintained to the level of the articular surface of the radius.

The deep fascia of the extensor carpi ulnaris sheath remains attached to the periosteum of the ulna and contributes to the stabilization of the ulna during the healing process. The large cancellous surface of the resected distal ulna will adhere securely to the ulnar sling mechanism without the need for sutures or fixation. (The *ulnar sling mechanism* includes the ligamentous structures that begin at the ulnarmost aspect of the distal radius and continue to the ulnar [superficial] part of the extensor carpi ulnaris sheath. The triangular fibrocartilage complex and its palmar and dorsal reflections are included, as are the ulnotriquetral ligament, the ulnolunate ligament, and the DRUJ capsule.) Soft tissue interposition is not necessary. Close the skin incision and apply a bulky dressing, incorporating a plaster splint to immobilize the wrist. Since the elbow is not included, pronation and supination are not limited.

The radius sulcus joint presents two situations that can affect the outcome of a matched ulnar arthroplasty adversely (1). Occasionally the slope of the sulcus of the radius is reversed. When seen on a posteroanterior film, the proximal portion of the radius sulcus protrudes more ulnarward than the distal portion. Thus, the slope of the radius sulcus joint in this case may be considered to be directed from proximal ulnar to distal radial. When the joint is sloped in this fashion, the proximal portion of the sulcus joint must be removed with a rongeur to prevent its impingement on the ulna (2).

Flaring of the edges of the radius sulcus joint frequently occurs. These radial flares occur more commonly dorsally than palmarly and may be normal for a particular individual or represent secondary degenerative osteophytic formations. They can be palpated directly intraoperatively and may be significant. If they protrude ulnarward they should be removed with a rongeur to prevent impingement of the ulna on the palmar or dorsal flares at the extremes of supination or pronation, respectively.

## POSTOPERATIVE MANAGEMENT

Remove the bulky dressing and splint 7 days postoperatively; the wrist is mobilized completely.

## COMPLICATIONS

Few complications occurred after matched ulnar arthroplasty in 88 patients (97 wrists) over a 21-year period (9,10). The most common preoperative diagnoses were rheumatoid disease in 34 wrists (35%) and ulnar impaction syndrome in 25 wrists (26%). Additional diagnoses included degenerative disease of the DRUJ (four wrists), ulnar impingement following Darrach resection (three wrists), Colles' fractures (12 wrists), premature closure of the distal ulnar epiphysis following fracture (one wrist), DRUJ dislocation or subluxation (three wrists), and Madelung's deformity (two wrists).

A wound infection occurred in one patient, but it responded well to immobilization and antibiotic therapy. Three patients experienced symptoms of radioulnar impingement secondary to periosteal bone spur formation at the site of the previous ulnar head resection. These patients responded well to excision of the spurs. One patient required reoperation for removal of a neuroma *in situ* of the dorsal sensory branch of the ulnar nerve. Eight patients developed triquetral impingement ligament tear (11) a mean of 34 months after matched ulnar arthroplasty; two of these patients had undergone a concomitant ulnar step-lengthening osteotomy as well. All of these patients demonstrated excellent range of motion and were pain free following triquetral impingement ligament tear repair.

## MODIFIED DISTAL RADIOULNAR JOINT ARTHROPLASTY FOR DEGENERATIVE ARTHRITIS

Patients who demonstrate degenerative arthritis of the DRUJ but have adequate cartilage on the distal half of the ulnar head may be treated with a modified DRUJ arthroplasty without the need for a formal matched ulnar arthroplasty. Thirty to fifty percent coverage of the articular surface of the distal half of the ulnar head with adequate cartilage is necessary to obtain satisfactory results with this procedure.

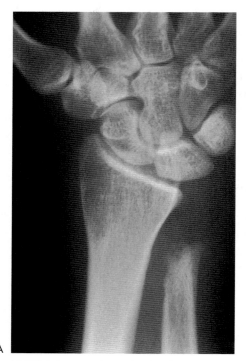
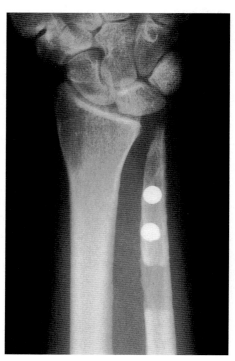

A

B

**FIGURE 6.   A:** A short ulna resulting in radial impingement produces a significantly symptomatic wrist in this female patient. **B:** The only adequate solution to this problem is a step-cut lengthening of the ulna to bring it up to the ulnar sling mechanism and to reshape the distal end of the ulna at the time of osteotomy to match the shape of the radius. In essence, the result is conversion from the ulnar resection to a matched ulnar arthroplasty. It is not necessary to reattach soft tissue to the distal ulna.

In these patients, a longitudinal dorsoulnar incision is used rather than a transverse incision, because a matched ulnar arthroplasty may be required in the future. Spreading technique is used to preserve the dorsal ulnar nerve and dorsal veins. The DRUJ capsule is opened proximally, as the degenerative arthritic process almost always occurs proximally with subsequent distal progression.

The proximal half of the articular surface of the ulna is typically devoid of cartilage with osteophyte formation and a hyperemic, eburnated appearance consistent with periostitis. A dental rongeur is used to remove the entire proximal articular surface while preserving the healthy cartilage on the distal half of the articular head of the ulna. This is performed for the entire articular circumference from full pronation to full supination of the radius on the ulna. The skin incision is closed and a bulky dressing is applied; 2 days after surgery, this dressing is removed and full mobilization is begun.

This modified DRUJ arthroplasty has been employed over the past 15 years with excellent results. All patients have maintained full pronation-supination and complete relief of symptoms on follow-up. None of these patients has required a subsequent matched ulnar arthroplasty.

## MATCHED ULNAR RESECTION FOR ULNAR IMPINGEMENT

Symptoms secondary to ulnar impingement, in which the distal end of a shortened ulna contacts or impinges on the radius during the range of pronation-supination, can be managed by performing a step-cut ulnar lengthening osteotomy followed by a matched resection. This problem is frequently seen as a consequence of an overzealous Darrach resection in which the remaining distal ulna is left without a support mechanism. In this situation, the unstable distal ulna is free to impinge on the radius. After appropriate lengthening and lag screw or plate fixation to restore the distal ulna to the level of the distal radius, a matched resection is performed in the manner described (Fig. 6).

## RECOMMENDED READING

1. Bell, M. J., Hill, R. J.: Ulnar impingement syndrome. *J. Bone Joint Surg.*, 67B: 126–129, 1985.
2. Black, R. M., Boswick, J. A., Wiedel, J.: Dislocation of the wrist in rheumatoid arthritis: the relationship to distal ulna resection. *Clin. Orthop.*, 124: 184–188, 1977.
3. Bowers, W. H.: The distal radioulnar joint. In: *Operative Hand Surgery*, 4th ed., edited by D. P. Green, R. N. Hotchkiss, and W. C. Pederson, Churchill Livingstone, New York, pp. 986–1032, 1999.
4. Darrach, W.: Anterior dislocation of the head of the ulna. *Ann. Surg.*, 56: 802–803, 1912.
5. Goncalves, D.: Correction of disorders of the distal radioulnar joint by artificial pseudoarthrosis of the ulna. *J. Bone Joint Surg.*, 56B: 462–464, 1974.
6. Goldner, J. L., Hayes, M. G.: Stabilization of the remaining ulna using one-half of the extensor carpi ulnaris tendon after resection of the distal ulna. *Orthop. Trans.*, 3: 330–331, 1979.
7. Minami, A., Ogino, T., Minami, M.: Treatment of distal radioulnar joint disorders. *J. Hand Surg.*, 12A: 189–196, 1987.
8. Watson, H. K., Brown, R. E.: Ulnar impingement syndrome after Darrach procedure: treatment by advancement lengthening osteotomy of the ulna. *J. Hand Surg.*, 14A: 302–306, 1989.
9. Watson, H. K., Gabuzdo, G. M.: Matched distal ulna resection for posttraumatic disorders of the distal radioulnar joint. *J. Hand Surg.*, 17A: 724–730, 1992.
10. Watson, H. K., Ryu, J., Burgess, R. C.: Matched distal ulnar resection. *J. Hand Surg.*, 11A: 812–817, 1986.
11. Watson, H. K., Weinzweig, J.: Triquetral Impingement Ligament Tear [TILT] syndrome. *J. Hand Surg.*, 24B: 350–358, 1999.

# PART X

# Rheumatoid Arthritis

# 29

# Synovectomy and Tendon Reconstruction

## Andrew L. Terrono and Lewis H. Millender*

## INDICATIONS/CONTRAINDICATIONS

Frequently performed operations for patients with rheumatoid arthritis affecting the digital extensor tendons and wrist joint are dorsal tenosynovectomy, wrist joint synovectomy, extensor tendon reconstruction, and reconstruction of the distal radioulnar joint (DRUJ). This chapter addresses the operative indications, surgical techniques, and expected outcomes of each of these procedures.

### Dorsal Tenosynovectomy

Dorsal tenosynovectomy is indicated for wrists with tenosynovitis that persists despite several months' adequate medical treatment, which includes systemic medications plus one or two steroid injections. An even more compelling indication is aggressive disease in a patient who has an enlarging mass despite adequate treatment. An absolute indication for surgery is a tendon rupture, because one rupture often foretells a second. Patients with mild disease under good control tolerate dorsal tenosynovitis well without tendon rupture, thus careful observation should be considered instead of surgery.

### Synovectomy

The indications for synovectomy remain controversial; no long-term studies have shown that this procedure changes the natural history of the disease. This is certainly true for the wrist joint, in which the surgeon's technical ability to carry

---

*Deceased.

out a complete synovectomy is limited because of the anatomic configuration of the joint.

The indications for synovectomy, therefore, are few. Wrist synovectomy is recommended for patients whose arthritis is under relatively good medical control and whose radiographs show minimal changes in the radiocarpal joint, but who continue to have isolated synovitis despite two to three steroid injections over a 6- to 9-month period. If other wrist surgery, such as dorsal tenosynovectomy or distal ulnar excision, is being considered and there is clinical evidence of radiocarpal synovitis, especially with pain, a synovectomy is performed even on patients whose radiographs reveal more advanced destruction.

Indications for isolated radioulnar synovectomy are more limited. Radioulnar joint synovitis causes destruction of the triangular fibrocartilage complex (TFCC) very early during the disease, leading to instability of the distal ulna with relation to the distal radius. Destruction of the TFCC is an indication for distal ulna excision with reconstruction of the DRUJ.

### Extensor Tendon Reconstruction

Tendon rupture necessitates extensor tendon reconstruction. Tendon ruptures are secondary to direct invasion, attrition, or ischemia. Most frequently, patients with dorsal tenosynovitis or caput ulnae syndrome (1) suddenly notice the inability to extend a single digit, usually one of the two ulnar digits. Sometimes when there is a rupture of the extensor digiti minimi (extensor digiti quinti) the patient may not discern any dysfunction or may note only that the control of the digit is not normal. Extensor pollicis longus (EPL) rupture, which occurs frequently, may go unnoticed until a physician discovers it.

When a tendon rupture occurs, prompt exploration, tenosynovectomy, and removal of osteophytes as needed are advisable to prevent additional tendon ruptures. When a rupture is detected on routine examination, treatment depends on the situation. Often, a ruptured extensor digiti minimi or ruptured EPL is seen without dorsal tenosynovitis and is secondary to attrition rupture. In such a case, when no functional impairment exists, no treatment is needed.

### Reconstruction of the Distal Radioulnar Joint

Involvement of the radioulnar joint by rheumatoid arthritis is one of the most frequent findings in the rheumatoid hand; it may cause significant disability. For this reason, distal ulna excision, with reconstruction of the triangular fibrocartilage and DRUJ, is a frequently indicated operative procedure.

The most compelling reason for surgery is a painful dislocated or subluxed distal ulna with limited rotation and tendon ruptures. Another indication is a dislocated distal ulna with persistent pain unresponsive to nonoperative treatment without extensor tendon ruptures. Painless limited rotation is a relative indication and surgery is recommended only if it impairs a patient's function. Minimal loss of rotation, especially pronation, is compensated for by shoulder abduction, and may not lead to functional impairment.

### Tendon Transfers to Restore Wrist Balance

Tendon transfers to restore wrist balance are indicated in patients undergoing dorsal wrist surgery who have a passively correctable radial deviation deformity. In these cases, the extensor carpi radialis longus (ECRL) tendon is transferred to the extensor carpi ulnaris (ECU) insertion. This transfer may be helpful in preventing further deformity when simultaneous metacarpophalangeal (MP) joint surgery (either extensor realignment or arthroplasty) or wrist synovectomy is performed (4).

## PREOPERATIVE PLANNING

Begin by asking the patient to describe all problems, including pain and functional deficits—specifically, what he or she cannot do but would like to be able to do.

Perform a physical examination of the entire upper extremity. Record active and passive range of motion of the digits, wrist, forearm, elbow, and shoulder. Seek out areas of tenosynovitis, synovitis, tenderness, and instability.

Take routine neutral posteroanterior, lateral, and oblique radiographs, including the wrist and hand, to evaluate the MP, radiocarpal, and distal radioulnar joints.

Because dorsal tenosynovitis is painless, its major clinical significance is its propensity to cause tendon rupture. The configuration of swelling is usually oblong along the direction of the extensor tendons and may move with the extensor tendons. Tenosynovectomy is performed to prevent tendon rupture.

Synovitis associated with rheumatoid arthritis usually causes pain that helps differentiate it from tenosynovitis. Radiocarpal synovitis may present with a painful dorsal wrist mass; the synovium, however, may not be palpable. Synovitis is suspected when flexion and extension cause pain and the radiocarpal joint is tender. There should not be a fixed deformity, and radiographs should show minimal changes. If there is a passively correctable radial deviation deformity, add an ECRL tendon transfer.

Synovitis involving the DRUJ invades the ulnar styloid, the ulnar head, and TFCC early in the disease, destroying the joint and the supporting structures. The DRUJ is tender and rotation is limited. Radiographs show only mild changes and extensor tendon function is intact.

### Extensor Tendon Surgery

The diagnosis of tendon rupture is made by the absence of the tenodesis effect, a difference between active and passive MP joint motion, and the inability to maintain a corrected position of digital MP joint extension, often with associated dorsal tenosynovitis. Seek out sources of attrition ruptures such as the distal ulna or Lister's tubercle of the radius. Evaluate the number of ruptures and sources for tendon transfer (extensor indicis proprius [EIP], wrist extensor if a simultaneous wrist fusion is performed, EPL if thumb fusion is performed), or graft (such as the palmaris longus). Passive MP joint motion should be good; if not, consider simultaneous MP arthroplasty. If the cause is attrition rupture on the distal ulna, perform reconstruction of the DRUJ simultaneously. Use radiographs to evaluate the patient for sources of attrition ruptures or a need for a simultaneous procedure (wrist fusion, DRUJ reconstruction, MP arthroplasty).

### Reconstruction of the Distal Radioulnar Joint

The DRUJ often has synovitis and is incongruous; it causes the patient to have pain with rotation and palpation. The distal ulna often is unstable, snaps during rotation, and is prominent. A supination deformity of the carpus that often is seen in conjunction with the final result of synovitis of the DRUJ is the caput ulnae syndrome (1), manifested by dorsal dislocation of the distal ulna, supination deformity of the carpus, and frequent tendon ruptures. Radiographs document these changes and are helpful in evaluating the wrist for ulnar translocation (Fig. 1). Often, there is a small shelf of bone supporting the lunate (Fig. 2). Sometimes this shelf of bone

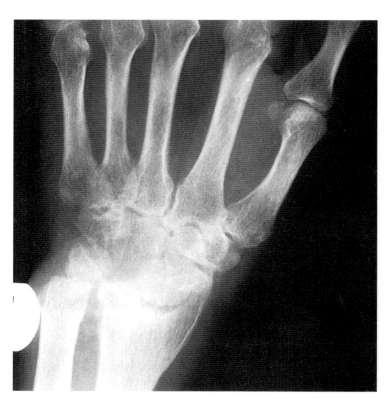

**FIGURE 1.** Radiograph showing ulnar carpal impingement with carpal erosion into the radius without ulnar translocation.

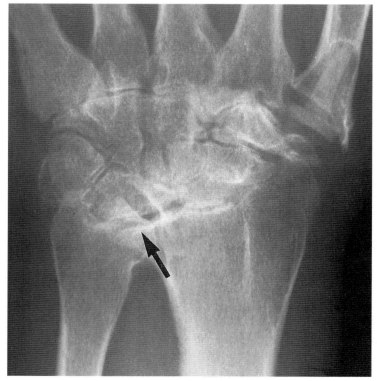

**FIGURE 2.** Preoperative radiograph showing a severely involved distal radioulnar joint. The lunate is ulnarly translocated, but there is a bony shelf (*arrow*) supporting it.

cannot be seen until after the distal ulna is excised (7). If the radius no longer supplies any support to the lunate, a partial or total radiocarpal fusion is performed (9).

### Tendon Transfers to Restore Wrist Balance

The most important part of the preoperative planning is to ensure that the radial deviation deformity is passively correctable and that the ECRL and extensor carpi radialis brevis are working. Otherwise, plan as you would for the other surgery that is being performed (4).

## SURGERY

### Dorsal Tenosynovectomy

Use a dorsal longitudinal incision (Fig. 3A). Take the incision to the level of the dorsal retinaculum, and form radial and ulnar skin flaps as required for the pro-

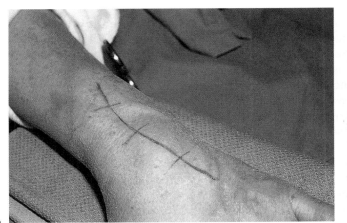

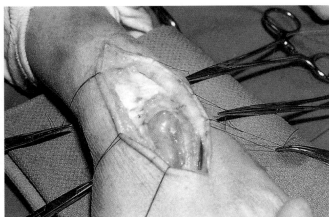

A                                                                                    B

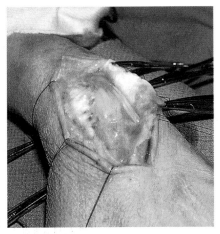

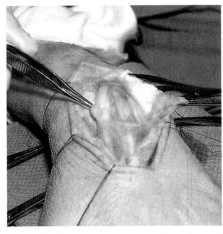

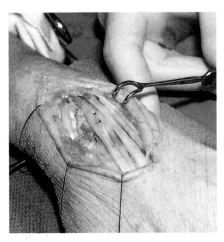

C                                                                                  D,E

**FIGURE 3. A:** Dorsal tenosynovitis is seen bulging distal to the extensor retinaculum. Extensor tendons are intact. A midline incision is marked out. **B:** Once the skin has been incised, raise thick flaps at the level of the extensor retinaculum. Put skin retraction sutures in place. Tenosynovitis is evident distal to the retinaculum. **C:** Open the extensor retinaculum in the fourth compartment and expose the tendons; make incisions proximal and distal to the retinaculum to facilitate this maneuver. **D:** Perform tenosynovectomy. Tenosynovium invaded the extensor tendon in this patient; wrist synovitis was not present, and the distal radioulnar joint was uninvolved. **E:** Remove the involved tissue by a longitudinal incision in the tendon. Then repair the tendon. After the involved tissue is removed, relocate the extensor retinaculum under the extensor tendons.

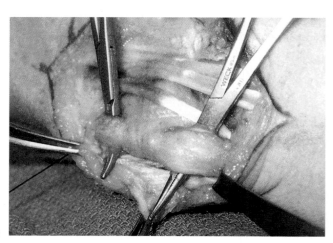

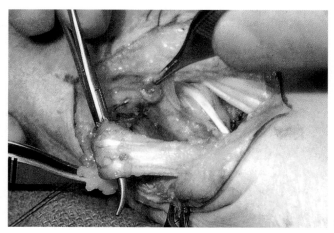

**FIGURE 4.** This patient is undergoing dorsal wrist surgery. **A:** Reflect the retinaculum; the extensor carpi ulnaris subsheath is seen clearly. **B:** The subsheath was opened in this patient to treat the abundant tenosynovitis.

posed surgery. The dorsal branches of the radial and ulnar sensory nerves frequently are seen as the flaps are formed; note and protect them. Section transverse communicating veins. Preserve longitudinal veins. After the skin flaps are formed, place retraction sutures in the skin edges (Fig. 3B).

Make a longitudinal incision into the fourth or sixth extensor compartment; we prefer to enter the fourth compartment. Raise radial and ulnar flaps (see Chapter 1). Make transverse incisions proximal and distal to the retinaculum, allowing the retinaculum to be reflected as a flap as the vertical septum between each compartment is opened (Fig. 3C). Identify the EPL tendon and open the septum. If there is evidence of tenosynovitis around the wrist extensor tendons, open the second compartment. Usually if only part of the septum is incised, the surgeon can evaluate the wrist extensor tendons. If there is no evidence of tenosynovitis, the tendons are not disturbed. In routine dorsal tenosynovectomy, the first compartment is not opened unless there is clinical evidence of involvement (Fig. 3D, E).

After the radial tendons are exposed, incise the vertical septum separating the fourth and fifth compartments, exposing the extensor digiti quinti tendon. Carefully dissect the retinaculum off the radioulnar joint until the subsheath of the ECU is identified (Fig. 4A). If the ECU is subluxed palmarly, careful dissection is necessary to isolate and expose both the tendon sheath and tendon. In these cases, leave the ulnar retinacular flap attached to the septum between the fifth and sixth compartments to use later to relocate the ECU tendon dorsally. Open the ECU sheath, perform a tenosynovectomy with sharp dissection, and open the subsheath if necessary to perform the tenosynovectomy (Fig. 4B). When there is invasive tenosynovitis, open the roof of the tendon longitudinally to remove diseased tissue (Fig. 3E). Remove as much of the tissue as possible; adherent tissue is sometimes impossible to remove. Repair frayed tendons; when imminent rupture is apparent, carry out side-to-side suture.

After completion of the tenosynovectomy, place the retinaculum deep to the tendons (Fig. 3E). Relocate the ECU to restore wrist balance by leaving the ECU in its unopened subsheath; when the ends of the retinaculum are sutured, using 3–0 monofilament polyglyconate (MPG) suture, the ECU is relocated. If the ECU is subluxed palmarly, pass the ulnar retinacular flap (which has been left attached to the vertical septum between the fifth and sixth compartments) palmar to the ECU tendon; loop it around the ECU and suture it dorsally. This loop of ulnar retinaculum relocates the palmarly subluxed ECU. Bowstringing of the tendons is not a significant problem when the entire retinaculum is placed under the

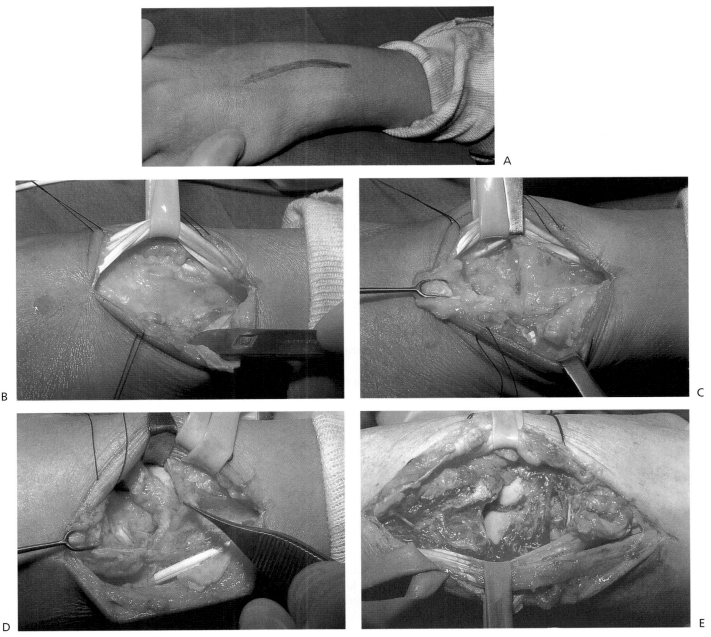

**FIGURE 5.  A:** Dorsal wrist synovitis is barely visible. There is no significant dorsal tenosynovitis. Midline incision is marked out. **B:** Open the extensor retinaculum in the fourth compartment as described; retract the tendons. Bulging dorsal synovitis is seen in this photograph. **C:** Make a transverse incision in the wrist capsule over the entire proximal row, and make a distally based capsular flap (retracted in skin hook). **D:** Perform synovectomy. **E:** After synovectomy, there is minimal cartilage loss; note partial scapholunate interosseous ligament destruction. Perform a tight capsular closure to restrict motion and help prevent later instability and pain.

tendons. If there is concern about bowstringing in the unusual patient with good wrist extension, the retinaculum is split and one portion placed over the tendons.

## Synovectomy

The exposure for a synovectomy is the same as for dorsal tenosynovectomy, which usually is performed at the same time (Fig. 5A, B).

Open the radiocarpal joint for radiocarpal joint synovectomy by making a transverse capsular incision over the entire proximal carpal row. Elevate a distally based flap to expose the midcarpal joints (Fig. 5C). Leave approximately 3 mm of capsule attached to the radius for closure. Note synovium bulging from the proximal and midcarpal joints. Traction applied to the hand distracts the joints and allows the synovectomy to be performed with a rongeur.

Use a small blunt periosteal elevator to provide better exposure within the joint. Curet periarticular erosions. If the triangular fibrocartilage is intact, remove synovium from between the triquetrum and the triangular fibrocartilage (Fig. 5D).

Expose the DRUJ through a longitudinal incision proximal to the triangular fibrocartilage. Rotate the forearm to provide exposure as the synovectomy is performed. Remove bony spurs from the distal ulna, and curet periarticular erosions.

After synovectomy is completed, close the capsular incisions. If there is evidence of major interosseous ligament disruption, such as tears of the scapholunate or lunotriquetrial ligaments, perform a tight capsular closure (Fig. 5E). Suture the dorsal capsule with 2–0 MPG suture to allow only 20° to 30° flexion. Prolonged splinting (4 to 6 weeks) in 10° extension is used to limit the range of wrist flexion and extension. If there is a tendency for the radioulnar joint to be unstable, hold the forearm in full supination while the DRUJ capsule is closed and splinted in that position; maintain the splint for 4 to 6 weeks to allow for more stability.

## Extensor Tendon Reconstruction

In patients treated for tendon rupture, perform complete dorsal tenosynovectomy; depending on the type and number of tendon ruptures, choose tendon transfer or graft. After dorsal tenosynovectomy, carry out retinacular reconstruction (see above), distal radioulnar reconstruction (see below), and tendon reconstruction (Fig. 6A). For a single rupture of the extensor communis, perform end-to-side transfer of the ruptured tendon into an intact extensor tendon.

Pass the ruptured tendon through a longitudinal slit in the intact tendon; suture it with 3–0 braided nonabsorbable suture to the intact tendon and then back to itself to reestablish the normal cascade. When treating rupture of the tendons to the fourth and fifth digit, transfer the EIP to the common extensor tendon of the fourth and fifth digits, excluding the extensor digiti minimi. Harvest the EIP through a transverse incision over the index finger MP joint; the EIP will be ulnar to the extensor digitorum communis and is detached at the extensor hood (Fig. 6B). Close the extensor hood with 4–0 MPG suture if a defect is present.

The EIP tendon is freed to the retinaculum to allow a straight line of pull to its transferred position. Pass the shorter of the two ruptured tendons through a longitudinal slit in the other tendon; suture it with 3–0 MPG suture to the other tendon and back to itself to reestablish the normal cascade. Then suture the EIP tendon using a Pulvertaft interlace technique (Fig. 6C, D) (3–0 MPG suture) in slightly more extension than the normal cascade.

In cases of rupture of the EPL with a functional deficit, we use the EIP for the motor. Harvest it as described above and suture it to the extensor mechanism using an interlace weave (3–0 MPG suture) at the MP joint of the thumb (Fig. 6D). Suture it tightly with the thumb in full extension and the wrist in neutral position.

In more complicated cases or if independent tendon function is desired, use an intercalary graft (Fig. 6A, D). If the palmaris longus is available, harvest it (Fig. 7A). Dissect the proximal and distal tendons free and apply traction for several minutes. The proximal muscle, usually functional, proves to be an adequate motor. Attach the distal stumps to each other in the end-to-side technique as described above, in the appropriate cascade (Fig. 7B). Connect the intercalary graft to the distal tendon stumps, as a group, by an interlace weave. Then attach

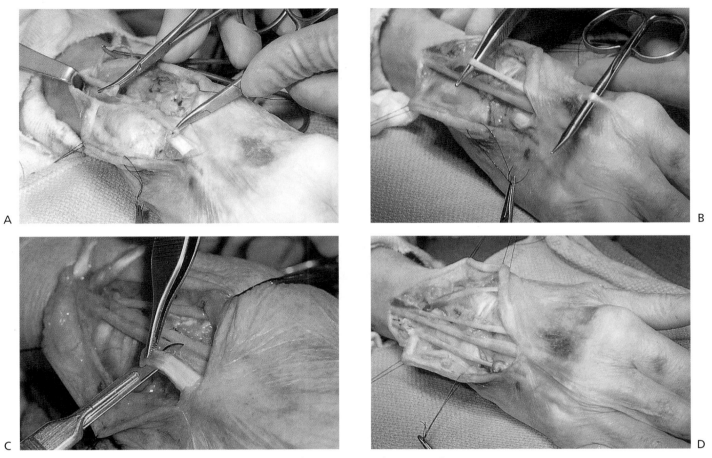

**FIGURE 6. A:** Retract the dorsal retinaculum to expose the extensor tendons. Note the extensor tendon rupture to the ulnar digits, with a gap between the proximal and distal stumps without evidence of tenosynovitis. There is also a rupture of the extensor pollicis longus tendon. **B:** Harvest extensor indicis proprius prior to transfer. It is transected at the metacarpophalangeal joint level and passed subcutaneously to the extensor of thumb at the metacarpophalangeal joint level. **C:** Distal stump of finger extensor. Make a transverse slit to pass the transfer through. **D:** Tendon reconstruction is complete. A palmaris longus intercalary graft was used to reconstruct the extensor tendons to the small and ring fingers. The extensor indicis proprius is used for the extensor pollicis longus tendon reconstruction. Because the patient had limited metacarpophalangeal joint motion after arthroplasty, the extensor indicis proprius, with its normal excursion, was used for the thumb, and an intercalary graft was used for the ulnar digits.

the graft to the proximal tendon in slightly more extension than normal, using an interlace weave technique (3) (Fig. 7C). We usually do not use the flexor digitorum sublimis for transfers in these cases.

At the conclusion of the procedure, deflate the tourniquet, obtain hemostasis, and, if indicated, use a Penrose drain for 24 hours. Support the hand in a bulky compressive dressing with palmar and dorsal splints in 30° extension and the MP joints in 20° to 30° flexion (Fig. 7D).

## Reconstruction of the Distal Radioulnar Joint

The same approach used for dorsal tenosynovectomy is used for distal ulnar excision (Fig. 8A, B). Reflect the extensor retinaculum and open the sixth compartment (Fig. 8C, D). Make a longitudinal incision directly over the distal ulna. Using sharp subperiosteal dissection, reflect the capsule and triangular fibrocartilage from the distal ulna and protect them.

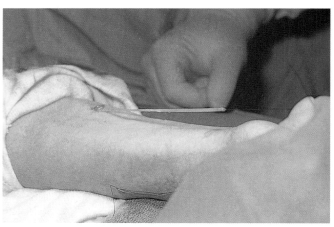

**FIGURE 7. A:** If there is a gap in the extensor tendons with a good motor, use an intercalary tendon graft. Harvest palmaris longus tendon graft. **B:** Weave together the distal stumps as described. Then weave the distal graft, using an interlace weave. **C:** The proximal juncture is done using the interlace weave technique in slightly more extension than the normal cascade. **D:** A bulky compressive hand dressing is applied, with splints supporting the wrist in 30° of extension and the metacarpophalangeal joints in 30° flexion.

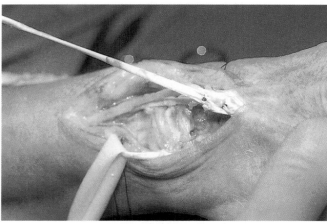

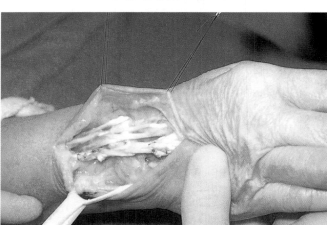

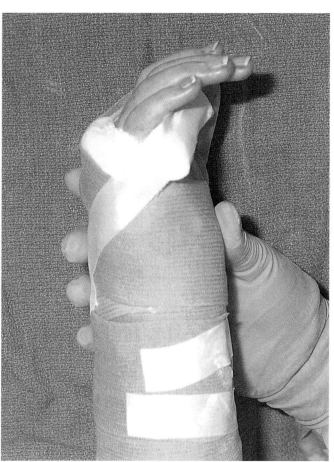

Place small bone retractors around the ulna. Section the distal ulna using a saw, osteotome, or bone cutter. Use a towel clip to apply traction to the bone while releasing the soft tissue attachments. Resect approximately 2 cm of bone to be just proximal to the sigmoid notch. Smooth the cut surface of ulna with a rongeur. If excessive bone is resected, stability of the distal ulna is compromised (Fig. 8E–G).

After the bone is removed, carry out synovectomy of the joint. Preserve the triangular fibrocartilage and carefully reconstruct it to ensure radioulnar stability. The TFCC frequently is eroded and partially destroyed; with careful dissection, however, the TFCC can be freed (Fig. 8H). Suture it with 2–0 or 3–0 MPG suture

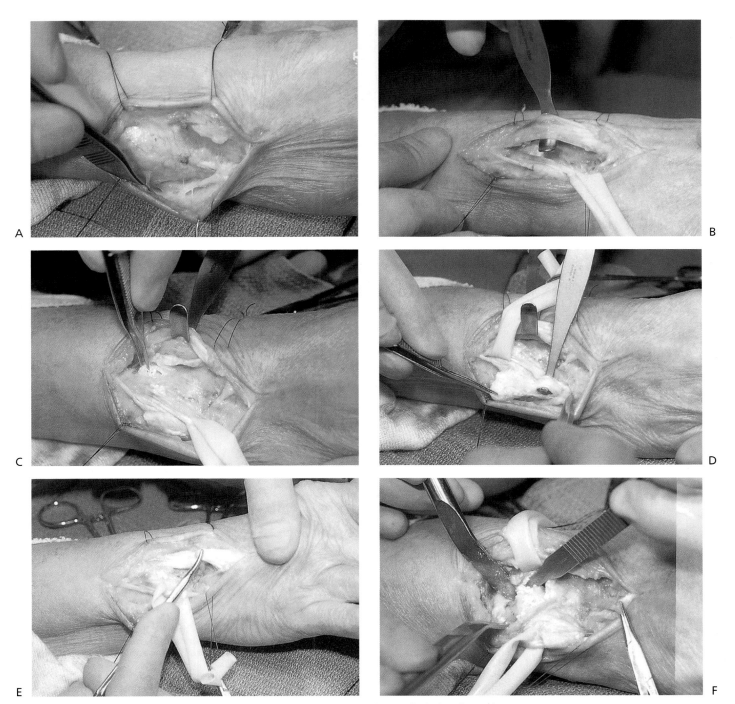

**FIGURE 8. A:** Make a skin incision to the level of the retinaculum and raise thick skin flaps. Place skin retraction sutures. Protect the dorsal sensory nerves in the flaps as shown. **B:** Open the fourth compartment, incise the proximal and distal margins of the retinaculum, and raise radial and ulnar retinacular flaps. Incise the vertical septa between compartments. Place traction on the fourth compartment's tendons. Place a Penrose drain around the extensor digitorum quinti tendon. **C:** Capsular erosion is seen secondary to the distal ulnar aspect, which caused the attrition rupture. **D:** The sheath over the extensor carpi ulnaris (retractor) is opened, but the subsheath is not. **E:** The distal tendon stumps are visible. **F:** Expose the distal ulna by subperiosteal dissection. *(continued.)*

to the dorsal ulnar periosteum of the radius and the radioulnar capsule (Fig. 8I, J). Following this repair, tightly suture the dorsal radioulnar capsule to stabilize the ulna. If there is sufficient tissue it can be imbricated for additional support. Close the capsule with the wrist in supination (Fig. 8K). At the end of the procedure, full rotation should be possible.

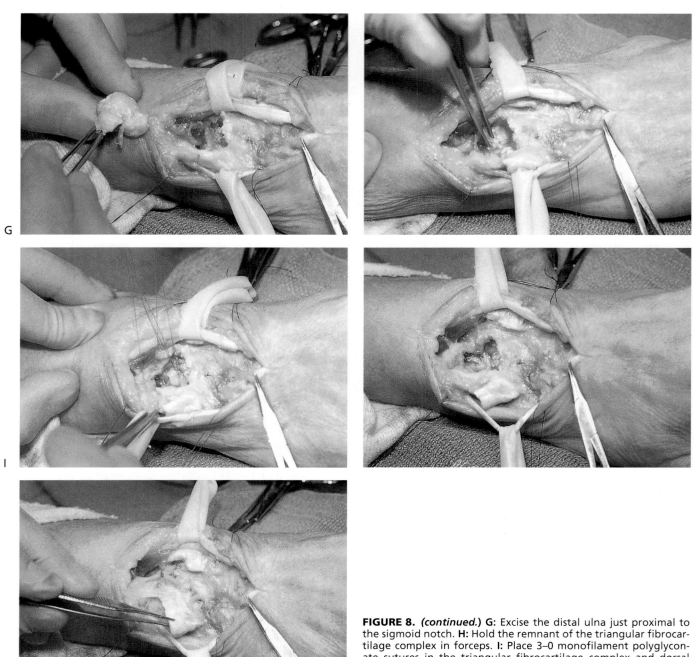

**FIGURE 8.** *(continued.)* **G:** Excise the distal ulna just proximal to the sigmoid notch. **H:** Hold the remnant of the triangular fibrocartilage complex in forceps. **I:** Place 3–0 monofilament polyglyconate sutures in the triangular fibrocartilage complex and dorsal ulnar periosteum of the radius. **J:** Hold the forearm in slight supination and tie the sutures. **K:** Close the periosteum and capsule over the distal ulna.

When there is an inadequate triangular fibrocartilage, raise a portion of palmar capsule (2) to reconstruct the ligament. Expose the palmar capsule through the space provided by the resected ulna. Carefully raise a distally based flap of palmar capsule to protect the ulnar neurovascular bundle. Make the drill holes in the dorsal distal ulna using a 0.045-in. K-wire. Place horizontal mattress sutures (3–0 MPG) in the proximal capsular flap. Hold the ulna reduced with dorsal pressure and tie these sutures over the drill holes.

Another method is to use a distally based strip of the ECU tendon as a tenodesis to the distal ulna to help in the reconstruction (8,12). Split the ECU longitudinally in half from the base of the fifth metacarpal to the musculotendinous junction.

Make a $\frac{1}{8}$-in. hole in the dorsal cortex of the distal ulna, leaving a bridge of bone distally large enough to prevent fracture. Pass the free end of the distally based ECU tendon slip through the dorsal cortex. Hold the ulna reduced, and suture the ECU to itself with an interlace weave (3–0 MPG suture).

After retinacular and ECU relocation, closure and dressings are completed for dorsal tenosynovectomy.

### Tendon Transfers to Restore Wrist Balance

Transfer the ECRL to the ECU to help restore wrist balance (4). After other dorsal wrist surgery is completed, detach the ECRL from the second metacarpal. Reroute the tendon palmar to the finger extensors. Hold the wrist in 10° ulnar deviation and slight extension and suture the ECRL to the insertion of the ECU tendon at the fifth metacarpal using an end-to-side weave (3–0 MPG suture). Perform closure as dictated by other procedures being performed. Place the wrist in a splint in neutral or slight ulnar deviation.

## POSTOPERATIVE MANAGEMENT

If a Penrose drain has been inserted, change the dressing in 24 hours. Otherwise, it is changed in several days.

### Dorsal Tenosynovectomy

For uncomplicated dorsal tenosynovectomy, splint the wrist in slight extension for 2 weeks, but have the patient initiate digital motion in 1 to 2 days. To prevent an extension lag, intermittently splint the digits in 20° to 30° flexion until active extension is possible. Formal therapy is needed only for patients who are having significant pain or who still do not have full active extension at 10 to 14 days. We expect the patients to regain full digital motion in 7 to 10 days and have minimal recurrence of dorsal tenosynovitis.

### Synovectomy

Apply a short-arm anteroposterior splint. Generally, immobilize the wrist for 2 to 3 weeks. When there is minimal joint destruction, good capsular tissues, no ligament injury, and a good closure, start guarded rotation and wrist motion between 2 and 3 weeks. Maintain splints for 8 weeks. If there was significant instability of the carpus, splint the radiocarpal joint continuously for 4 more weeks to restrict motion.

Wrist motion is expected to be decreased, with approximately 30° to 40° flexion and extension. This helps to provide stability and prevent later deformity. Rotation usually returns close to normal by 6 to 8 weeks. There may be some delay in progression of the disease after synovectomy, but not as dramatic as after tenosynovectomy.

### Extensor Tendon Reconstruction

Postoperatively, splint the digits in 20° to 30° flexion for several days until pain and swelling have subsided. Hold the wrist in 30° extension. Change the dressing, protect the MP joints, and encourage proximal interphalangeal (PIP) joint motion. If a good intertendinous weave is achieved, have the patient begin controlled supervised exercises at 7 to 10 days.

Use active assisted motion. Instruct the patient to relax the digits and allow the MP joints to flex. The MP joints usually flex about 15° to 25°, depending on the tightness of the transfer. The patient then is instructed to extend the digits actively. The patient learns to activate the transfer quickly. Between exercise periods, have the patient hold the MP joints in extension, but encourage PIP joint motion. If the patient is having trouble actively extending the MP joints at 3 to 4 weeks, tape the PIP joints in a fully flexed position and perform active flexion and extension of the MP joints. At 3 or 4 weeks after reconstruction, introduce more aggressive exercises, depending on the progress. Use dynamic extension splints occasionally if progress is slow or if the repair needs to be protected.

We expect active extension to be within 20° of full extension and flexion to be 60°, depending on the patient's other problems (i.e., MP arthroplasty, number of ruptures).

### Reconstruction of the Distal Radioulnar Joint

Postoperative management for reconstruction of the DRUJ is similar to that following radioulnar synovectomy. If there has been adequate soft tissue reconstruction, short-arm anteroposterior splints will provide adequate protection; guarded rotation is started approximately 2 weeks following surgery. When there is significant radioulnar instability the forearm is immobilized in supination for 4 weeks to prevent instability. Rotation is started, and the patient is splinted between exercise periods in neutral rotation for 4 more weeks.

Patients often need hand therapy following this procedure; in some cases, prolonged exercises are required to regain motion. Pain and a "clunking" sensation are common for several weeks following the procedure; this usually resolves within 8 to 10 weeks.

We expect the patient to have full painless rotation by 8 to 10 weeks and no further attrition ruptures on the ulna.

### Tendon Transfers to Restore Wrist Balance

As tendon transfer is always done as a secondary procedure, the primary procedure dictates postoperative management. Splint the wrist in neutral or slight ulnar deviation for 4 weeks. Start intermittent active assisted range-of-motion exercises with splinting in between exercise periods for 4 more weeks. The transfer helps maintain neutral wrist position. Patients are expected to lose most of their radial deviation.

## COMPLICATIONS

### Skin

The two major skin complications are injury to the sensory nerves and skin slough (Fig. 9). If the surgeon is careful when raising the flaps, there should not be a major nerve injury. When one of the small terminal branches is injured, patients have minimal hypesthesia in a small area distal to the injury. Injury to a major branch of the radial or ulnar nerve can result in a major sensory loss, but even more troublesome is the painful dysesthetic area over the dorsum of the hand.

Fortunately, dorsal skin sloughs are uncommon. They are major complications exposing the extensor tendons, resulting in infection, tendon necrosis, and adhesions. Skin sloughs are seen in patients with tissue-paper–thin skin and are associated with long-standing use of steroids. Hematoma formation also can be a big

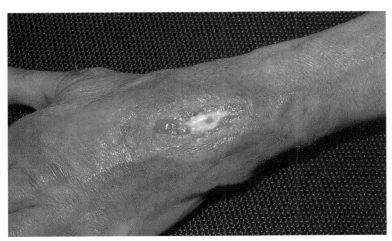

**FIGURE 9.** This patient had a dorsal tenosynovectomy and subsequent dorsal skin slough 2 weeks before this photograph was taken. Extensor tendons are exposed. A pigskin homograft was used, and the skin healed by 5 weeks after surgery. A 30° extension lag was associated with the tendon adhesions.

factor in causing skin slough. To avoid it, use skin retraction sutures, handle the skin as little and as gently as possible, and deflate the tourniquet before skin closure. If there is any concern about bleeding, use a Penrose or small suction drain for 24 hours. In patients who have fragile skin, be especially careful with the skin closure. Evert the skin edges, avoid a tight closure, and change the dressing at 24 hours to evaluate for hematoma, bleeding, or skin problems.

Skin sloughs are difficult to treat. We have used dressing changes with or without homographs with reasonable results.

## Dorsal Tenosynovectomy

Complications following dorsal tenosynovectomy are infrequent. Occasionally, adhesions will result in an extensor lag at the MP joint level or loss of active digital flexion. Hand therapy is adjusted to emphasize flexion or extension as necessary. Dynamic extensor or flexor splints are used in these cases. These complications occur more frequently in patients whose tendons are in poor condition at surgery or in patients with multiple joint involvement.

## Synovectomy

Surgical complications following synovectomy are uncommon. The most serious problem is limited rotation and persistent pain at the radioulnar joint. When patients have difficulty regaining rotation, hand therapy is begun. It is common for patients to have persistent rotational pain for 6 to 8 weeks after synovectomy. Persistent wrist pain is possible following synovectomy, with the potential for recurrent synovitis and further destruction. Limited wrist flexion and extension are to be expected; advise patients of these outcomes before surgery. In loose wrists, especially when there is ligament destruction, limited motion is a goal.

## Extensor Tendon Reconstruction

Complications following tendon reconstruction are relatively frequent because of the severity of the condition plus the need to temper postoperative exercises.

Limited active extension and flexion are common outcomes, proportional to the number of tendons ruptured, the type of transfers used, and the severity of joint destruction. When patients have significant MP joint extensor lag following reconstruction, it is preferable to maintain prolonged MP joint extension and try to preserve extension even if there is loss of MP joint flexion. This is especially true when the patient has good PIP joint motion.

### Reconstruction of the Distal Radioulnar Joint

The most frequent complication following distal ulnar excision, painful and limited forearm rotation, often responds to prolonged splinting plus a gentle exercise program. No surgery is indicated for several months unless a definite cause for the problem is apparent. If symptoms do not remit in several months and there is significant disability, exploration is appropriate. If the problem is impingement of the distal ulna on the radius, additional bone is resected. If there is instability with subluxation, the ECU can be used to increase stability as described under the Surgical Technique section.

Symptomatic ulnar translocation in these patients has not been a problem. If it does occur, radiocarpal fusion, leaving the minimally involved midcarpal joints alone, is a good solution.

### Tendon Transfers to Restore Wrist Balance

The only complication of tendon transfers to restore wrist balance is failure to maintain a corrected position. Progression of the disease can lead to further wrist destruction and deformity.

## ACKNOWLEDGMENT

The authors thank Richard Mottla of the New England Baptist Hospital Medical Media Department for his excellent photography.

## RECOMMENDED READING

1. Backdahl, M.: The caput ulnae syndrome in rheumatoid arthritis: a study of morphology, abnormal anatomy and clinical picture. *Acta Rheumatol. Scand.*, 5: 1–75, 1963.
2. Blatt, G.: Capsulodesis in reconstructive hand surgery. *Hand Clin.*, 3(1): 81–102, 1987.
3. Bora, F. W., Osterman, A. L., Thomas, V. J., Maitin, E. C., Polineni, S.: The treatment of ruptures of multiple extensor tendons at the wrist level by free tendon graft in the rheumatoid patient. *J. Hand Surg.*, 12A: 1038–1040, 1987.
4. Clayton, M. L., Ferlic, D. C.: Tendon transfer for radial rotation of the wrist in rheumatoid arthritis. *Clin. Orthop.*, 100: 176–185, 1974.
5. Darrach, W.: Anterior dislocation of the head of the ulna. *Ann. Surg.*, 56: 802–803, 1912.
6. Feldon, P. G., Millender, L. H., Nalebuff, E. A.: Rheumatoid arthritis in the hand and wrist. In: *Operative Hand Surgery*, edited by D. P. Green, Churchill Livingstone, New York, 1993.
7. Gainor, B. J., Schaberg, J.: The rheumatoid wrist after resection of the distal ulna. *J. Hand Surg.*, 10A: 837–844, 1985.
8. Leslie, B. M., Carlson, G., Ruby, L. K.: Results of extensor carpi ulnaris tenodesis in the rheumatoid wrist undergoing distal ulnar excision. *J. Hand Surg.*, 15A: 547–551, 1990.
9. Linscheid, R. L., Dobyns, J. H.: Radiolunate arthrodesis. *J. Hand Surg.*, 10A: 821–829, 1985.
10. Linscheid, R. L., Dobyns, J. H.: Rheumatoid arthritis of the wrist. *Orthop. Clin. North Am.*, 2: 649–665, 1971.
11. Millender, L. H., Nalebuff, E. A.: Preventive surgery—tenosynovectomy and synovectomy. *Orthop. Clin. North Am.*, 6: 709–732, 1975.
12. O'Donovan, T. M., Ruby, L. K.: The distal radialulnar joint in rheumatoid arthritis. *Hand Clin.*, 5(2): 249–256, 1989.
13. Shapiro, J. S., Rodts, T., Labanauskas, I., Payne, T.: Early synovectomy versus late arthroplasty of the rheumatoid wrist: a comparative study. *J. Hand Surg.*, 10A: 430, 1985.
14. Thirupathi, R. G., Ferlic, D. C., Clayton, M. L.: Dorsal wrist synovectomy in rheumatoid arthritis—a long term study. *J. Hand Surg.*, 8: 848–856, 1983.

# 30

# Combined Radiocarpal Arthrodesis and Midcarpal (Lunocapitate) Arthroplasty

Julio Taleisnik

## INDICATIONS/CONTRAINDICATIONS

This procedure consists of an arthrodesis between the radius, scaphoid, and lunate, combined with an arthroplasty between the lunate and capitate. The distal radioulnar joint also is commonly involved, and its treatment should be included as part of the operation. This procedure is indicated for patients with rheumatoid arthritis of the wrist and with clinical and radiographic findings for which a pan-arthrodesis or the insertion of a total wrist implant may be considered.

These patients are beyond the stage at which a synovectomy or a partial arthrodesis alone, across either radiocarpal or midcarpal joints, may be considered. The traditional approach at this stage of the disease is to perform a pan-arthrodesis (5,6,8,11,13), or, when preserving motion is important, an arthroplasty, with or without the use of a prosthesis (1,2,7,9,10,12,16). All arthroplasties traditionally have been devised for the articulation between the radius and the carpus, although this joint is inherently less stable than the midcarpal joint and subject to greater destruction and instability by the rheumatoid arthritic process. Therefore, the ideal surgical procedure at the unstable radiocarpal joint is not its replacement, but rather its stabilization by a radioscapholunate fusion. Conversely, the midcarpal joint remains usually aligned and recognizable even in advanced, severe rheumatoid arthritis deformity, with erosive or destructive changes that are limited to just the head of the capitate, involved earlier and more severely than the triquetrohamate or the scaphotrapeziotrapezoid joints. When this situation is present, the head of the capitate may be excised and replaced with a small silicone condylar implant, originally designed for the trapeziometacarpal joint (17). A partial but functional range of motion thus is preserved at the midcarpal level.

When there are no contraindications, we prefer this operation to arthrodesis or arthroplasty because it is reliable, durable, and consistent in providing painless, stable, and limited but functional motion. This procedure may be used exceptionally for degenerative or posttraumatic conditions.

The use of a silicone implant within the carpus may be questioned by some. I used a silicone condyle as part of this operation long before silicone particle synovitis was reported (15), and thus far have not observed such a reaction in any of my patients. This probably is due to the stable load-bearing column provided by the partial arthrodesis, sparing the implant unusual wear. Since the other choices for these wrists would be a pan-arthrodesis or the insertion of a much larger (and less stable) implant, the use of a small condyle has been preferred whenever possible, in spite of the remote risk of particle synovitis. The main attraction of this technique is its salvageability. If the need arises, the silicone condyle may be removed to be replaced by a biological implant, such as a soft tissue "anchovy," or be easily converted to a pan-arthrodesis. In addition, because the scaphoid and trapezium remain intact, the patient retains a stable base for the thumb, and the surgeon finds all options for the treatment of the severe rheumatoid involvement of the scaphotrapeziometacarpal joints still available.

There are two contraindications to this technique (17): wrists with extensive preexistent midcarpal osseous ankylosis, making the prospects of regaining midcarpal motion remote; and wrists with severe resorption of scaphoid and lunate, leaving very little bone stock for arthrodesis to the radius. Pan-arthrodeses or arthroplasties should be considered for these patients. Selecting one of these techniques depends on multiple factors, among which are functional requirements, the need to use crutches or canes for ambulation, the patient's age, and the involvement and salvageability of other joints, such as the opposite wrist and the ipsilateral elbow. Evaluation of the condition of the trapeziometacarpal joint is also important when considering the use of an endoprosthesis, because of the potential loss of support to the thumb ray, as the trapezium is left to articulate against the implant and either resorbs or migrates proximally. This becomes an unsalvageable problem and the source of severe additional disability for these patients who are already severely disabled.

## PREOPERATIVE PLANNING

Patients with rheumatoid arthritis should be considered for this operation. Clinically, they present with painful, limited motion of the wrist. They complain of weakness and an unstable sensation in the wrist when attempting to grasp with any degree of strength, lift, support their body weight on crutches, or use a cane during ambulation. Examination may disclose synovitis, deformity, crepitation, or any combination of the three. Range of motion, although painful, may be minimally limited.

Routine radiographs show destruction, dislocation, or severe destabilization (ulnar translation, palmar subluxation, scapholunate dissociation) at the level of the radioscapholunate joint. Midcarpal architecture and alignment are preserved, although radiographic involvement of the lunocapitate articulation is present. In most cases, the distal radioulnar joint is destroyed, subluxed, or dislocated.

Ancillary or special diagnostic procedures are not necessary.

## SURGERY

With the patient supine, the entire upper extremity is draped free and placed on a hand table; the forearm is pronated and the dorsum of the wrist is exposed. The ipsilateral iliac crest area is prepped and draped as well, for there may be a need for bone to graft into the radiocarpal joint, in addition to that obtained locally, from the carpus, the distal ulna, and the distal radius.

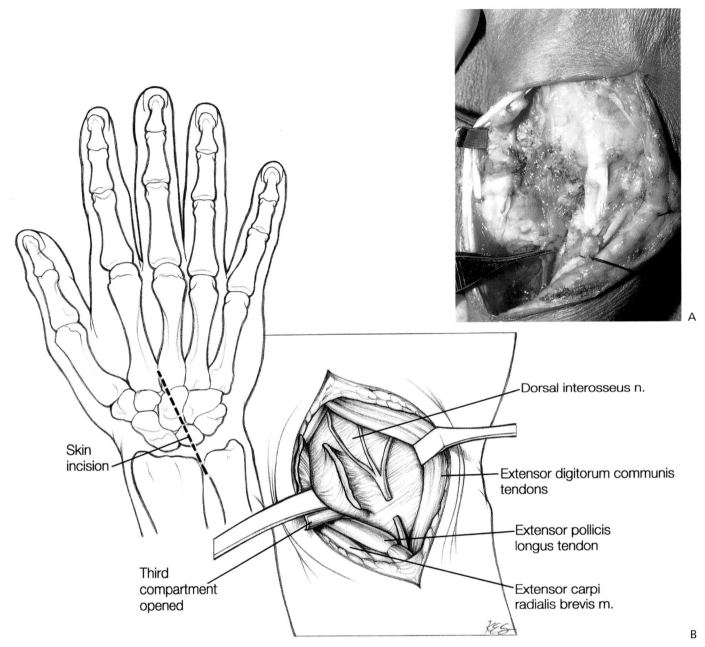

**FIGURE 1.** **A** and **B:** The dorsal retinaculum has been divided along the roof of the tunnel for the extensor pollicis longus tendon. The dorsal capsule is exposed between the third and fourth dorsal wrist compartments. The extensor carpi radialis brevis tendon is seen. The dorsal interosseous neurovascular bundle is identified, coagulated, and divided.

## Technique

A straight incision is preferred, obliquely placed along the dorsum of the wrist, between the radial side of the base of the third metacarpal and the neck of the ulna. Once the extensor retinaculum is exposed, further dissection depends on the presence or absence of extensor tenosynovitis. When there is no synovitis of the extensor compartments, the skin flaps are elevated just enough to expose the tunnel of the extensor pollicis longus tendon. This tendon is unroofed and retracted radially. The dorsal interosseous neurovascular bundle is exposed routinely, cauterized, and divided (Fig. 1). The joint and the distal radius are exposed subcapsu-

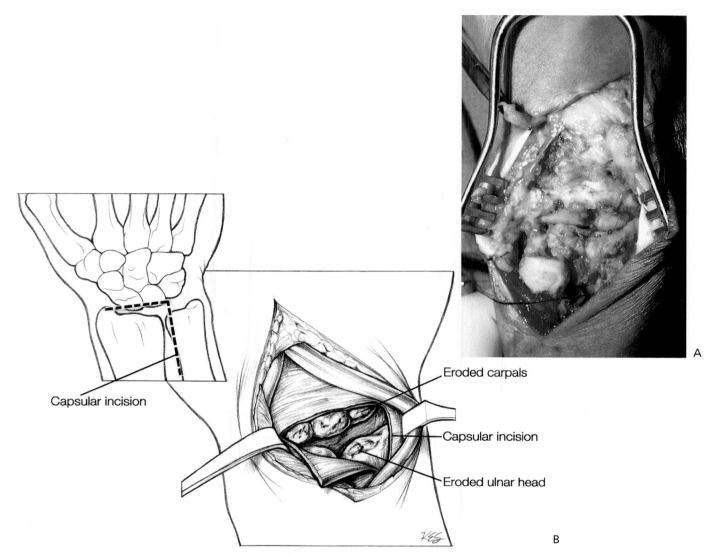

Capsular incision

Eroded carpals

Capsular incision

Eroded ulnar head

A

B

**FIGURE 2. A** and **B:** The ulnar head is exposed using a longitudinal capsular incision. The capsular incision is completed, into an L, with a horizontal limb along the radiocarpal joint. The destroyed surfaces of scaphoid and lunate are visualized faintly.

larly and subperiosteally. In most patients, the ulna can be reached from this approach (Fig. 2). Rarely is a second retinacular incision needed. When there is extensor tenosynovitis and a dorsal tenosynovectomy is necessary, both skin flaps are developed to expose all extensor tendon compartments involved. The dorsal retinaculum is divided longitudinally along the extensor carpi ulnaris. Because the radiocarpal relationship will be restored by an arthrodesis, there is no need to create retinacular flaps in anticipation of a stabilization of the extensor carpi ulnaris tendon. The retinaculum is elevated in a radial direction by dividing the septae that anchor it, which are located between the extensor compartments. This creates a retinacular flap based radially, which may be used at the end of the operation to reinforce capsular closure beneath the extensor tendons or to be replaced dorsal to the tendons. Alternatively, the retinacular flap may be divided into two, one distal to reinforce capsular closure, and a second more proximal to be replaced dorsal to the extensor tendons.

The distal radioulnar joint may be treated next. Most frequently, a hemiresection interposition technique is used (3). Bone obtained from the excised ulnar head may be used as a bone graft for the radiocarpal arthrodesis. The pronator

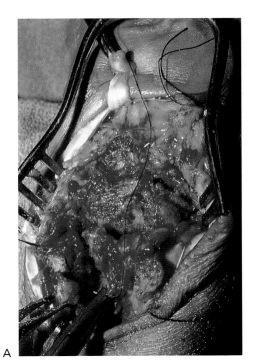

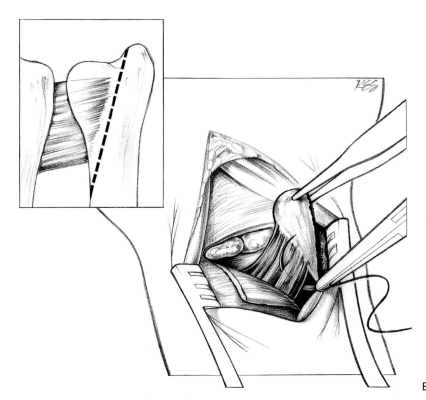

**FIGURE 3.** **A** and **B:** The ulnar head has been excised. The pronator quadratus is brought up into the radioulnar gap and is tagged for later reinsertion.

quadratus, which is exposed as the seat of the ulna is excised, is tagged at this point for later attachment to the remaining ulnar shaft (Fig. 3).

The distal radius and the scaphoid and lunate are exposed at this point. One of two situations may present: When scaphoid and lunate are dissociated, which is usually the case, their contiguous surfaces are excised, and both bones are retracted away from each other to facilitate access to the head of the capitate; when the scapholunate ligaments are preserved, both bones are tilted into dorsiflexion to expose the head of the capitate.

The head of the capitate with the proximal pole of the hamate are sawed off, leaving behind a transverse cut surface (Figs. 4, 5). Cancellous bone is shelled out from the body of the capitate until a space is created that is large enough to accept the shortened stem of a silicone condylar implant. There are 13 sizes available; numbers 11 to 13 are used most often (Fig. 6). The implant must be seated flush against the cut surfaces of capitate and hamate (Fig. 7). It then is reduced under the scaphoid and lunate.

The articular surface of the radius and the corresponding surfaces of the scaphoid and lunate are excised to expose underlying cancellous bone. When present, the scapholunate gap is packed with bone chips from the head of the capitate or the distal ulna and is fixed with a 0.045-in. K-wire inserted transversely from lateral to medial. The assembled scapholunate unit is manipulated into neutral from dorsipalmar flexion, restoring the normal alignment of the midcarpal joint, in which the dorsal pole of the lunate covers the head of the capitate (Fig. 8). Two 0.045- or 0.054-in. K-wires are introduced along the scaphoid, from distal to proximal, until the tips appear on the surface of its proximal pole. Two other similar K-wires are inserted from distal to proximal across the triquetrum and lunate, until their tips show on the proximal surface of the lunate. All wires should miss the condylar implant. When the reassembled carpus fits well against the radius, the wires are advanced through the radius. Bone chips

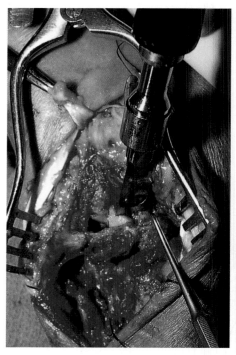

**FIGURE 4.** Lunate and scaphoid are retracted to expose the head of the capitate and proximal pole of the hamate, about to be excised.

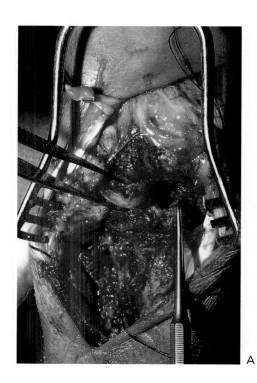

A

Head of capitate removed

Proximal pole of hamate removed

Pronator quadratus tagged

Proximal row carpals pulled proximally

B

**FIGURE 5.** A and B: The head of the capitate is shown being removed. Lunate and scaphoid are retracted proximally.

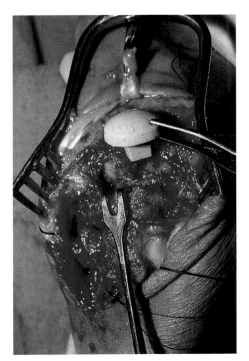

**FIGURE 6.** A suitable size condylar implant, its stem shortened, is shown about to be inserted into a cavity created within the body of the capitate.

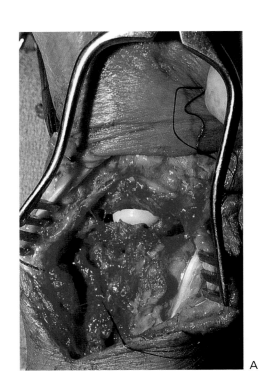

A

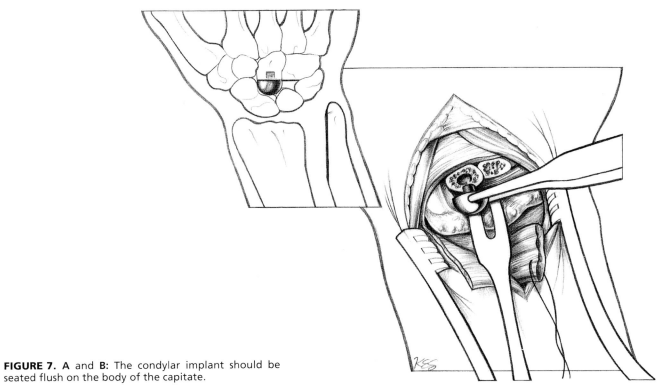

B

**FIGURE 7.** A and B: The condylar implant should be seated flush on the body of the capitate.

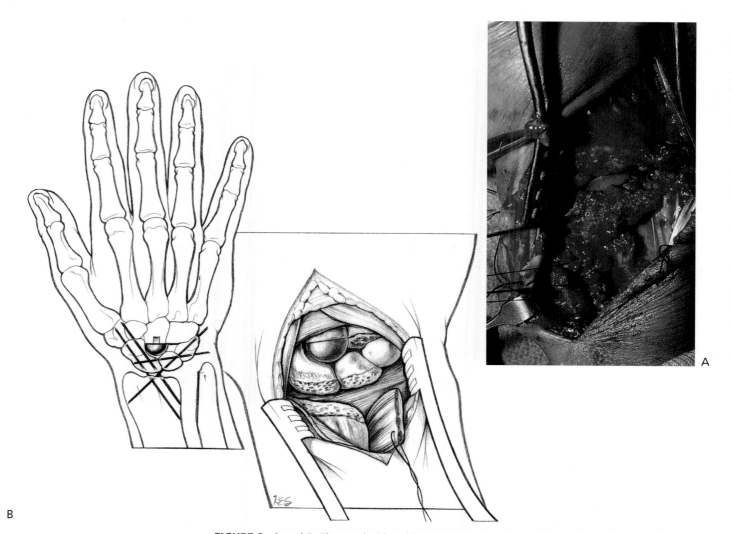

**FIGURE 8. A** and **B:** The scaphoid and lunate are replaced over the capitate. Scaphoid, lunate, and radius are decorticated to expose cancellous bone. A single K-wire is used to secure the scapholunate unit. Multiple sutures are passed through the cortex of the remaining ulna to reattach the pronator quadratus.

from the head and body of the capitate and from the excised ulnar head are used to pack all interstices.

When lunate and scaphoid bone stock is precarious, or in the presence of large subchondral cysts, additional bone graft is required, which may be obtained from the distal radius or from the ipsilateral iliac crest. All wire ends are cut under the skin. Just before closure, treatment of the distal radioulnar joint is completed. When the head of the ulna is excised, I prefer reinforcing the soft tissue stabilization of the ulnar stump; this is done by reattaching the pronator quadratus with nonabsorbable sutures inserted through holes drilled through the dorsal cortex of the ulna, and by a careful capsular repair (Fig. 8). Closure is completed in layers.

## POSTOPERATIVE MANAGEMENT

Immediate postoperative immobilization is provided with a well-padded compression-type dressing that includes the hand and wrist, to above the elbow. This is reinforced with plaster splints. I rarely have utilized suction drains, although these may be used when indicated. At 3 to 5 days following operation, all dressings are changed.

Exercises to maintain range of motion of the shoulder and all digits are stressed. Long-arm immobilization is continued, usually in semisupination, mostly because of the discomfort arising from the distal radioulnar arthroplasty but also to allow for stabilization of the distal ulna.

Sutures are removed at 10 or 11 days after the operation. At this time a short-arm plaster gauntlet is applied, extended laterally and medially to above the elbow, and well molded around the humeral epicondyles, allowing limited elbow flexion/extension while maintaining control of pronation/supination. Short-arm immobilization is used after the fourth postoperative week, until the fusion appears radiographically solid, usually at 8 weeks following the operation. All K-wires are removed at this time. The patient is provided with a removable splint for the wrist, and is instructed to remove it several times daily to exercise the wrist. It is useful to proceed with this exercise program under the direction and supervision of hand therapists.

In my experience, relief of pain and restoration of joint stability have been uniform. Patients may expect to retain on an average most of the preoperative ranges of wrist extension and ulnar deviation. Palmar flexion is most disturbed, and an average loss of approximately 15° of palmar flexion is anticipated. In my experience, the most striking change has been a gain in radial deviation, almost double that which was present preoperatively, which I believe is due to improved radiocarpal alignment. The range of motion that is possible with this technique is excellent for some patients, but for others can be disappointing. The disappointment, however, is more the surgeon's than the patient's; patients are usually delighted with the limited, but painless and stable, motion. Biomechanical studies of normal functional wrist motion (4,14) have demonstrated that most activities may be accomplished with a range from 35° of extension to 5° to 10° of flexion, and from 15° of ulnar deviation to 10° of radial deviation. This flexion/extension range is reached, or surpassed, by the vast majority of patients.

Lamberta and coauthors (10) proposed a rating system based on a 100-point score sheet. Wrist balance, motion, relief of pain, and percentage of change in grip strength were evaluated. Balance was given a 30-point value (15 points assessed to flexion/extension, and 15 points to radioulnar deviation), motion 25 points, pain relief 35, and grip strength 10. A result was "excellent" if the score was higher than 70 points. Using this method, all wrists following this operation have been scored as "excellent." I believe that the reason for this is the emphasis that this scoring method places on pain relief and balance (or stability), which together account for 65 points.

## COMPLICATIONS

Other than the complications inherent in all operations (i.e., infection) or the surgical approach itself (i.e., cutaneous nerve injury), complications intrinsic to this procedure are the following:

1. *Nonunion of the radiocarpal arthrodesis*: This is infrequent; in my experience, only one patient developed a painless nonunion between radius and scaphoid. Should this become symptomatic, it could be treated by a bone graft to the nonunited site.
2. *Particle synovitis surrounding the midcarpal silicone implant*: This is a theoretical possibility, not observed thus far in more than 15 years of experience. If and when particle synovitis occurs, I would remove the silicone implant, débride the bone graft cysts and pseudocysts, and fill the space with an "anchovy" filler.
3. *Tear or break of the condylar implant, between the head and stem*: This was seen during a routine radiographic follow-up 6 years postoperatively, in a

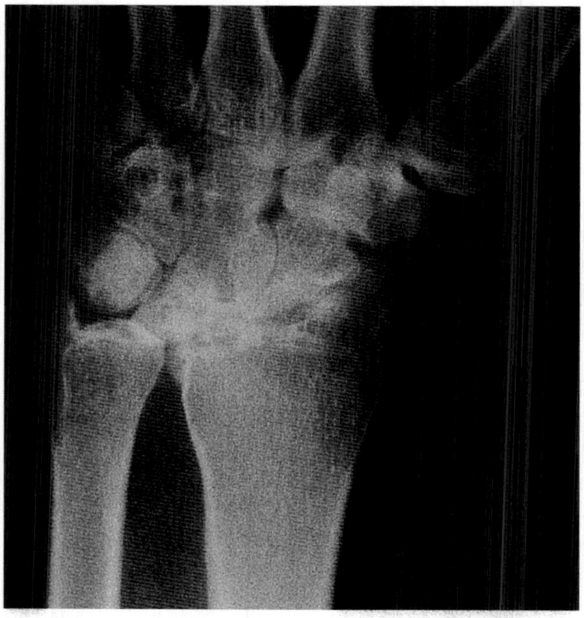

**FIGURE 9.** Preoperative radiograph.

patient who had remained symptom-free. One potential problem here would be particle synovitis, which may be treated as outlined above. Abnormal subluxation or dislocation of the distal carpal row on the arthrodesed scapholunate unit is also conceivable, in which case carpal alignment should be restored and the radiocarpal fusion extended to include the midcarpal joint.

## ILLUSTRATIVE CASE FOR TECHNIQUE

The patient was 38 years old when first examined in 1984 for complaints of pain, weakness, and limitation of motion referred to both wrists, particularly the nondominant left. Rheumatoid arthritis had been diagnosed in 1974. On examination, there was a minimal amount of palpable synovitis. Crepitation during motions of the wrist and forearm rotation was severe and accompanied by pain. The wrist extended 35°, flexed 37°, and deviated 15° ulnarly and 15° radially. Pronation was 80% of normal and supination 70%.

Radiographs showed significant erosive and destructive changes between radius, scaphoid, and lunate (Fig. 9). The midcarpal joint, although narrow, was preserved. There were minimal radiographic changes at the distal radioulnar level. This is the type of wrist for which a pan-arthrodesis would be indicated in a young, active patient such as this, except for the involvement of the opposite, dominant wrist, a previous total elbow arthroplasty performed on the right side, and early rheumatoid changes of the left elbow. Preservation of some pain-free motion and restoration of stability were deemed important. A radioscapholunate arthrodesis was performed, the head of the capitate and proximal pole of the scaphoid excised, and a condylar implant inserted (Fig. 10). The ulnar head was excised. The patient's postoperative course was uneventful. Six months later, the right wrist was treated by a radioscapholunate arthrodesis and excision of the distal ulna. The midcarpal joint was found to be serviceable and was left intact after synovectomy. When last examined in 1992, 8 years following the operation, the patient was free of pain. The range of extension of the left wrist was 35°, flexion 32°, ulnar deviation 15°, and radial deviation 15°. Pronation was full and supination was 80% of normal. Radiographs showed maintenance of a serviceable mid-

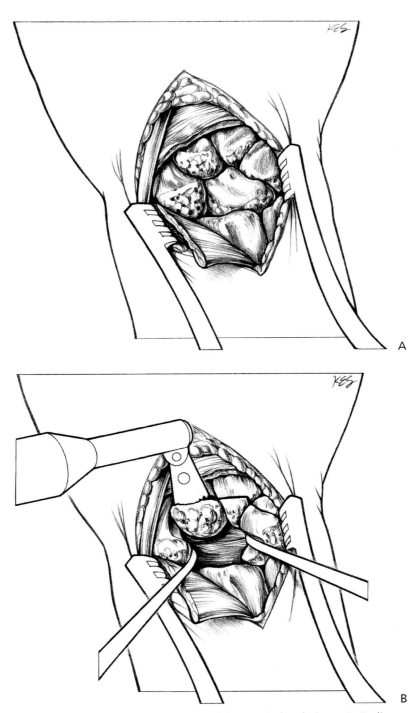

**FIGURE 10.** Schematic representation of the surgical technique. **A:** Radio-carpal and midcarpal joints are exposed. Erosive changes of the articular surfaces are depicted. **B:** There is usually a dissociation between scaphoid and lunate, facilitating exposure and excision of the head of the capitate and of the proximal pole of the hamate. (*continued.*)

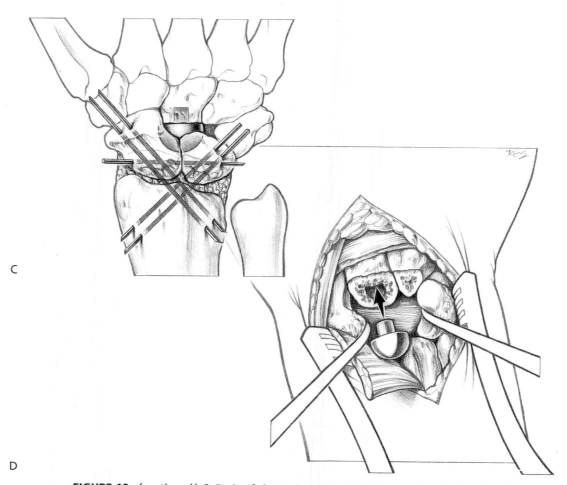

C

D

**FIGURE 10.** *(continued.)* **C:** Body of the capitate is prepared to receive the shortened stem of a condylar implant. **D:** Arthrodesis between radius, scaphoid, and lunate is completed. The assembled scapholunate unit should be rotated enough to cover most of the condylar implant. [From Taleisnik, J.: Combined radiocarpal arthrodesis and midcarpal (lunocapitate) arthroplasty for the treatment of rheumatoid arthritis of the wrist. *J. Hand Surg.*, 12A: 1–8, 1987, with permission.]

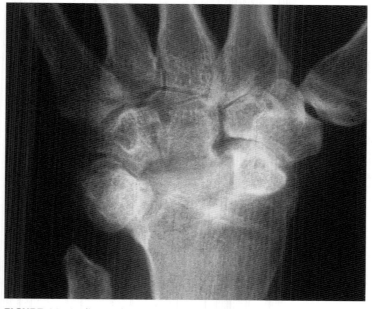

**FIGURE 11.** Radiograph 8 years postoperative.

carpal condylar arthroplasty, a solid radioscapholunate arthrodesis, and a satisfactory stable excision of the distal ulna (Fig. 11).

## RECOMMENDED READING

1. Allieu, Y., Asencio, G., Brahin B., et al.: First results of arthroplasty of the wrist by Swanson's implant. Twenty-five cases. *Ann. Chir. Main*, 1: 307, 1982.
2. Beckenbaugh, R. D., Linscheid, R. L.: Total wrist arthroplasty: a preliminary report. *J. Hand Surg.*, 2: 337, 1977.
3. Bowers, W. H.: Distal radioulnar joint arthroplasty. The hemiresection interposition technique. *J. Hand Surg.*, 10A: 169, 1985.
4. Brumfield, R. H., Champoux, J. A.: A biomechanical study of normal functional wrist motion. *Clin. Orthop.*, 187: 23, 1984.
5. Carroll, R. E., Dick, H. M.: Arthrodesis of the wrist for rheumatoid arthritis. *J. Bone Joint Surg.*, 53A: 1365, 1971.
6. Clayton, M. L., Ferlic, D. C.: Arthrodesis of the arthritic wrist. *Clin. Orthop.*, 187: 89, 1984.
7. Engkvist, O., Johansson, S. H., Ohlsen, L., Skoog, T.: Reconstruction of articular cartilage using autologous perichondrial grafts. A preliminary report. *Scand. J. Plast. Reconstr. Surg. Hand Surg.*, 9: 203, 1975.
8. Haddad, R. J., Riordan, D. C.: Arthrodesis of the wrist. *J. Bone Joint Surg.*, 49A: 950, 1967.
9. Kulick, R. G., De Fiore, J. C., Staub, L. R., Ranawat, C. S.: Long-term results of dorsal stabilization in the rheumatoid wrist. *J. Hand Surg.*, 6: 272, 1981.
10. Lamberta, F. J., Ferlic, D. C., Clayton, M. L.: Volz total wrist arthroplasty in rheumatoid arthritis: a preliminary report. *J. Hand Surg.*, 5: 245, 1980.
11. Mannerfelt, L., Malmsten, M.: Arthrodesis of the wrist in rheumatoid arthritis: a technique without external fixation. *Scand. J. Plast. Reconstr. Surg. Hand Surg.*, 5: 124, 1971.
12. Meuli, H. Ch.: Meuli total wrist arthroplasty. *Clin. Orthop.*, 187: 107, 1984.
13. Millender, L. H., Nalebuff, E. A.: Arthrodesis of the rheumatoid wrist. *J. Bone Joint Surg.*, 55A: 1026, 1973.
14. Palmer, A. K., Werner, F. W., Murphy, D., Glisson, R.: Functional wrist motion: a biomechanical study. *J. Hand Surg.*, 10A: 39, 1985.
15. Smith, R. J., Atkinson, R. E., Jupiter, J.: Silicone synovitis of the wrist. *J. Hand Surg.*, 10A: 47, 1985.
16. Swanson, A. B., de Groot Swanson, G., Maupin, B. K.: Flexible implant arthroplasty of the radiocarpal joint: surgical technique and long-term study. *Clin. Orthop.*, 187: 94, 1984.
17. Taleisnik, J.: Combined radiocarpal arthrodesis and midcarpal (lunocapitate) arthroplasty for the treatment of rheumatoid arthritis of the wrist. *J. Hand Surg.*, 12A: 1–8, 1987.

# 31

# Arthrodesis of the Rheumatoid Wrist

Andrew L. Terrono, Paul Feldon,
and Lewis H. Millender*

## INDICATIONS/CONTRAINDICATIONS

Although the radiologic appearance of the wrist joint influences the type of reconstruction, the indications for surgery are clinical. Absolute indications include disabling pain that is unresponsive to nonoperative treatment coupled with deformity or instability that impedes hand function. A painless, well-aligned wrist with minimal motion provides good function regardless of the radiologic appearance and rarely requires operative treatment.

When it has been determined that nonoperative treatment (including splinting, steroid injections, and systemic medication) have failed, surgery should be considered. Frequently, even with minimal wrist motion and moderate wrist joint destruction, most of the discomfort and functional disability is associated with problems of the distal radioulnar joint (DRUJ). In these cases, distal ulna surgery without radiocarpal reconstruction is advised. Radioulnar reconstruction is less disabling than radiocarpal fusion and is effective in these patients. However, when pain is located in both joints, appropriate radiocarpal and DRUJ reconstruction is necessary.

Occasionally, patients require simultaneous wrist arthrodesis and metacarpophalangeal (MP) joint arthroplasty. They should meet the indications for wrist fusion as well as MP joint arthroplasty. The wrist should have minimal deformity and not need to be dislocated to expose the joint surfaces and/or reduce the joint (see Fig. 3A). By realigning a deformed wrist, correcting deviation, and eliminating wrist pain, the results of the MP joint arthroplasty are improved (4). This less extensive exposure allows the MP joint arthroplasty to be carried out with minimal risk of excessive postoperative swelling and the attendant risk of skin slough

---

*Deceased.

or other complications. A contraindication for the procedure is extensive deformity that requires wrist dislocation and major dissection.

In most cases total wrist fusion is the recommended procedure for radiocarpal reconstruction. It is a safe, well-established procedure with few complications. It is a definitive operation that provides a pain-free, well-aligned, and stable wrist that improves hand function.

## PREOPERATIVE PLANNING

The patient is asked to describe all problems, including pain and functional deficits, and to identify specifically what physical activities cannot be done, as well as what activities are desired.

Physical examination of the entire upper extremity is performed. Range of motion, active and passive, of the digits, wrist, forearm, elbow, and shoulder are recorded. Areas of tenosynovitis, synovitis, crepitus, tenderness, and instability are sought.

On physical examination of the wrist one determines if pain is due primarily to radiocarpal and/or radioulnar joint abnormalities. The radiocarpal joint should be tender and painful when evaluated. Synovitis is not seen in all cases. If the wrist is the major source of problems and is well aligned, the MP joints are evaluated for the need for simultaneous MP joint arthroplasty. When a wrist fusion is performed, a DRUJ reconstruction is done simultaneously, if indicated.

The elbow and shoulder are evaluated completely as well. If the elbow and shoulder have very limited flexion and the flexed wrist allows the hand to get to the mouth, then shoulder and elbow function are addressed first. The wrist is fused in slight flexion in these patients.

Radiographs, using neutral posteroanterior, lateral, and oblique views and including the hand to evaluate the MP joints, are obtained. However, radiographs do not correlate well in all cases with the clinical picture. The radiographs may show severe destruction when symptoms are minimal. The DRUJ also is evaluated. If an intramedullary rod is going to be used, the metacarpals and distal half of the radius are evaluated for deformity and medullary diameter to judge rod size and whether intramedullary fixation is possible.

## SURGERY

The wrist is exposed under tourniquet control using a longitudinal dorsal incision, usually centered in the midline of the wrist (Fig. 1C). The incision is taken to the level of the dorsal retinaculum, and radial and ulnar skin flaps are formed as required for the proposed surgery. The dorsal branches of the radial and ulnar sensory nerves, frequently seen as the flaps, are formed (Fig. 1E), noted and protected with this approach. Transverse communicating veins are sectioned. Longitudinal veins are preserved. After skin flaps are formed, retraction sutures (3–0 silk) are placed in the skin edges.

A longitudinal incision is made into the fourth or sixth extensor compartment. In this instance, preferring to enter the fourth compartment, radial and ulnar flaps are raised (Fig. 1F). Transverse incisions are made proximal and distal to the retinaculum, allowing the retinaculum to be reflected as a flap as the vertical septum between each compartment is opened. Tenosynovectomy and distal ulnar excision are performed before arthrodesis (see Chapter 29). The radiocarpal joint is exposed using a transverse capsular incision over the entire proximal carpal row, leaving 3 mm of capsule attached to the radius for closure. A distally based capsular flap is constructed and preserved for closure. If palmar dislocation of the carpus is needed to prepare the joint surfaces and allow proper wrist alignment, the radial capsule is incised (Fig. 1H). If there is any difficulty exposing the

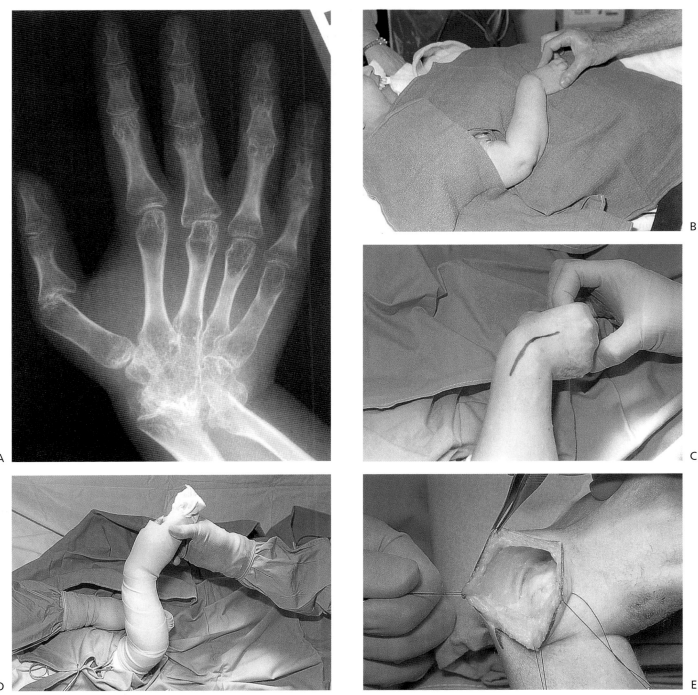

**FIGURE 1.** This patient is a 16-year-old girl who has had juvenile rheumatoid arthritis for 13 years. She presents with a painful deformed wrist, distal radioulnar joint, radiohumeral joint, and only 20° of rotation. **A:** Preoperative radiograph showing wrist destruction and deformity with small medullary canals of the radius and metacarpals. **B:** Wrist deformity, flexion, and ulnar deviation is seen. Because of limited shoulder, elbow, and forearm motion, surgery was performed with the arm resting on the abdomen. **C:** Midline dorsal longitudinal incision is marked. **D:** Tourniquet control is used. **E:** Full-thickness skin flaps are raised on the extensor retinaculum. Skin retraction sutures are placed to retract the skin gently. The dorsal sensory branch of the radial nerve is seen in the flap and protected. (*continued.*)

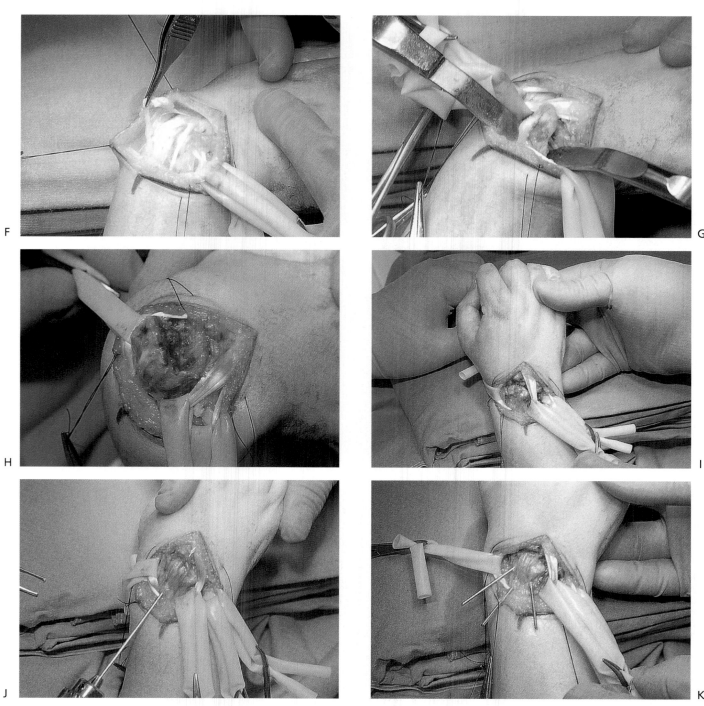

**FIGURE 1.** *(continued.)* **F:** The extensor retinaculum is incised in the fourth compartment, and radial and ulnar flaps are raised. Tenosynovectomy is performed. **G:** Penrose drains are used to retract the extensor tendons. The distal ulnar is exposed and distal excision performed. The subsheath in the palmarly subluxed extensor carpi ulnaris tendon is not opened since there is no synovitis. **H:** The radius is exposed completely. This is facilitated by release of the first compartment. The surfaces of the carpal bones and radius are prepared at this time. **I:** The hand can be aligned on the radius. **J:** Oblique 0.062 K-wires were positioned so that their exit from the radius was seen. Intramedullary fixation could not be used because of the small canal diameter. **K:** Three 0.062 K-wires are used to stabilize the wrist fusion. *(continued.)*

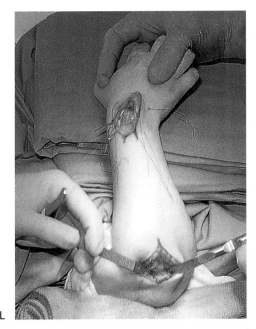

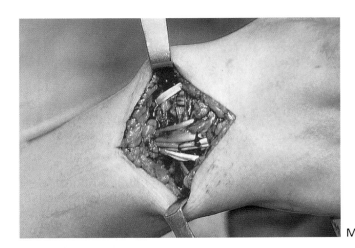

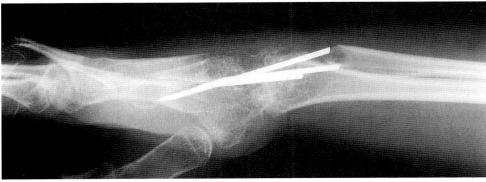

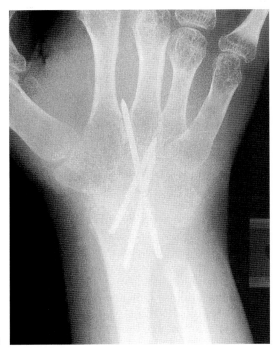

**FIGURE 1. (continued.) L:** Radial head resection is performed at same time as wrist reconstruction. **M:** The capsule retinaculum is closed with 3–0 monofilament polyglyconate suture. The retinaculum is put under the extensor tendons. **N** and **O:** Postoperative radiographs showing wrist alignment and K-wire position.

radius, the first extensor compartment tendons are released and retracted before the radial capsule is released from the radial styloid to facilitate exposure and to avoid injury. Rongeurs are used to carry out the synovectomy. Cartilage and sclerotic bone are removed from the radius and carpal bones. This includes the radius; the proximal, distal, and intracarpal surfaces of the scaphoid, lunate, and triquetrum; and the proximal surfaces of the capitate and hamate. The scaphotrapezial, trapezoid, and carpometacarpal joints are not included routinely. The amount of bone removed depends on the degree of deformity and destruction present. When there is significant palmar and ulnar erosion of the radius secondary to palmar subluxation of the carpus, more dorsal and radial bone needs to be removed to correct the deformity and realign the wrist. When there is extensive destruction of the proximal carpal row, these bones can be removed and used for bone graft, and the distal carpus can be fused to the radius. Iliac bone graft is not used routinely; however, local bone grafts (metacarpal heads, distal ulnar) are used when available.

After alignment is restored and the radius and carpus are prepared, internal fixation is carried out. Traditionally, we have used a Steinmann pin introduced into the carpus. The radius is perforated with an awl to identify the medullary canal. The medullary canal of the radius is sized by preoperative radiographs and by passing rods down the canal to determine the appropriate rod to be used. The rod is drilled from the carpus distally between the second and third metacarpal bones to penetrate the skin between the dorsal aspects of the MP joints (3). This helps to avoid neurovascular injury. The wrist is reduced and the pin is tapped into the radius under direct vision, then countersunk deep between the metacarpal bones. A staple or other fixation can be used to add stability. This method has provided excellent stability and allowed patients to be out of splints in 4 to 6 weeks. Alternatively, if there is severe instability with carpal bone destruction, the MP joint is destroyed, or a simultaneous MP joint arthroplasty is going to be performed, the rod is introduced into the long finger metacarpal to increase the stability. In this case, the size of the metacarpal determines the rod size. If an MP joint arthroplasty is indicated, the rod is introduced distally through the joint; otherwise, it is introduced through the dorsal aspect of the metacarpal. In either case, the distal end of the rod must be countersunk.

Occasionally, we use a modification of this technique. Two relatively thin Steinmann pins (5/64" to 9/64", usually 3/32" or 7/64" in diameter) are used instead of one large Steinmann pin. The subchondral bone of the radius is perforated with an awl to identify the medullary canal and allow insertion of the Steinmann pins. A small window in the dorsal cortex of the radius allows the pins to be seen entering the radius (Fig. 2B, C). Pins are inserted distally through the dorsal aspect of the second and third web spaces (to avoid damage to the neurovascular structures of the palm), between the metacarpals, across the carpus, and into the radius (Fig. 2A). The pins are thin enough to allow adjustment of the final position by bending the rods. If slightly more extension is desired the wrist is positioned after rod placement. The thinner pins also minimize the potential for compression of the intrinsic muscles. While the wrist is held in the appropriate position, the pins are tapped into position. Drilling is avoided to protect the soft tissues and to minimize perforation of the radius. Rotational stability is provided by this "stacked pin" effect (Fig. 2D, E) (2).

If intramedullary fixation of the radius is not possible, other techniques are used. Instead of the intramedullary technique, a few smaller pins are placed from the radius into the carpus (Fig. 1J) or from the index metacarpal into the carpus (6). These techniques are especially useful in patients with juvenile rheumatoid arthritis who have small medullary canals. Additional advantages include the fact that the carpus does not have to be dislocated to introduce the pin in a retrograde fashion, and wrist position can be varied as needed.

## Combined Wrist Arthrodesis and Metacarpophalangeal Joint Arthroplasty

The following technique merges the procedures into one operation (Fig. 3). The wrist joint is exposed in a similar method to that of routine wrist fusion, through a small radiocarpal incision without wrist dislocation. Distal ulna excision is performed. The wrist capsule is opened and synovectomy, débridement, and preparation for fusion carried out.

Without dislocating the wrist, the joint surfaces are prepared and a standard MP joint arthroplasty is performed. Metacarpal heads are used for bone graft. Before inserting the prosthesis, a Steinmann pin is introduced into the long finger metacarpal (Fig. 3E) and tapped across the carpus into the medullary canal of the radius under direct vision. The pin is tapped deeply into the metacarpal to allow room for the prosthesis. Intraoperative radiographs are obtained to document pin position.

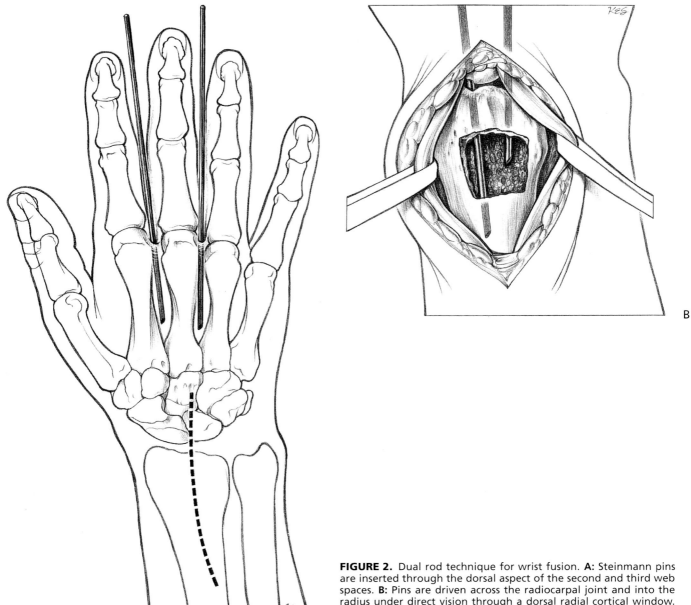

**FIGURE 2.** Dual rod technique for wrist fusion. **A:** Steinmann pins are inserted through the dorsal aspect of the second and third web spaces. **B:** Pins are driven across the radiocarpal joint and into the radius under direct vision through a dorsal radial cortical window. (*continued.*)

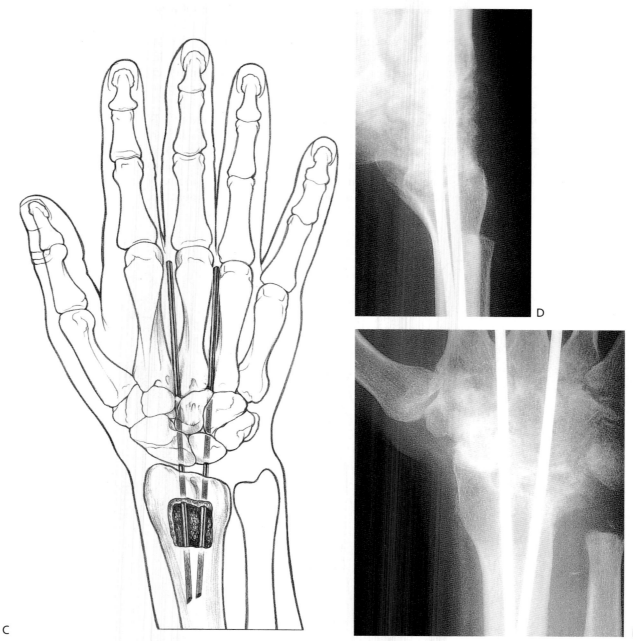

**FIGURE 2. (continued.) C:** The "stacked pin" effect provides rotational stability while allowing adjustment of final position. **D** and **E:** Final radiographs after radial carpal fusion using the dual rod technique with distal ulnar resection.

A small plug of bone is tapped into the canal to prevent distal migration of the pin. Additional fixation can be used if more stability is needed. After this is completed the MP joint arthroplasty is completed (Fig. 3J, K).

## Closure

In all cases in which pins are left in place, intraoperative radiographs or fluoroscopy are used to see the entire rod to make sure it is properly located and that the wrist position is appropriate (neutral to 10° of extension). The capsule is closed using 2–0 or 3–0 monofilament polyglyconate suture.

At the conclusion of the procedure the tourniquet is deflated, hemostasis is obtained, and a Penrose drain is used for 24 hours as needed. The entire retinaculum is sutured with 3–0 or 4–0 monofilament polyglyconate suture, deep to the tendons. The skin is approximated using interrupted 5–0 nylon sutures. A bulky compression dressing is applied, including palmar and dorsal short-arm plaster splints. The dressing is modified if other procedures have been performed.

## POSTOPERATIVE MANAGEMENT

Postoperative management consists of short-arm palmar and dorsal splints unless there is a need to protect the radioulnar joint, in which case a long-arm splint is used. The digits are splinted in extension until active extension is possible, to prevent an extension lag. Formal therapy is needed only for patients who have significant pain. Patients usually regain full finger motion in 7 to 10 days. If there is firm fixation the wrist is taken out of the splints at 2 weeks to bathe, and usually the splints are discarded in 4 to 6 weeks. When the patient has undergone simultaneous wrist fusion plus MP joint arthroplasty the digits are splinted for 7 to 14 days depending on the capsular reconstruction. A dynamic splint is fabricated at this point. If the Steinmann pin does not cause discomfort, it is not

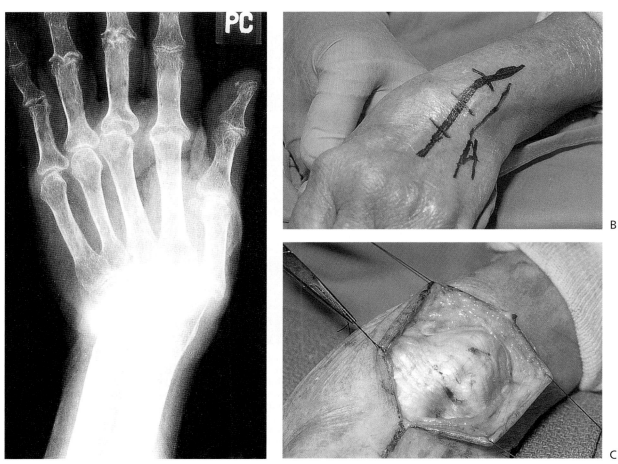

A                                                                                                    B

                                                                                                     C

**FIGURE 3.** This patient had radiocarpal pain and wrist destruction plus metacarpophalangeal involvement. Therefore, simultaneous wrist fusion and metacarpophalangeal arthroplasty were performed. **A:** Preoperative radiograph showing wrist and index metacarpophalangeal joint destruction. **B:** Midline incision marked out, previous incision for distal ulnar excision seen. Note minimal wrist deformity. **C:** Thick skin flaps raised on the extensor retinaculum. (*continued.*)

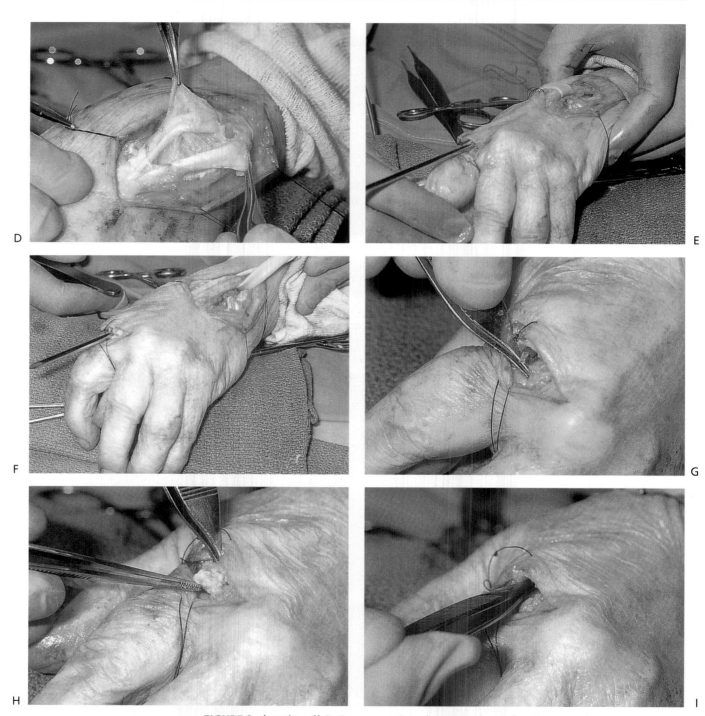

**FIGURE 3.** (*continued.*) **D**: Extensor retinaculum incised over fourth compartment and tenosyn-ovectomy performed. **E**: After wrist joint is exposed, bone is prepared using a rongeur. The metacarpophalangeal arthroplasty is performed. Before a prosthesis is inserted, a Steinmann pin is sized, then placed into the medullary canal of the index finger metacarpal and tapped until it is seen at the proximal carpus. **F**: The radius had been perforated to locate the medullary canal. The wrist is held reduced. The pin is driven into the medullary canal of the radius under direct vision. **G**: The pin is countersunk so that the prosthesis will fit. **H**: A plug of bone is inserted into the metacarpal medullary canal to help prevent distal pin migration. **I**: The bone plug is inserted in its entirety. (*continued.*)

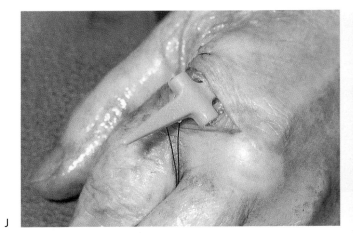

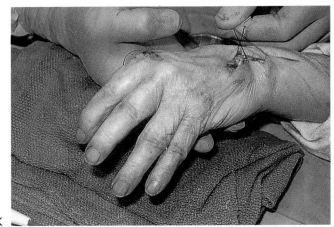

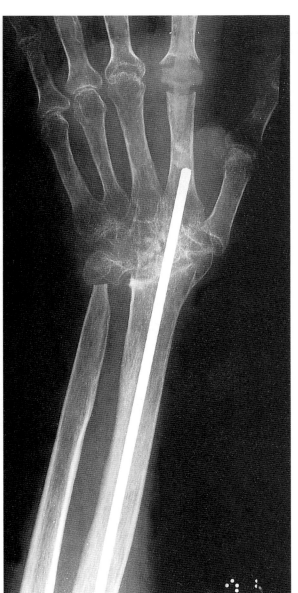

**FIGURE 3.** (*continued.*) **J**: Trial prosthesis is inserted to ensure complete seating of the prosthesis. **K**: Prosthesis is inserted and wounds closed. **L**: Postoperative radiograph with index metacarpophalangeal joint arthroplasty and bone plug distal to rod in index metacarpal.

removed. However, when the dual rod technique is used, the pins usually are removed under local anesthesia, using a "vise grip," between 4 and 6 months. When pins are introduced from the radius or from the base of the index metacarpal, they require removal after the fusion has healed.

We expect excellent pain relief and stability with good alignment, which provides a stable platform for hand function. Function usually is substantially improved. Wrist fusion in proper alignment also helps prevent ulnar deviation and failure of MP arthroplasties.

## COMPLICATIONS

Intraoperative complications are uncommon. Perforation of the palmar cortex of the radius (Fig. 4) does occur; however, it can be prevented by careful preoperative evaluation of the radius and intraoperative posteroanterior and lateral radiographs showing the entire pin. Complications following wrist arthrodesis are also

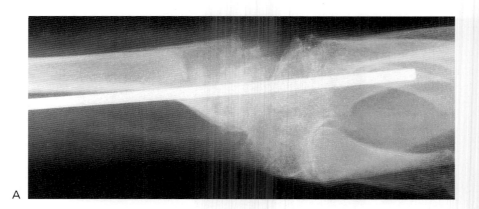

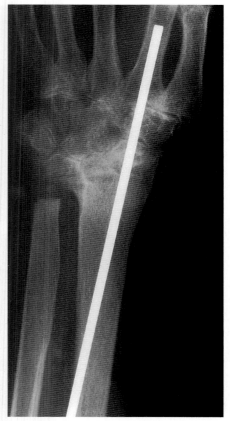

**FIGURE 4. A and B:** Inadvertent perforation of the Steinmann pin through the palmar cortex of the radius. A small window in the dorsal cortex of the radius and/or intraoperative radiographs showing the entire rod in both planes may have prevented this.

uncommon. Distal migration of the Steinmann pin requiring early removal has been the most frequent complication. Sometimes a pseudarthrosis results, but is usually painless. Other Steinmann pin complications have been observed, including breakage of the pins (Fig. 5).

## ILLUSTRATIVE CASE FOR TECHNIQUE

A 16-year-old girl presented with a 13-year history of juvenile rheumatoid arthritis. She complained of a painful deformed wrist with limited motion and a painful radiohumeral joint with only 20° of rotation (Fig. 1B). She had enough shoulder and elbow flexion to get her hand to her mouth even if the wrist was straight. Finger extensors and flexors were working, and the MP joints were satisfactory.

Preoperative radiographs showed a deformed dislocated wrist with small medullary canals of the radius and metacarpals (Fig. 1A). The distal ulnar was dislocated and eroded. The radiohumeral joint also was involved.

She had a dislocated radiocarpal joint with bone loss and narrow medullary canals of the radius and metacarpals with intact MP joint and tendons. The DRUJ was involved, as well as the radiohumeral joint. Therefore, she needed a wrist fusion to provide a stable platform for hand function. Other reconstructive options were not appropriate because of the severe deformity and bone loss. Because of the small medullary canals, intramedullary pins could not be used. DRUJ reconstruction and radial head excision were indicated to restore rotation.

A radiocarpal fusion, using radius to carpal pins with DRUJ reconstruction and radial head excision, was performed (Fig. 1B–M). Rehabilitation without formal

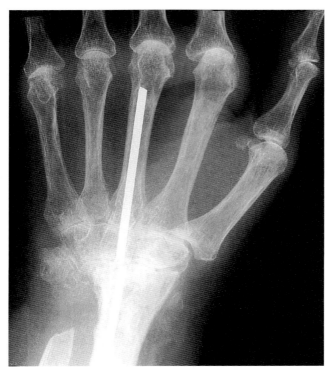

**FIGURE 5.** Fracture of the Steinmann pin can occur. This may be secondary to persistent nonunion.

hand therapy was done as described above. At 8 weeks, solid fusion was noted (Fig. 1N, O), and pins were removed. Her function was improved, and pain relief was excellent. She had 60° of pronation and 55° of supination.

## ACKNOWLEDGMENT

The authors thank Richard Mottla of the New England Baptist Hospital Medical Media Department for his excellent photography.

## RECOMMENDED READING

1. Ely, L. W.: Study of the joint tuberculosis. *Surg. Gynecol. Obstet.*, 10: 561–572, 1910.
2. Feldon, P., Terrono, A. L., Millender, L. H., Nalebuff, E. A.: Rheumatoid arthritis and other connective tissue diseases. In: *Operative Hand Surgery*, 4th ed., edited by D. P. Green, R. N. Hotchkiss, and W. C. Pederson, Churchill Livingstone, New York, pp. 1651–1739, 1999.
3. Millender, L. H., Nalebuff, E. A.: Arthrodesis of the rheumatoid wrist—an evaluation of sixty patients and a description of a different surgical technique. *J. Bone Joint Surg.*, 55A: 1026–1034, 1973.
4. Millender, L. H., Phillips, C.: Combined wrist arthrodesis and metacarpophalangeal joint arthroplasty in rheumatoid arthritis. *Orthopedics*, 1: 43–48, 1978.
5. Smith-Peterson, M. N., AuFranc, O. E., Corrsen, C. B.: Useful surgical procedures for rheumatoid arthritis involving joints of the upper extremity. *Arch. Surg.*, 46: 764–770, 1943.
6. Viegas, S. F., Rimoldi, R., Patterson, R.: Modified technique of intramedullary fixation for wrist arthrodesis. *J. Hand Surg.*, 14A: 618–623, 1989.

# 32

# Total Wrist Arthroplasty

Robert D. Beckenbaugh

## INDICATIONS/CONTRAINDICATIONS

Arthrodesis of the wrist is a reconstructive procedure that provides pain relief and stability with a reasonable level of function for patients with painful wrist arthritis. In patients with single joint upper extremity disease the presence of satisfactory digital, elbow, and shoulder range of motion generally precludes the necessity of the motion-providing operation of total wrist arthroplasty. Certain occupations, however, despite other normal upper extremity functions, may have special requirements for motion (e.g., musicians or mechanics who require wrist flexion to perform their jobs). The major indication for total wrist arthroplasty, however, is in patients with rheumatoid arthritis who have general destructive arthritis involving all joints of the upper extremity, coupled with limitation of forearm rotation, elbow flexion, and shoulder motion as well as deformity and limited motion of the digits. In these patients eliminating wrist motion may diminish rather than improve overall upper extremity function. The capability of performing radial deviation and some flexion enhances a patient's functional capacity. In these instances, the procedure of total wrist arthroplasty may be selected over the traditional procedure of wrist arthrodesis.

Prior to performing a total wrist arthroplasty, the surgeon explains to the patient that the procedure of total wrist replacement may necessitate further operative reconstructive procedures such as revision for imbalance or loosening. Although the procedure provides pain relief with motion, it is a higher-risk operation than the more traditional procedure of arthrodesis. Arthrodesis generally provides relief of pain (although with absence of motion) with little risk of additional complications or the need for further surgery. Therefore, it is often appropriate to consider arthroplasty a high-risk, high-reward procedure (1,5).

The only contraindication to total wrist arthroplasty is infection. It may be performed in the presence of very advanced destructive arthritis with absence of considerable bone stock. In rare instances in cases of juvenile rheumatoid arthritis, the medullary canal of the radius may be so deficient as to preclude the possibility of performing total wrist arthroplasty. In some cases in which severe palmar sub-

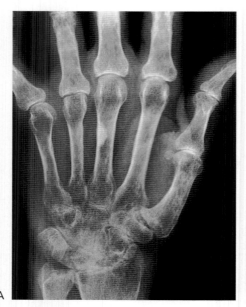
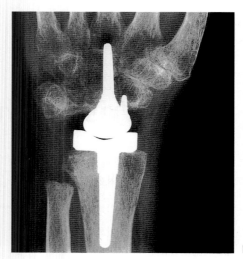

A                                                                B

**FIGURE 1. A:** Preoperative radiograph. **B:** Van Leeuwen technique. Note that distal stem tip just crosses the carpometacarpal joint to strengthen resistance to dorsal "breakout." Note preservation of more of proximal carpus.

luxation is present, the wrist extensors may have ruptured rather than dislocated to the radial side of the forearm. In these instances the wrist extensors must be repairable or reconstructible with adjacent tendon transfers, as the procedure of total wrist arthroplasty requires the presence of functioning radial wrist extensors.

## PREOPERATIVE PLANNING

The biaxial wrist is available in three sizes: large, medium, and small. Templates with 6% magnification factors are available for preoperative planning. Routine anteroposterior and true lateral radiographs of the wrist are taken, and the templates are placed over the radiographs to identify the largest prostheses that will fit within the boundaries of the cortical margins of the shaft of the third metacarpal and the distal radius. In general, the largest available prosthesis is inserted. Utilizing the templates, the amount of bone to be resected and the location of the bone resection are estimated. In cases of very advanced destructive wrist arthritis and collapse, it may be necessary to insert the prostheses directly into the base of the third metacarpal. In general, however, the plan is to place the stem of the distal component into the distal half of the body of the capitate, preserving the distal half of the distal carpal row. Van Leeuwen has described a modification of the technique in which small components are used with preservation of the majority of the capitate. This results in the distal stem tip being located at the carpal metacarpal joint (Fig. 1A and B). No cement is used. He believes that this decreases distal component loosening and dorsal migration (6). The distal ulna is resected in total wrist arthroplasty in all cases to allow proper placement of the radial components, which would otherwise impinge upon the distal ulna if not removed during the procedure.

## BIAXIAL WRIST DEVICE

The device has an offset stem on the radial component to allow for ulnar displacement of the prosthesis center of rotation, located in the palmar third of the head of

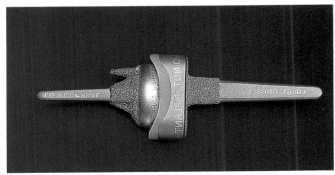

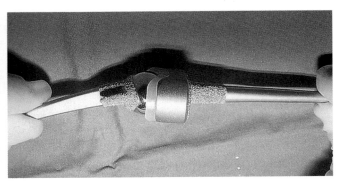

**FIGURE 2. A:** Biaxial wrist device. The device has an offset stem on the radial component to allow for ulnar displacement of the prosthesis and center of rotation, located in the palmar third of the head of the capitate. **B:** On the lateral view, one can see that the radial stem is displaced dorsally from the prosthetic articulation to lower the center of rotation to its more physiologic position.

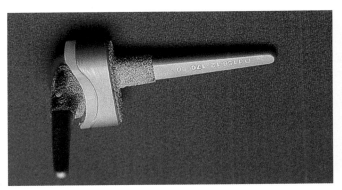

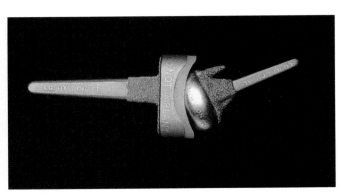

**FIGURE 3.** The articulating surfaces allow 80° **(A)** of both flexion and extension of the wrist within the prosthetic confines as well as 30° **(B)** of radial and ulnar deviation.

the capitate. On the lateral view, one can see that the radial stem is displaced dorsally from the prosthetic articulation to lower the center of rotation to its more physiologic position (Fig. 2). In addition, on the lateral view a curvature in the stem of the metacarpal component can be seen that allows insertion following the natural curve of the shaft of the metacarpal. The distal component has a stud for fixation of the trapezoid to help control rotation, and both components have a porous coating surface, applied to the area immediately adjacent to the articulating surfaces, to enhance fixation, with or without the use of bone cement.

The articulating surfaces allow 80° of flexion and extension of the wrist within the prosthetic confines, as well as 30° of radial and ulnar deviation; however, these excess ranges of motion should be avoided in the clinical setting (Fig. 3).

## SURGERY

Surgery is performed under general or regional anesthesia with tourniquet control. In standard cases, the arm is positioned on a hand operating table and draping is performed above the elbow to allow for forearm rotation. In patients with advanced rheumatoid arthritis and severe shoulder and elbow disease, evaluate range of motion before draping. It may not be possible to perform the procedure on the hand table because of significant limitations of abduction and internal rotation of the shoulder and/or extension of the elbow. In those cases, it may be preferable for the patient to be in a supine position with the hand placed across the abdomen.

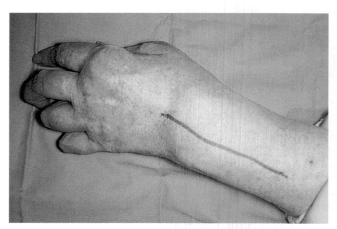

**FIGURE 4.** The incision is outlined directly centered over the dorsum of the wrist in a straight longitudinal fashion.

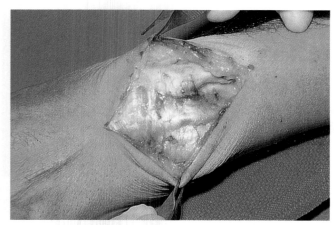

**FIGURE 5.** The subcutaneous dissection is performed, preserving the subcutaneous fat and the neurovascular structures intact, making the flaps as thick as possible.

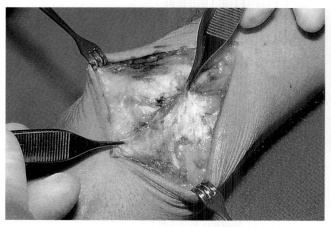

**FIGURE 6.** The retinaculum is split longitudinally through the fourth dorsal compartment.

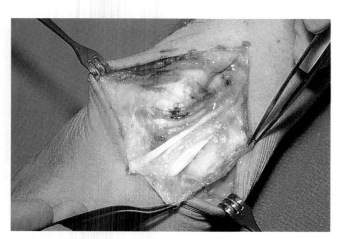

**FIGURE 7.** The retinaculum is retracted medially and laterally to expose the tendons of the fourth dorsal compartment, and a local dorsal extensor tenosynovectomy is performed.

### Technique

The incision is outlined directly centered over the dorsum of the wrist in a straight longitudinal fashion (Fig. 4). Avoid dorsal zigzag, S-shaped, and transverse incisions in this procedure, as they are associated with higher incidences of skin edge slough. Transverse incisions are not extensile, as may become necessary in revision surgery. Hypertrophic scarring in patients with longitudinal incisions over the dorsum of the wrist has not been a problem (see Chapter 1).

The skin and subcutaneous tissues are elevated directly to the retinaculum over the centrum of the dorsum of the wrist. Perform the subcutaneous dissection, preserve the subcutaneous fat with the neurovascular structures intact, and make the flaps as thick as possible (Fig. 5).

Split the retinaculum longitudinally through the fourth dorsal compartment (Fig. 6). Retract the retinaculum medially and laterally to expose the tendons of the fourth dorsal compartment, and perform a local dorsal extensor tenosynovectomy (Fig. 7).

Release the extensor digiti quinti minimi tendon from the retinaculum; the extensor carpi ulnaris tendon may be exposed and retracted at this time (Fig. 8).

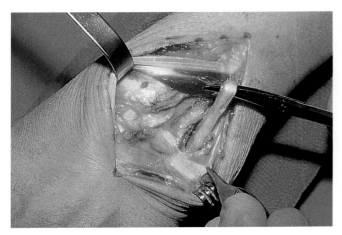

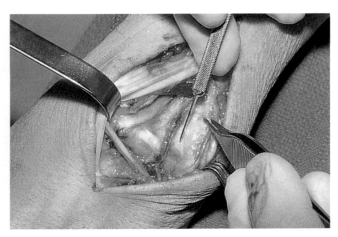

**FIGURE 8.** The extensor digiti quinti proprius tendon is released from the retinaculum, and the extensor carpi ulnaris tendon may be exposed and retracted.

**FIGURE 9.** The periosteum of the distal ulna is incised sharply, and, subperiosteally, the distal ulna is exposed.

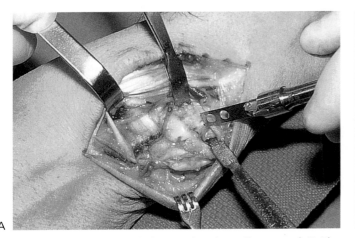

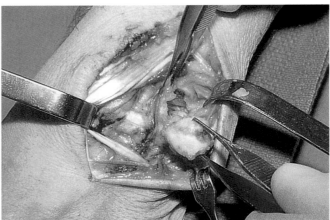

A

B

**FIGURE 10. A:** The distal ulna is subperiosteally resected. **B:** The resection level is made at the area just proximal to the sigmoid notch of the radius.

The periosteum of the distal ulna is incised sharply, and subperiosteally the distal ulna is exposed (Fig. 9) and resected. The resection level is made at the area just proximal to the sigmoid notch of the radius, according to the preoperative planning, at the level just proximal to the proposed resection of the distal radius (Fig. 10). The exposure radially involves release of the extensor pollicis longus and then development of the dorsal flap over the radial wrist extensors (Fig. 11).

Expose the tendons in the first dorsal compartment subperiosteally and retract them during later resection of the distal radial bone. It is essential to expose and retract these tendons directly to prevent damage to them during resection of the radial articular surface (Fig. 12).

At this point, expose the dorsum of the wrist capsule by retracting the tendons of the second and third dorsal compartments radially and the fourth and fifth dorsal compartments ulnarly. Then make a T-shaped incision in the dorsal wrist capsule, extending from the base of the third metacarpal longitudinally and transversely across the level of the radiocarpal joint (Fig. 13). The medial and lateral capsular flaps of tissue are elevated sharply distally to expose the dorsum of the carpus (Fig. 14).

Use a sagittal saw to resect the distal end of the radius transverse to the long axis of the radius (Fig. 15), and to resect the bone distally through the middle to

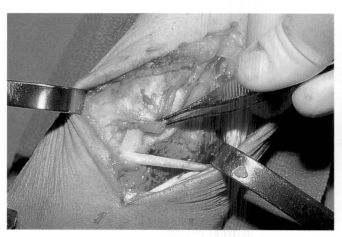
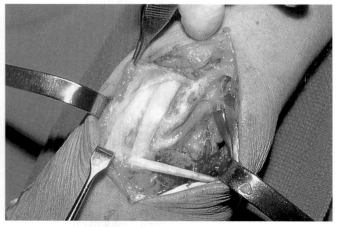

A

B

**FIGURE 11.** **A:** The exposure radially involves release of the extensor pollicis longus. **B:** Development of the dorsal flap over the radial wrist extensors.

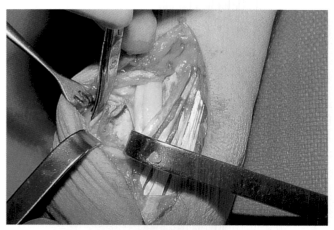
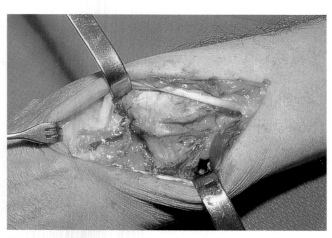

**FIGURE 12.** Subperiosteally, the tendons in the first dorsal compartment are exposed; they are retracted during later resection of the distal radial bone.

**FIGURE 13.** The dorsum of the wrist capsule is exposed by retracting the tendons of the second and third dorsal compartments radially and the fourth and fifth dorsal compartments ulnarly.

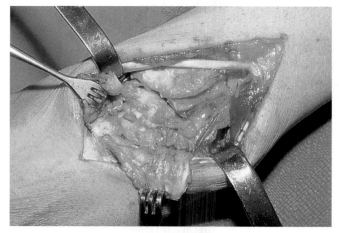
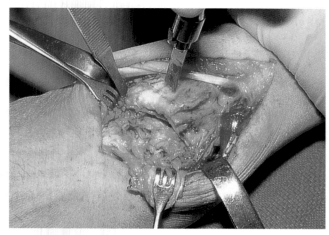

**FIGURE 14.** The medial and lateral capsular flaps of tissue are elevated sharply distally to expose the dorsum of the carpus.

**FIGURE 15.** A sagittal saw is used to resect the distal end of the radius transverse to the long axis of the radius.

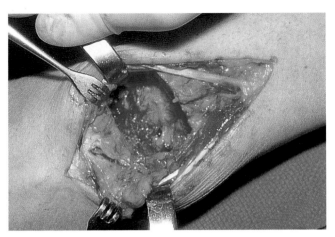

FIGURE 16. The sagittal saw also is used to resect the bone distally through the middle to distal third of the remnants of the distal carpal row.

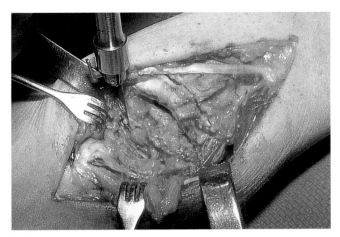

FIGURE 17. The carpal bones are resected sharply, leaving the palmar capsule intact.

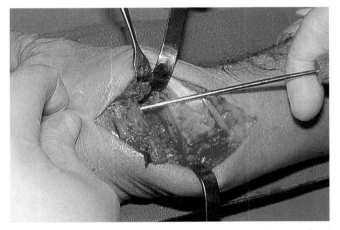

FIGURE 18. The next step is to identify the level of the shaft of the third metacarpal and place the starting awl down the medullary canal of the third metacarpal.

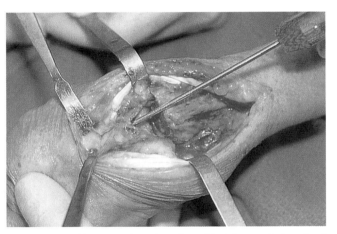

FIGURE 19. This procedure can be aided by a slight distal extension of the incision to allow subperiosteal exposure of the shaft of the third metacarpal (shown here exposed between two Hohmann retractors).

distal third of the remnants of the distal carpal row (Fig. 16). The carpal bones are resected sharply, leaving the palmar capsule intact if possible; if it is severely destroyed, or eroded by synovium, the flexor tendons may be seen in the palmar portion of the wound (Fig. 17).

The next step is to identify the location of the shaft of the third metacarpal and to place the starting awl down the medullary canal of the third metacarpal (Fig. 18). This procedure, which can be difficult (with perforation of the shaft of the third metacarpal), is aided tremendously by a slight distal extension of the incision to allow exposure of the shaft of the third metacarpal, as shown here between the two Hohmann retractors. This direct visualization of the third metacarpal greatly increases the ease of proper centering of the awls in the intramedullary canal of the third metacarpal, eliminating the possibility of perforating the metacarpal shaft during placement. It is highly recommended for all arthroplasty procedures (Fig. 19).

The blunt awl provided with the instrumentation is used to confirm the presence of the awl within the medullary canal by placing it down the reamed medullary canal until it reaches the metacarpal head cortex (Fig. 20). It is seen by distance

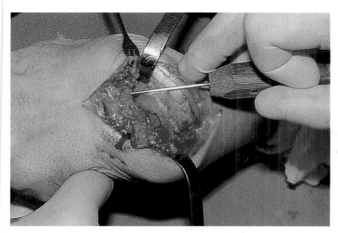

**FIGURE 20.** The blunt awl provided with instrumentation is used to identify the presence of the awl within the medullary canal by placing it down the reamed medullary canal until it reaches the metacarpal head cortex.

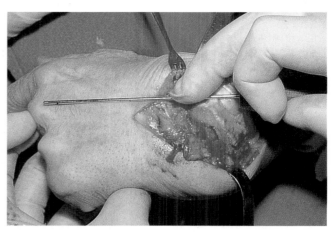

**FIGURE 21.** The photo shows the distance measurement to touch the base of the inner cortical margin of the head of the third metacarpal.

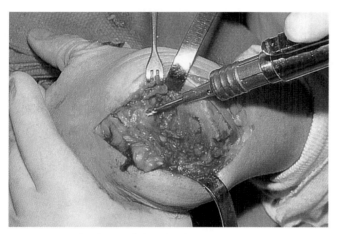

**FIGURE 22.** The base of the third metacarpal and sometimes the cortical bone of the capitate need to be expanded by the use of a power burr to allow placement of the prosthesis if the larger size is used.

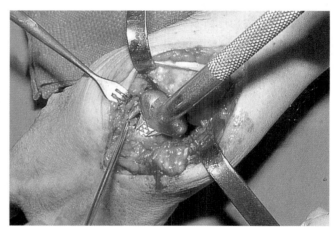

**FIGURE 23.** The distal reamer is used in a repetitive fashion to prepare a carpentry match fit for the distal component. There is a stud on the radial side of this component that is sharp enough to be driven into the trapezoid by simple impaction. In extremely dense bone situations, it may be necessary to use a small awl to start this hole in the base of the trapezoid and/or second metacarpal if the carpus have all been resected.

measurement to touch the base of the inner cortical margin of the head of the third metacarpal (Fig. 21).

After identifying and confirming the intramedullary presence in the third metacarpal, the canal is expanded gradually by various reamers to accept the largest possible size implant. The base of the third metacarpal and sometimes the cortical bone of the capitate need to be expanded by the use of a power burr to allow placement of the prostheses if the larger size is used (Fig. 22).

The distal reamer, which has impacting and cutting edges, is used in a repetitive fashion to prepare a carpentry match fit for the distal component. There is a stud on the radial side of this component that is sharp enough to be driven into the trapezoid by simple impaction. In extremely dense bone situations, it may be necessary to use a small awl to start this hole in the base of the trapezoid and/or second metacarpal if the carpus have all been resected (Fig. 23).

After reaming and impaction are completed, the semi-oval impacting reamer shaped in the form of the metacarpal component should seat nicely into the pre-

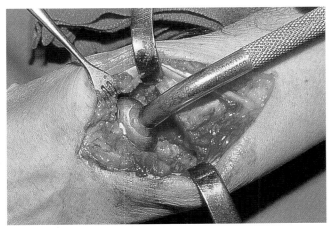

**FIGURE 24.** After the reaming and impaction is completed, the semi-oval impacting reamer shaped in the form of the metacarpal component should seat nicely into the prepared curved distal cortical and cancellous margin of the base of the remnant carpus.

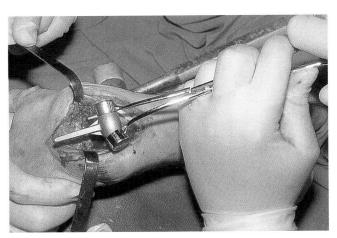

**FIGURE 25.** Utilizing a special holding instrument, the trial distal component is inserted.

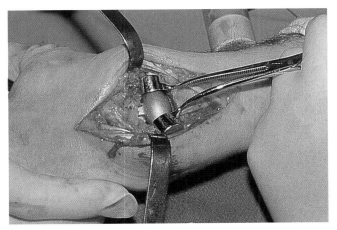

**FIGURE 26.** Care is taken to be certain that the ellipsoidal articulating surface is oriented in the same transverse plane as that of the dorsal metacarpals, avoiding any tendency toward rotation of the component (pronation or supination with regard to the plane of the metacarpals).

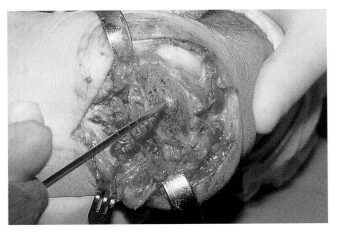

**FIGURE 27.** Utilizing the larger awls down, the narrower proximal medullary canal of the radius tends to self-center the stem of this component.

pared curved distal cortical and cancellous margin of the base of the remnant carpus (Fig. 24).

Using a special holding instrument, the trial distal component is inserted (Fig. 25). The trial component, which has no porous surfacing, should fit slightly snugly into the medullary canal of the third metacarpal and basal carpus. Care is taken to make sure that the ellipsoidal articulating surface is oriented in the same transverse plane as that of the dorsal metacarpals, avoiding any tendency toward rotation of the component (pronation or supination with regard to the plane of the metacarpals) (Fig. 26).

Attention is turned to the distal resected surface of the radius; using the smallest awl, the medullary canal of the radius is identified and enlarged starting at the central portion of the distal radial canal. When the larger awls are used, the narrower proximal medullary canal of the radius tends to self-center the orientation of the stem of this component (Fig. 27).

At this point, medullary canal bone is impacted with the reamers that are of equal size to the stemmed components. In the majority of cases in this situation, bone is impacted into the medullary canal of the radius; it is not removed (Fig. 28).

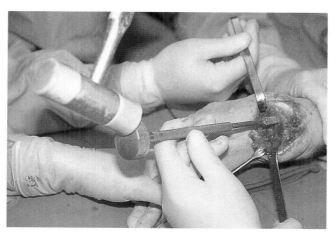

**FIGURE 28.** The medullary canal bone is impacted with the reamers that are of equal size to the component stems.

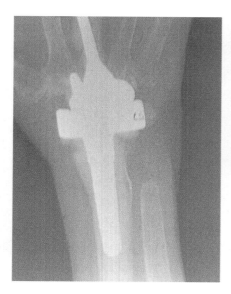

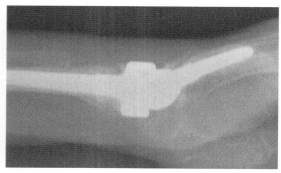

**FIGURE 29.** The properly seated *radial* component tends to be straight due to the natural confines of the cortical bone of the distal radius. In patients with osteoporosis, however, as demonstrated in these radiographs, the medullary canal may be relatively larger, and proper centering of the radial stem within the radial medullary canal will need to be confirmed with intraoperative radiographs.

The properly seated radial component will tend to be straight due to the natural confines of the cortical bone of the distal radius. In patients with a large amount of osteoporosis, however, the medullary canal may be relatively larger and proper centering of the radial stem within the radial medullary canal will need to be confirmed with intraoperative radiographs (Fig. 29).

Take care in impacting the radial component that the transversely oriented polyethylene cup is parallel to the transverse plane of the radius. Pronation and supination of the radial component is tolerable from a functional standpoint due to the few degrees of freedom allowed in the articulation, but it may result in an increased wear pattern (Fig. 30).

Impact the radial trial component and articulate with the distal trial component and the tension test as described later (Fig. 31).

A small periosteal elevator may be used to disimpact the radial trial component (Fig. 32).

The articulating surfaces of the permanent component have a porous coated base 1 mm thick at the bases of the metacarpal and radial components (Fig. 33). In addition, the thickness of the polyethylene buildup is slightly greater than in the

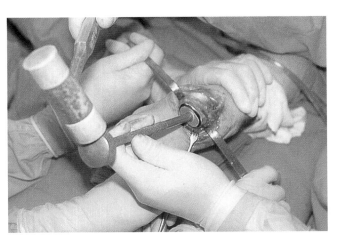

FIGURE 30. Care is taken when impacting the radial component that the transversely oriented polyethylene cup is parallel to the transverse plane of the radius.

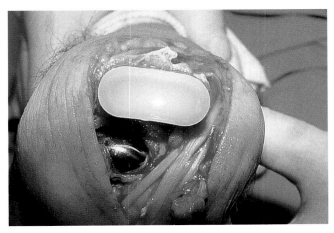

FIGURE 31. The radial trial component is impacted.

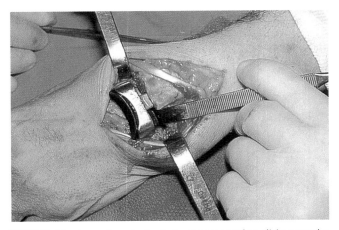

FIGURE 32. A small periosteal elevator is used to disimpact the radial trial component.

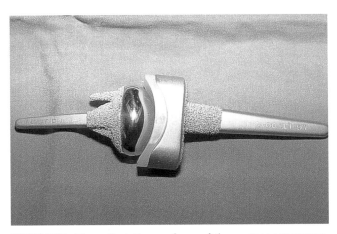

FIGURE 33. The articulating surfaces of the permanent component have a porous coated base of 1-mm thickness at the bases of the metacarpal and radial components.

trial Delrin component. As a result, the tension in this true prosthetic insertion will be slightly greater (approximately 2.5 mm increased length) than that of the trial components. The real components thus will have a snugger fit than the trials, which generally is desirable. In those situations when the fitting is so tight that it is difficult to achieve articulation of the trial components due to the tightness of the soft tissues, an additional 1 or 2 mm of bone should be removed from the distal radius prior to insertion of the real components. In general, when selecting the level of resection of the distal radius and the distal carpus, the maximum amount of radius should be retained that will allow a flat articulating surface at the resected distal end of the radius in the anteroposterior and medial-lateral planes, and the distal half of the distal carpal row should be preserved. In certain situations of advanced destructive arthrosis and previous proximal migration and subluxation, more bone resection may be required. The goal is to achieve a segmental resection just shorter than the width of the articulated prostheses (2.5 cm for the large prostheses).

Take radiographs after insertion of the trial components to verify the proper intramedullary position of the components (Fig. 34).

Methylmethacrylate cement is mixed and used in fixation of the distal component for the metacarpal component in all cases except for those with very hard

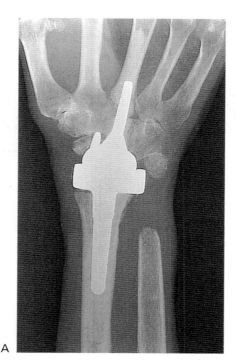

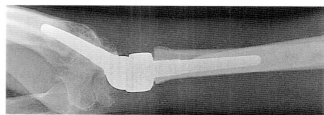

A

B

**FIGURE 34. A** and **B:** Radiographs are taken after insertion of the trial components to verify the proper intramedullary position of the component, as well as after cementation as shown here.

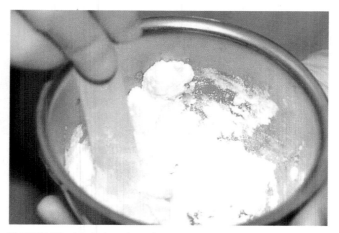

**FIGURE 35.** Methylmethacrylate cement is mixed and used in fixation of the distal component in all patients for the metacarpal component, except in those patients with very hard cancellous bone structures (young rheumatoid or posttraumatic patients).

cancellous bone structures (young rheumatoid or posttraumatic patients) (Fig. 35). Use a straight hemostat or the intermediate awl to expand the distal plastic end of a 12-cc syringe with a metallic control holder (Fig. 36). Pack cement into the plastic injection syringe in a more sticky state for the distal component than is used in lower extremity joint replacement surgery (Fig. 37).

Insert small portions of cancellous bone (from the bone resected previously from the carpus) into the base of the medullary canal of the third metacarpal. Impact into the medullary canal with the large medullary reamer or awl (Fig. 38). This provides a cement block in the middle of the long finger medullary shaft to allow for later metacarpophalangeal arthroplasty, if necessary. The cement is injected in a slightly more liquid state into the third medullary canal (Fig. 39). Using the special impactor, the component is impacted into the base of the third

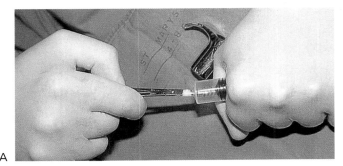
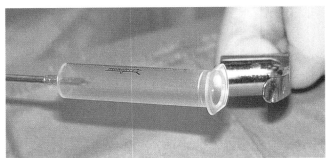

FIGURE 36. A straight hemostat (A) or an intermediate-size awl (B) is used to expand the distal plastic end of a 12-cc syringe with a metallic control holder.

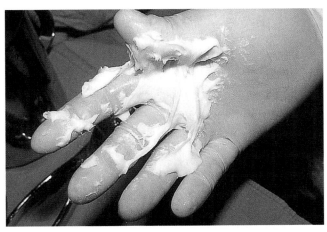

FIGURE 37. The cement is packed into the plastic injection syringe for the distal component in a more sticky state than is used in lower extremity joint implant surgery.

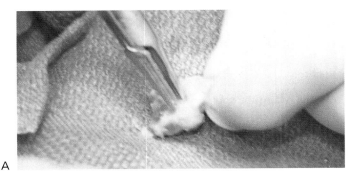
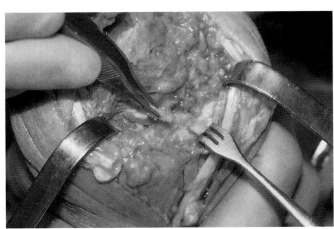
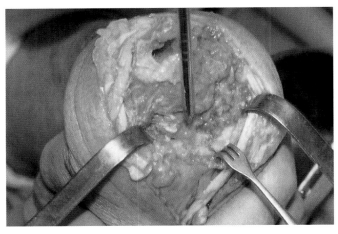

FIGURE 38. Small portions of cancellous bone (A) from the bone resected previously from the carpus are inserted (B) into the base of the medullary canal of the third metacarpal and (C) impacted into the medullary canal with the large medullary reamer. This provides a cement block in the middle of the long finger medullary shaft to allow for later metacarpophalangeal arthroplasty as necessary.

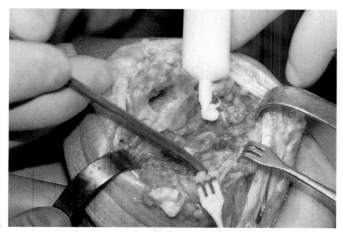

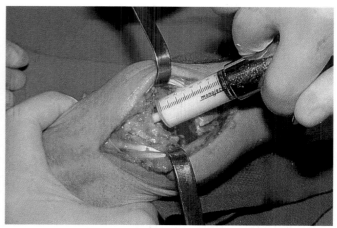

A                                                                          B

**FIGURE 39.** **A** and **B:** The cement is injected in a slightly more liquid state into the medullary canal.

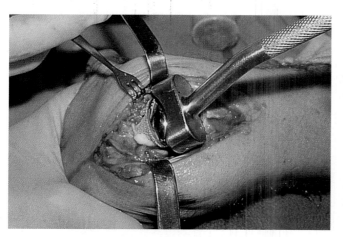

**FIGURE 40.** Utilizing the special impactor, the component is impacted into the base of the third metacarpal.

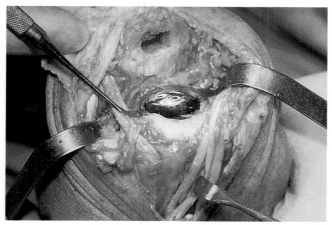

**FIGURE 41.** As the porous beading at the base of the metacarpal component is generally somewhat proud, this area is covered with methylmethacrylate cement.

metacarpal (Fig. 40). The porous beading at the base of the metacarpal component is generally prominent, and the exposed portion is covered with the methylmethacrylate cement (Fig. 41).

The radial component is not cemented, but simply impacted with the special impactor. A press-fit is very easy to achieve. In those patients who have had previous arthroplasty involving the medullary canal of the radius, cement may be necessary but, as stress shielding occurs, avoid cementing of the radial component if possible (Fig. 42).

After inserting the components the joint is articulated and tested through an easy range of motion. Identify whether there is impinging bone in radial or ulnar deviation over the bases of the carpals. If so, resect the bone causing the impingement (Fig. 43).

Test tension by distraction. If distraction is not possible, the fit is considered tight. If the distal component can be distracted to allow placement of a small probe within the articulating surface, fit is considered moderate. If the distal metacarpal component can be distracted beyond the level of the polyethylene articulating surface, it is considered a loose fit. As described below, the tightness of the fit determines the amount of postoperative immobilization (Fig. 44).

The capsule, which was previously elevated, is closed over the prosthesis (Fig. 45). If the capsule was attenuated on initial elevation, synovium is retained to

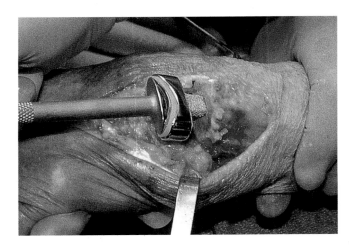

**FIGURE 42.** In those patients who have had previous arthroplasty involving the medullary canal of the radius, cement may be necessary on occasion; however, stress shielding does occur, and cementing of the radial component is avoided if possible.

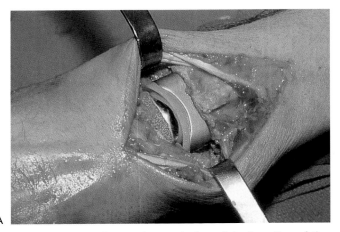

A

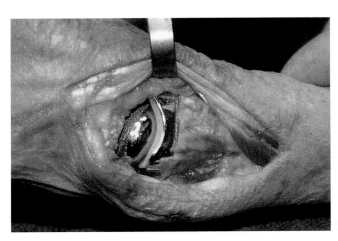

B

**FIGURE 43. A** and **B:** At the conclusion of the insertion of the components, the joint is articulated and tested through an easy range of motion. Determination is made whether there is impinging bone in radial and ulnar deviation over the bases of the carpals; if this is the case, bone is resected.

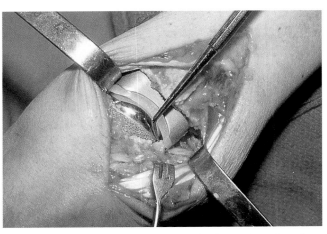

A

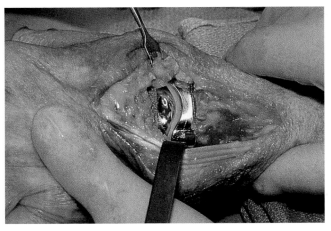

B

**FIGURE 44. A** and **B:** Tension is tested by distraction. If no distraction is possible, there is a tight fit **(B).** If the distal component can be distracted to allow placement of a small probe within the articulating surface, the fit is considered moderate **(A).** In a loose fit, the distal component can be pulled beyond the margin of the proximal component.

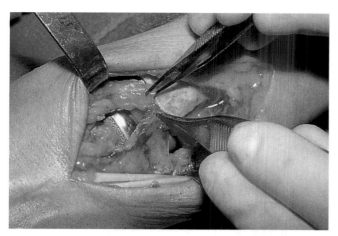

**FIGURE 45.** The capsule, which was previously elevated, is closed over the prosthesis.

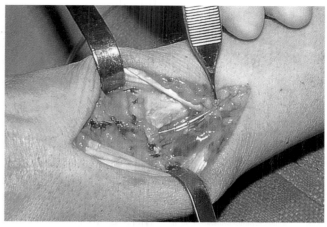

**FIGURE 46.** If closure is not possible over the prosthesis, a portion of the retinaculum is divided from the dorsal retinacular layer and used to cover the prosthesis. The entire retinaculum is never placed beneath the extensor tendons because, if this is done in wrist arthroplasty, the extensor tendons may sublux off to the radial or ulnar sides of the prosthesis during flexion of the wrist.

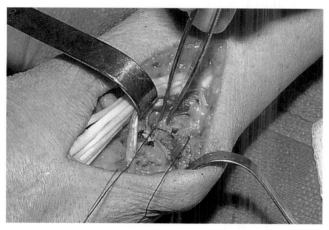

**FIGURE 47.** The periosteal soft tissues over the resected distal ulna are sutured firmly to the remnant soft tissues of the distal radius to stabilize the distal ulnar stump.

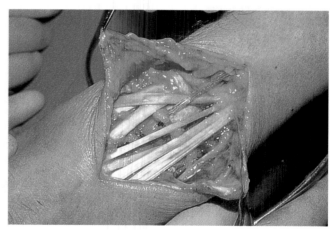

**FIGURE 48.** The extensor retinaculum, which was elevated from the first to the fifth or sixth dorsal compartment, is repaired as a single layer over the extensor tendons.

allow closure of the soft tissues over the prostheses (Fig. 46). If closure is not possible over the prosthesis, a portion of the retinaculum is divided from the dorsal retinacular layer and used to cover the prosthesis. The entire retinaculum is not placed beneath the extensor tendons. If this is done in wrist arthroplasty, subluxation of the extensor tendons off to the radial or ulnar side of the prosthesis during flexion of the wrist may occur.

The periosteal soft tissues over the resected distal ulna are sutured firmly to the remnant soft tissues of the distal radius to stabilize the distal ulna resection (Fig. 47).

The extensor retinaculum, which has been elevated from the first to the fifth or sixth dorsal compartments, is then repaired as a single layer over the extensor tendons. It is important to retain the extensor retinaculum to stabilize the tendons over the dorsum of the wrist (Fig. 48).

Repair is accomplished with absorbable sutures (Fig. 49). Skin repair is completed over deep and superficial suction drains (Fig. 50). A postoperative long-arm bulky dressing is applied with the forearm in supination (to protect ulna repair) and the wrist in slight dorsiflexion (Fig. 51).

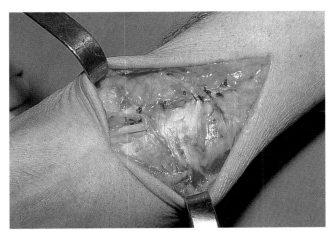

**FIGURE 49.** Repair is accomplished with absorbable sutures.

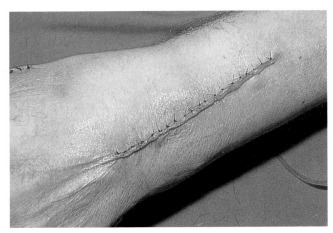

**FIGURE 50.** Skin repair is completed over deep and superficial suction drains.

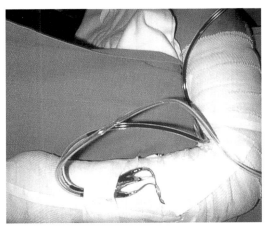

**FIGURE 51.** A postoperative long-arm bulky dressing is applied with the forearm in neutral rotation and the wrist in slight dorsiflexion.

## POSTOPERATIVE MANAGEMENT

Because of the distal ulna resection and stabilization, maintain the limb in a long-arm cast for 2 weeks. Then use a short-arm cast for a variable period of time as described, unless the soft tissue reconstruction of the ulna was tenuous. In this case, use of a long-arm cast is preferred. If the operative finding of the fit was described as tight (Fig. 44), the following protocol is used.

The wrist is tested with a gentle passive range of motion. If it is very stable with only 5° to 10° of palmar and dorsiflexion, apply a plastic splint and give the patient an 8-week regimen of gentle wrist mobilization exercises. Formal instruction in isometric strengthening of the wrist extensors is presented. The patient is asked to achieve a range of motion of no greater than 30° of dorsiflexion and 30° of palmar flexion. Minimal radial and ulnar deviation is advised. There is no instruction in active assisted range of motion of the wrist.

If, in a tight fit, more than 20° of motion is possible passively at the time of initial cast removal at 2 weeks, the wrist is placed in a cast for 2 additional weeks. The postoperative regime is reinstated. If the operative description is of a medium fit (in which the wrist may be partially distracted after insertion of the prostheses), a period of immobilization in a long-arm cast is continued for 6 weeks postoperatively. At that time the wrist is removed from the cast, placed in a plastic splint, and begun on a program of gentle active range of motion with isometric strengthening of the wrist extensors. Use protective splinting in the interim for an additional 6 weeks. If, at the time of surgery, there was a "loose" fit, the wrist is maintained in a cast for a total of 8 weeks postoperative; and upon removal of the cast, if the wrist has become snug and there is only 20° of passive gentle motion possible, a program of isometric strengthening and active exercises is begun. If the wrist appears to have more than 30° of flexion and extension at this time, an orthoplast last splint is worn without exercises for an additional 4 weeks.

Generally, at the end of 3 months, the patient is able to begin utilizing the wrist in a normal everyday functional fashion without additional splinting. The patient is cautioned against any impact activities or activities that cause either distraction or excessive dorsiflexion or palmar flexion of the prosthesis. Specifically, the patient is instructed not to participate in impact sports activities such as golf or tennis, not to use a hammer, not to use the wrist in a dorsiflexed position to assist in rising from a chair, and not to use the hand in a distraction fashion, such as pulling a heavy door open. Otherwise, activities are allowed, as tolerated, on a "common sense" basis.

## COMPLICATIONS

The major long-term complication of biaxial total wrist arthroplasty is loosening of the distal component. This occurs in a higher percentage in wrists that previously had silicone wrist arthroplasties. The anticipated failure rate due to distal component loosening is 20% after 5 years. While all wrists with loosening may not require reoperation, they are followed closely to make sure that the loosening process is not progressive. When loosening occurs, it does so in standard fashion, with palmar drifting of the distal component due to the stresses applied to it when the wrist is in a dorsiflexed position. These stresses cause the distal component to teeter-totter in a palmar direction with dorsal migration of the stem through the metacarpal shaft distally and palmar migration of the head of the prosthesis into the carpal canal proximally. This may result in some secondary carpal tunnel symptomatology, requiring release of a transverse carpal ligament.

It is loosening of the distal component, seen in the 5-year follow-ups, that leads us to recommend cementing the distal component for additional support except when there is very strong bone stock. In fact, for patients with bone deficiency (severe rheumatoid arthritis with or without steroid and/or metabolic drug therapy), specially designed prostheses with double or extended distal component stems have been developed (Fig. 52).

As mentioned in the section Preoperative Planning, van Leeuwen has attempted to decrease distal component loosening (dorsal breakout of the stem through the mid-metacarpal) by altering the technique of placement of the distal component. This method also has been used by Trail in Wrightington (3,6). Van Leeuwen's principle is to provide for a distal point of fixation at the carpal metacarpal joint area so that the stronger subchondral bone surfaces at the joint provide resistance to dorsal breakout. He does not use cement fixation (Fig. 1B). To accomplish this, small components are used and more of the capitate is preserved.

A rarely seen complication is dislocation of the prosthesis. Occasionally, if care is not taken during the application of a dressing in a loose fit, an immediate postoperative subluxation of the prosthetic components may occur. This can be remedied by simple manipulation and application of a cast. After 6 weeks of immobilization, the capsular structures stabilize the components.

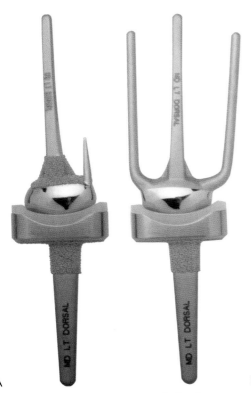

**FIGURE 52. A:** Long-stemmed distal compo-nent may be used in revision surgery or in pri-mary surgery in patients with bone deficiency/osteoporosis (rheumatoid arthritis on steroids). **B:** Triple-pronged component. Available for use in revision surgery. Rarely used in patients with special needs for motion and weak long meta-carpal secondary to previous failed arthroplasty (total wrist or silicone).

One out of 56 patients studied beyond 2 years experienced late dislocation of the prosthesis. This occurred secondary to rotation of the proximal component with wear of the captive polyethylene cup. Some patients have experienced carpal tunnel symptomatology. If this occurs early on, it is probably due to diminution in the size of the carpal canal from the prosthetic distal component or to primary rheumatoid tenosynovial proliferation. When carpal tunnel syndrome is seen within the first several months postoperative, release of the transverse carpal liga-ment is carried out. If carpal tunnel symptoms occur in a delayed fashion, it is necessary to look for loosening of the component and migration into the carpal canal or for excessive dorsiflexion of the wrist. In these situations, exploration, release of the transverse carpal ligament, palmar ligamentous repair or reconstruc-tion, or reposition of the distal component is necessary.

Revision surgery following total wrist arthroplasty with failure secondary to loosening or late subluxation includes revision with custom-designed distal components (Fig. 52) or, more often, conversion to a wrist fusion (4). This is relatively easy to accomplish with autogenous iliac bone graft with the assis-tance of cast or external or internal fixation devices (Fig. 53). Simmons et al. (2) recently have reported on the successful use of femoral head allograft in total wrist revision (2). The technique uses intramedullary rods placed in the metacarpals across the large allograft and into the medullary canal of the radius (Fig. 54).

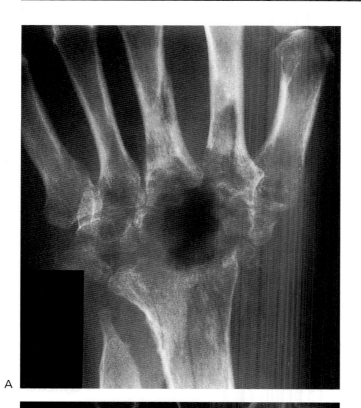

A

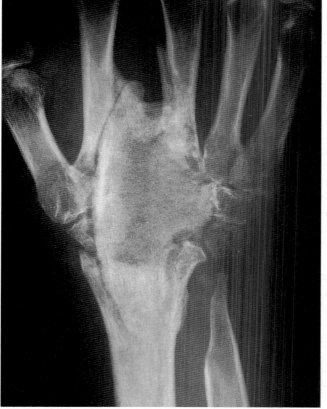

B

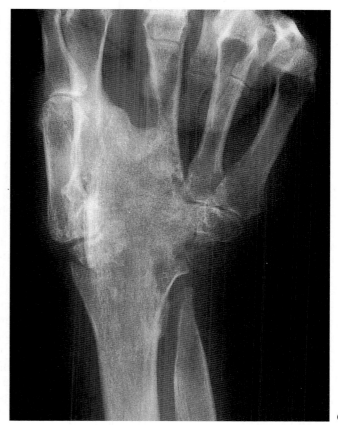

C

**FIGURE 53. A:** Large defect following removal of cemented Meuli wrist prosthesis. Note cracks in distal radius and long metacarpal. **B:** Defect was filled by a large corticocancellous graft from the iliac crest. Postoperative immobilization was achieved with cast only. **C:** One year post-arthrodesis, solid fusion with incorporation of bone graft is noted.

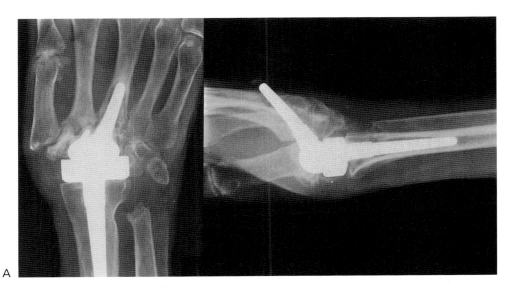

A

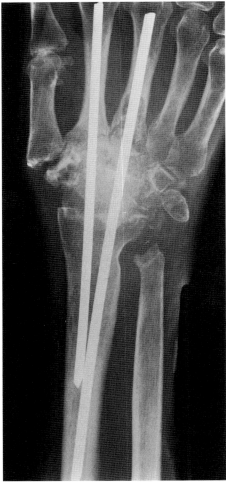

B

**FIGURE 54. A:** Preoperative failed total wrist arthroplasty with distal component loosening and pain. **B:** Revision to arthrodesis with femoral head allograft and intramedullary Steinmann pins.

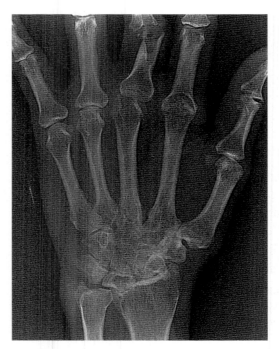

**FIGURE 55.** Preoperative radiograph demonstrating rheumatoid arthritis of the wrist.

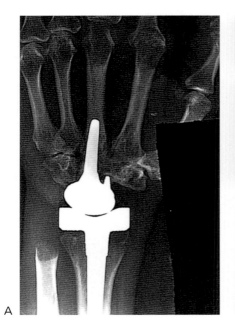

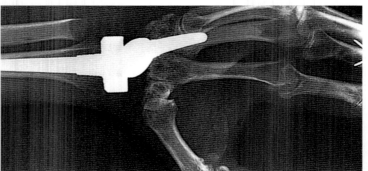

**FIGURE 56.** **A** and **B:** One-year postoperative radiographs.

## ILLUSTRATIVE CASE FOR TECHNIQUE

This 58-year-old woman presented with rheumatoid arthritis and painful wrist. She underwent total wrist arthroplasty. At 7 years postoperatively, she had well-balanced range of motion and excellent fixation of the components (Figs. 55–57).

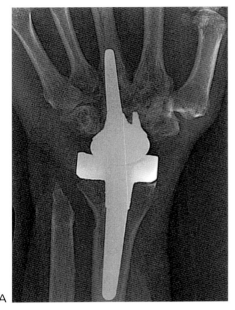

A

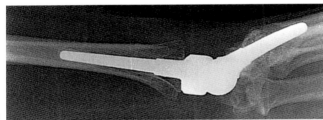

B

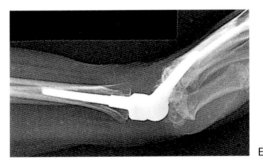

E

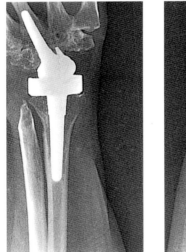

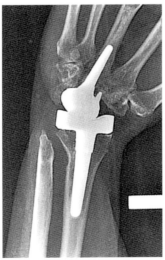

C,D

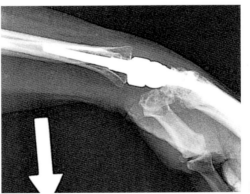

F

**FIGURE 57.  A–F:** Postoperative radiographs after 7 years. Radiographs indicate excellent biologic fixation of the proximal component and excellent cement fixation of the distal component as well as an excellent balanced range of motion of wrist.

## RECOMMENDED READING

1. Beckenbaugh, R. D., Linscheid, R. L.: Arthroplasty in the hand and wrist. In: *Operative Hand Surgery*, 3rd ed., vol. 1, edited by D. P. Green, Churchill Livingstone, New York, pp. 143–187, 1993.
2. Carlson, J. R., Simmons, B. P.: Wrist arthrodesis after failed wrist implant. *J. Hand Surg.*, 23(5): 893–898, 1998.
3. Courtman, N. H., Sochart, D. H., Trail, I. A., Stanley, J. K.: Biaxial wrist replacement. *J. Hand Surg.*, 24B(1): 32–34, 1999.
4. Rettig, M. E., Beckenbaugh, R. D.: Revision total wrist arthroplasty. *J. Hand Surg.*, 18A(5): 798–804, 1993.
5. Swanson, A. B., deGroot Swanson, G.: Implant arthroplasty in the carpal and radiocarpal joint. In: *The Wrist and Its Disorders*, edited by D. M. Lichtman, W. B. Saunders, Philadelphia, pp. 404–438, 1988.
6. van Leeuwen, N.: Presentation regarding Biaxial Total Wrist Arthroplasty. Presented at the 53rd annual meeting of the American Society for Surgery of the Hand, Minneapolis, MN, Sept. 1998.

PART **XI**

**Other Wrist Disorders**

# 33

# Radius Shortening in Kienböck's Disease

David M. Lichtman, Charlotte E. Alexander, and A. Herbert Alexander

---

## INDICATIONS/CONTRAINDICATIONS

The surgeon caring for a patient with Kienböck's disease (avascular necrosis of the lunate) is faced with multiple treatment options. An understanding of the natural history of the disease process is an essential first step in effective treatment. In general, Kienböck's disease is a progressive disorder, and intervention is based on our radiographic classification of the disease. The 1988 expanded classification is used (Table 1). Kienböck's disease may be treated by modalities that are stage and ulnar variance dependent. These are summarized in Table 2.

Patients with negative to neutral ulnar variance in stages I, II, and IIIA (before significant fixed deformity has occurred) are candidates for radial shortening. For stage I patients, however, we usually try a period of immobilization (at least 12 to 16 weeks) before proceeding with surgical treatment. Once significant carpal collapse occurs (stage IIIB), radial shortening will not address the carpal instability and we prefer to do a triscaphe fusion or a scaphocapitate fusion. For pancarpal arthrosis, we do a salvage procedure, usually proximal row carpectomy or wrist fusion.

Postoperative ulnocarpal abutment is a potential problem for patients who end up with a positive variance of greater than 1 mm. Therefore, lunate revascularization should be considered for patients with II or IIIA and ulnar-neutral or positive variance. Capitate shortening with capitate-hamate fusion is another option.

## PREOPERATIVE PLANNING

Ulnar variance is evaluated by obtaining posteroanterior (PA) radiographs of the wrist with the shoulder abducted 90°, the elbow flexed 90°, and the arm and fore-

**TABLE 1. 1988 EXPANDED CLASSIFICATION OF KIENBÖCK'S DISEASE**

Stage I: Normal radiograph. Increased uptake on bone scan. Magnetic resonance imaging study is diagnostic.
Stage II: Density changes with possible early collapse of the lunate radial border.
Stage III: Lunate collapse, capitate displaces proximately.
  A: Without fixed scaphoid rotation. Normal carpal alignment.
  B: With fixed scaphoid rotation and altered carpal architecture.
Stage IV: Severe lunate collapse with sclerosis and osteophyte formation in the remaining carpus.

**TABLE 2. TREATMENT ALGORITHM FOR KIENBÖCK'S DISEASE**

Stage I (ulnar-negative): Immobilization, possible radial shortening.
Stage I (ulnar-positive): Immobilization, possible lunate revascularization.
Stage II to IIIA (ulnar-negative): Radial shortening.
Stage II to IIIA (ulnar positive): Revascularization or capitate shortening.
Stage IIIB (negative/positive): Scaphocapitate fusion or triscaphe fusion.
Stage IV: Salvage (proximal row carpectomy or wrist fusion).

arm in neutral rotation (8). This position is easily achieved by having the patient seated in a chair alongside the radiograph table with the arm and forearm resting on the table. We measure ulnar variance as described by Gelberman et al. (3), in which a parallel line is extended from the ulnar border of the radial articular surface toward the ulna, and the distance between the distal carpal surface of the ulnar head and this line is measured (Fig. 1).

In addition to radiographs to determine ulnar variance, all patients have standard PA and lateral wrist radiographs. PA views of both wrists in neutral deviation, including the full length of the long metacarpal, are also obtained to quantitatively evaluate collapse of the lunate by measuring the carpal height ratio

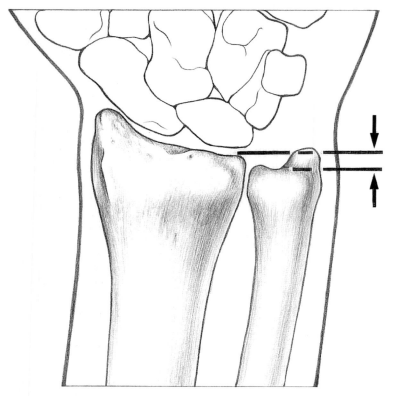

**FIGURE 1.** Measurement of ulnar variance.

as described by McMurtry and associates (4). This ratio is obtained by dividing the perpendicular distance from the base of the long metacarpal to the radial articular surface by the length of the long metacarpal. This radiograph is an important baseline study for postoperative evaluation of carpal collapse. If the metacarpals are not included on the x-ray, the alternate method to determine carpal height can be used instead (8).

## SURGERY

We prefer radial shortening to ulnar lengthening because it obviates the need for bone graft. There are minimal problems with irritation from hardware, and theoretically, a lower incidence of nonunion. We recommend that the amount of shortening be sufficient to create 1 mm of ulnar-positive variance but no greater than 4 mm to effectively unload the lunate and avoid distal radioulnar joint symptoms.

### Technique

Perform the procedure using regional or general anesthesia. With the patient in the supine position and the arm on a hand operating table, under tourniquet control, the distal third of the radius is exposed using a palmar approach as described by Henry (Fig. 2). A template or a seven- or eight-hole 3.5-mm AO dynamic compression plate is placed over the exposed radius to mark the approximate level of the osteotomy. The plate is contoured to allow placement of the plate and osteotomy as far distal as is possible on the radius. The plate is then secured to the radius proximally with screws in the hole just proximal to the proposed osteotomy site and in the most proximal hole to prevent rotation of the plate on the radius. The osteotomy

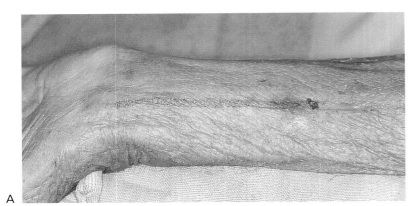

**FIGURE 2.** **A** and **B**: A 12- to 15-cm longitudinal incision along the radial border of the flexor carpi radialis is made, followed by Henry's palmar approach to the distal third of the radius. (This figure and Figs. 3–9 are of a left forearm; the hand is to the left.)

A

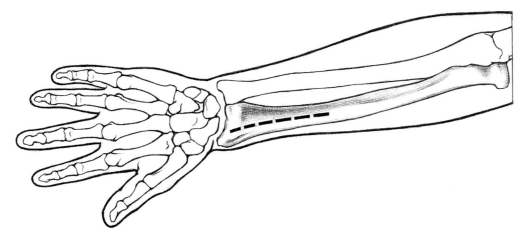

B

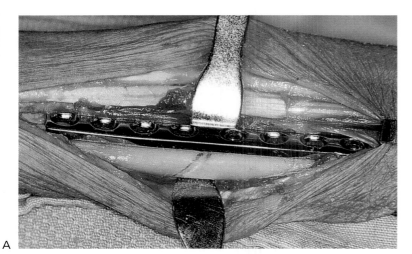

A

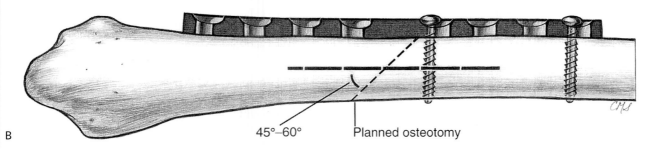

B

45°–60°    Planned osteotomy

**FIGURE 3. A** and **B**: A seven- or eight-hole 3.5-mm dynamic compression plate is contoured and secured to the radius with two proximal screws. One screw is adjacent to the proposed osteotomy site, and the other screw is the most proximal screw. The osteotomies are then marked on the radial border of the radius.

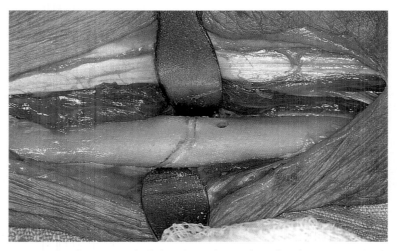

**FIGURE 4.** After removal of the plate, the marking for the osteotomies is completed.

is then marked on the radial aspect of the radius using a marking pen, electrocautery tip, or saw (Fig. 3). The plate is removed, and the marking for the osteotomies is completed using a millimeter ruler (Fig. 4). The amount of shortening to be performed is determined by measuring the amount of ulnar variance on a preoperative PA view of the wrist in neutral rotation and adding 1 mm (i.e., in a wrist with 2 mm of ulnar-negative variance the radius will be shortened 3 mm).

Before performing the osteotomy, a line is also drawn parallel to the long axis of the radius at the proposed site to help avoid rotation. We perform an oblique osteotomy because it allows interfragmentary compression as well as longitudinal com-

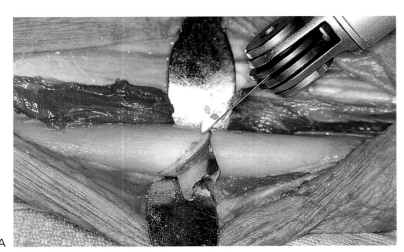

**FIGURE 5. A** and **B:** Parallel oblique osteotomies are performed using a microsagittal saw with a 9-mm blade. On the first osteotomy, the dorsal cortex is left intact, and a saw blade is left in the osteotomy to act as an alignment guide for the second saw cut.

A

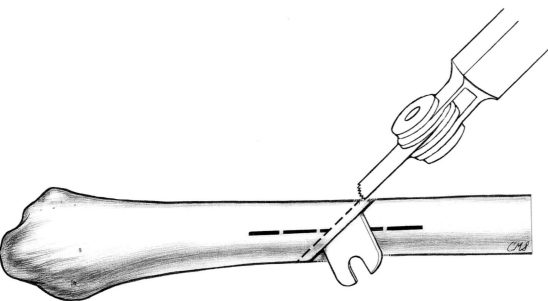

B

pression, and a larger area of bone contact at the osteotomy. The osteotomy should be oriented as obliquely as possible (at least 45° to the long axis of the radius) from proximal on the palmar surface to distal on the dorsal surface. A microsagittal saw is used to minimize the amount of bone removed with the actual saw cut. On first osteotomy, the dorsal radial cortex is left intact and a free saw blade is placed in the osteotomy to assist in creating parallel cuts (Fig. 5). There are commercially available guides for making parallel osteotomies but we have no experience with them.

After both osteotomies are completed and the piece of bone removed, the previously contoured plate is reattached securely, using the drill holes in the proximal fragment, and the bone ends aligned anatomically and held using bone-holding forceps. Use a 3.5-mm bit and guide to drill the gliding hole (near the cortex only) in the hole adjacent to the osteotomy on the distal end of the plate at an angle bisecting a perpendicular to the long axis of the radius and a perpendicular to the osteotomy (Fig. 6). Then place a screw in compression in the hole just distal to the gliding hole (Fig. 7). Place a 3.5-mm/2.5-mm insert drill sleeve in the 3.5-mm gliding hole; drill the far cortex (dorsal) using a 2.5-mm drill bit and place an interfragmentary screw (Fig. 8). Place a third screw distal to the osteotomy and then insert alternating screws using standard AO technique (Fig. 9). Before closure deflate the tourniquet and obtain hemostasis. Closure is routine.

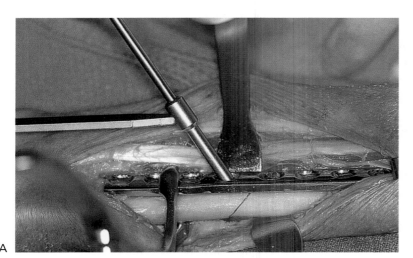

A

**FIGURE 6.** **A** and **B:** The plate is reattached, the radius reduced with a bone-holding clamp, and the 3.5-mm gliding hole drilled for the interfragmentary screw.

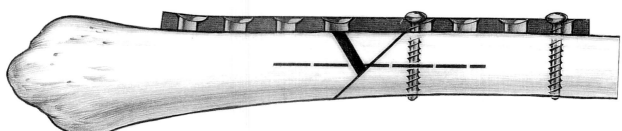

B

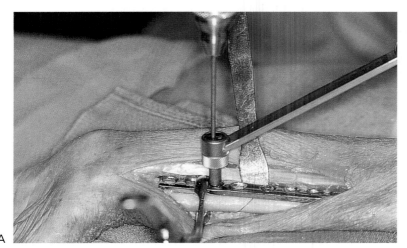

A

**FIGURE 7.** **A** and **B:** A screw is then placed in compression in the hole just distal to the hole to be used for an interfragmentary screw. Note the loaded guide is being used for drilling.

Screw loaded

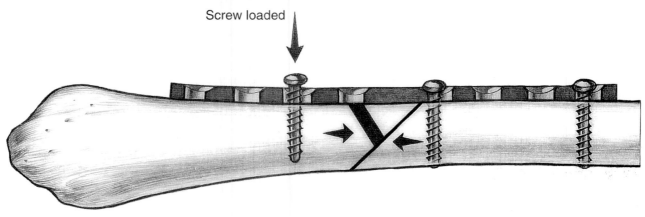

B

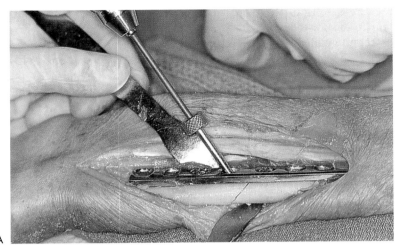

A

**FIGURE 8. A** and **B:** If the compression at the osteotomy site is felt to be adequate, the dorsal cortex is then drilled and tapped for placement of the interfragmentary screw.

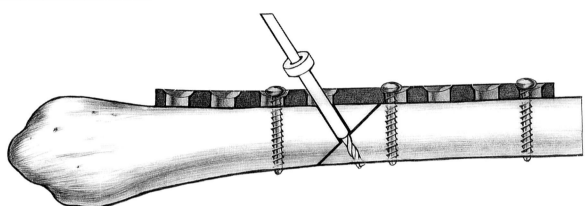

B

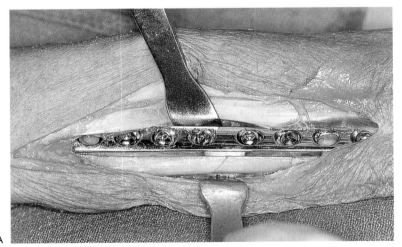

A

**FIGURE 9. A** and **B:** A third screw is placed distal to the osteotomy, and then alternating screws are inserted using standard AO technique.

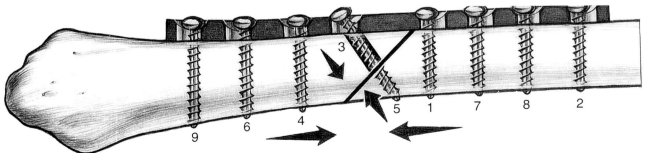

B

There are several surgical pitfalls to avoid when performing a radial shortening. First, it is important to ensure that the osteotomies are parallel and that both surfaces are flat. The second challenge is to approximate the osteotomy surfaces once the plate has been reattached proximally and is being held distally with a bone-holding forceps. Using bone-holding forceps, the surgeon ensures that the surfaces are approximated as closely as possible without angulation or rotational malalignment. If necessary, after placement of the first compression screw, more compression can be attained by a second loaded screw placed in compression. But this must be done before drilling the dorsal cortex and placing the interfragmentary screw. This second compression screw is placed in the second hole on the proximal radius opposite the first compression screw. Before tightening this screw, the other screws on the same side of the osteotomy must be loosened one quarter-turn to allow the plate to slide. This adds further compression and then the screws are retightened.

Avoid excessive shortening by starting each osteotomy cut on the inside of the line drawn to allow for bone removed by the actual saw cuts. An intraoperative radiograph taken before applying the interfragmentary screw may be helpful in fine-tuning the amount of bone resection. Under no circumstances should the radius be shortened more than 4 mm, as this has been associated with ulnocarpal impingement and patient dissatisfaction (5).

## POSTOPERATIVE MANAGEMENT

Place the affected limb in a short-arm cast for 8 weeks. The cast is used to immobilize the lunate rather than to protect the internal fixation. Instruct the patient in range-of-motion exercises of fingers and thumb. Obtain radiographs at monthly intervals until the osteotomy is healed. Radiographic union is usually achieved in the first 8 weeks postoperatively.

After removing the cast, begin range-of-motion and then grip-strengthening exercises. The patient usually returns to full activities by 3 months postoperatively. A palmar wrist splint may be required for certain activities for several months after cast removal if the patient still has some wrist pain with exertion. In the Nakamura et al. (6) study, 87% of their 23 patients followed for at least 1 year had no or only mild wrist pain with strenuous activity postoperatively. Range of motion and grip strength should be equal to or greater than preoperative values within 6 months. We advise our patients that they may experience mild residual wrist pain with strenuous activity.

## COMPLICATIONS

Reported postoperative complications include nonunion, failure of hardware, and division of the palmar cutaneous branch of the median nerve. Nonunion and hardware failure are treated with bone grafting and revision of internal fixation. Division of the palmar cutaneous branch may or may not be troublesome to the patient. Symptoms usually diminish with a desensitization program.

## ILLUSTRATIVE CASE FOR TECHNIQUE

A 26-year-old right-handed active duty infantryman had a fall, resulting in the gradual onset of right wrist pain. Radiographs were negative, and the patient was treated with a short-arm cast without relief of symptoms. Magnetic resonance imaging 4 months later revealed changes compatible with avascular necrosis of the lunate. Preoperative radiographs showed stage I or early stage II disease, with 3 mm of ulnar-negative variance (Fig. 10). Radial shortening was performed 9 months after the initial injury (Fig. 11). The osteotomy healed uneventfully and

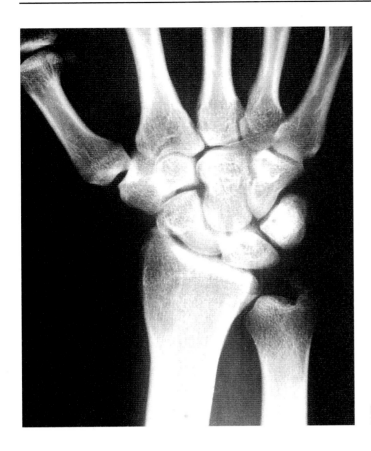

**FIGURE 10.** Preoperative posteroanterior view of early stage II Kienböck's disease with ulnar-negative variance.

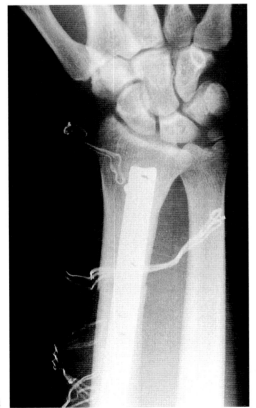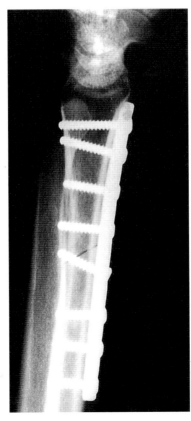

A,B

**FIGURE 11. A** and **B:** Intraoperative posteroanterior and lateral radiographs of radial shortening. Note that there appears to be about 2 mm of ulnar-positive variance. This is due to parallax and nonstandard positioning. Compare this to the variance in the same patient (Fig. 12A) following plate removal. This emphasizes the importance of obtaining the standard posteroanterior view of the wrist in neutral rotation, a view sometimes difficult to obtain in surgery.

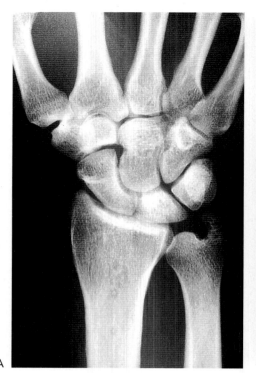
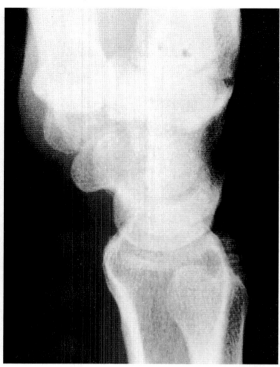

A

B

**FIGURE 12. A** and **B:** Posteroanterior in neutral rotation and lateral radiographs 2.5 years after radial shortening. There is no carpal collapse present.

the patient returned to full duty by 6 months postoperatively. The plate was removed, and at follow-up 2.5 years postoperatively, the patient is asymptomatic except for mild wrist pain with strenuous activity. Grip strength was 100 compared to 105 on the left using the Jamar dynamometer. Range of motion was normal except for a 10° decrease in wrist palmar flexion compared with the nonoperated extremity. Radiographs showed no change in the appearance of the lunate and no change in carpal height ratio (Fig. 12).

## RECOMMENDED READING

1. Alexander, A. H., Lichtman, D. M.: Kienböck's disease. In: *The Wrist and Its Disorders*, 2nd ed., edited by D. M. Lichtman, W. B. Saunders, Philadelphia, pp. 329–346, 1997.
2. Alexander, A. H., Lichtman, D. M.: The Kienböck's dilemma: how to cope. In: *International Symposium on the Wrist*, edited by R. Nakamura. Springer-Verlag, Tokyo, 1992.
3. Gelberman, R. H., Salamon, P. B., Jurist, J. M., Posch, J. L.: Ulnar variance in Kienböck's disease. *J. Bone Joint Surg.*, 57A: 674–676, 1975.
4. McMurtry, R. Y., Youm, Y., Flatt, A. E., Gillespie, T. E.: Kinematics of the wrist. *J. Bone Joint Surg.*, 60A: 423–431, 1978.
5. Nakamura, R., Horii, E., Imaeda, T.: Excessive radial shortening in Kienböck's disease. *J. Hand Surg.*, 15B: 46–48, 1990.
6. Nakamura, R., Imaeda, T., Miura, T.: Radial shortening for Kienböck's disease: factors affecting the operative result. *J. Hand Surg.*, 15B: 40–45, 1990.
7. Natrass, G., King, G., McMurtry, R., Brant, R., An alternative method for determination of the carpal height ratio. *J. Bone Joint Surg.* 76A: 88–94, 1994.
8. Palmer, A. K., Glisson, R. R., Werner, F. W.: Ulnar variance determination. *J. Hand Surg.*, 7: 376–379, 1982.
9. Weiss, A. P., Weiland, A. J., Moore, J. R., Wilgis, E. F.: Radial shortening for Kienböck's disease. *J. Bone Joint Surg.*, 73A: 384–391, 1991.

# 34

# Surgical Management of de Quervain's Disease

Marc E. Umlas and Richard H. Gelberman

## INDICATIONS/CONTRAINDICATIONS

Surgical release of the first dorsal compartment is indicated following failure of conservative treatment of de Quervain's disease. Patients are initially managed by a trial of splinting and corticosteroid injection of the first dorsal compartment. Repeat trials of nonoperative management, including up to three injections, are occasionally indicated. If the patient fails to improve, operative release is elected. There are no direct contraindications to surgery, but it behooves the surgeon to fully explore other possible local conditions (basal joint arthritis, triscaphoid arthritis, etc.) as explanations for failure of conservative management.

## PREOPERATIVE PLANNING

Initial patient evaluation includes history, physical examination, and plain radiographs of the wrist and hand. Patients present with complaints of pain and swelling over the dorsal radial aspect of the wrist. Wrist pain exacerbated by thumb motion is classic but inconsistently noted by the patient. A thorough occupational history is necessary, because chronic overuse has been implicated in the disease process. It is important to question the patient for associated conditions. Arons (2) in 1987 noted a high incidence of "generalized nonarticular rheumatism of the upper extremity" in patients presenting with de Quervain's disease. This included fasciitis, tendonitis, bursitis, and chronic ligament and muscle strain. A thorough medical history is important as well, with attention to concurrent rheumatologic diseases and diabetes.

Physical examination begins with an evaluation of both hands. Tenderness over the contents of the first dorsal compartment is elicited. Finkelstein's test is performed and is fairly specific for de Quervain's disease. To perform this test, have the patient place his thumb into the ipsilateral palm and grip the thumb tightly. Then place the patient's wrist into a position of forced ulnar deviation. Pain

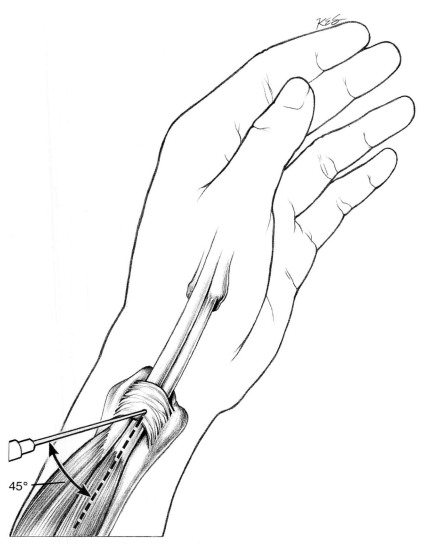

**FIGURE 1.** Injection of local anesthetic and steroid solution into the first dorsal compartment of the wrist.

directly over the first dorsal compartment signifies a positive test result. It is important to differentiate de Quervain's disease from both basal joint arthritis and triscaphoid arthritis. A basal joint grind test is performed, which is positive in basal joint arthritis and normally negative in de Quervain's disease. Triscaphoid arthritis is differentiated by direct palpation. A neurologic examination is performed to rule out concomitant carpal tunnel syndrome.

All patients have plain radiographs taken of the wrist and hand. Attention is drawn to bony abnormalities in the region of the first dorsal compartment. Additionally, basal joint arthritis and triscaphoid degenerative changes are noted.

Once the diagnosis has been made, the patient is treated nonoperatively. A trial of injection and splinting is initiated. The dorsal radial aspect of the wrist is prepped with Betadine. A mixture containing 40 mg of methylprednisolone acetate (Depo-Medrol; Upjohn, Kalamazoo, MI) and 1% solution of lidocaine without epinephrine is injected into the tendon sheath of the first dorsal compartment through a 22-gauge needle. The needle is introduced 1 cm proximal to the tip of the radial styloid process and angled distally at 45° to the longitudinal axis of the lateral aspect of the forearm (Fig. 1). Filling of the tendon sheath is noted distal to the annular ligament of the first dorsal compartment. The wrist is fitted with a polyethylene thumb spica splint with the wrist in 20° of dorsiflexion and the metacarpophalangeal and interphalangeal joints of thumb in extension. The patient, maintained in the splint for 3 weeks, is allowed to remove it for bathing. After 3 weeks of immobilization, unrestricted activity is allowed. A total of 6 weeks following injection must elapse before the success of the injection is judged. Failure of nonoperative management is indicated by persistence of first dorsal compartment tenderness, a positive Finkelstein's test, and continued restricted use of the hand because of persistent symptoms. Having failed a trial of conservative treatment, consisting of one to three injections, the patient is considered for operative release of the first dorsal compartment.

Witt et al. (13) reported 38% unsatisfactory results from steroid injection and splinting. No significant association between the outcome of nonoperative management and sex, hand dominance, age, or duration of symptoms was noted.

Patients referred for operative release are scheduled in the same day at the surgical unit of our hospital for release of the first dorsal wrist compartment under local anesthesia. They are informed about the nature of the procedure and possible complications, including numbness in the distribution of the radial sensory nerve, painful neuroma formation in the distribution of the radial sensory nerve, and failure of the operation to relieve symptoms of pain and tenderness.

## SURGERY

Proximal to the wrist, the tendons of the abductor pollicis longus (APL) and the extensor pollicis brevis (EPB) cross superficial to the tendons of the extensor carpi radialis brevis and longus to enter the first dorsal extensor compartment of the wrist (7) (Fig. 2). The tendons remain closely associated, with the EPB tendon slightly overlapping the APL on its dorsal aspect. Together they form the palmar aspect of the anatomic snuffbox. Lying within the anatomic snuffbox, the radial artery passes onto the dorsum of the hand deep to the tendons of the APL and EPB at the level of the radiocarpal joint. These tendons then separate distal to the first dorsal compartment. The EPB inserts onto the dorsum of the base of the proximal phalanx of the thumb and commonly provides a slip that joins the long extensor of the thumb. It extends the proximal phalanx in a plane orthogonal to the plane of the palm. Although the APL inserts on the anterolateral aspect of the base of the thumb metacarpal, it has been noted to be widely varied in its insertion. Lacey et al. (8) dissected 38 cadaveric forearms in 1951 and noted that only seven had a single APL insertion. They noted up to three aberrant slips of tendon with insertion occurring into the abductor pollicis brevis tendon, trapezium, palmar carpal ligament, and opponens pollicis tendon. The APL extends the thumb in the plane of the palm.

Several studies have demonstrated variations within the first dorsal compartment (3,5,6,9–11). Giles (5) reported on a series of 50 dissected wrists in which he found 56% with an accessory tendon of the APL; 2% with an accessory tendon of the EPB; 20% with tendons of the APL and EPB in separate compartments; 34% with tendons of the EPB lying in a separate canal in the distal part of the main compartment; 12% with the APL and its accessory tendon(s) lying in a separate canal; 14% with the tendon of the EPB lying in a separate canal in the distal part only associated with duplication of the APL; and 4% with the accessory tendon of the APL lying in a separate canal. Other anatomic studies have found similar results. Witt et al. (13) noted an increased incidence of separate compartments for the EPB and APL (73%) in patients who failed nonoperative management. This was much higher than the previously noted incidence in cadaveric studies. Failure of operative release has also been associated with failure to fully release all tendons within the first dorsal compartment.

The patient is positioned supine with the involved upper extremity placed on a hand table. An upper arm inflatable tourniquet cuff is placed. The skip prep and

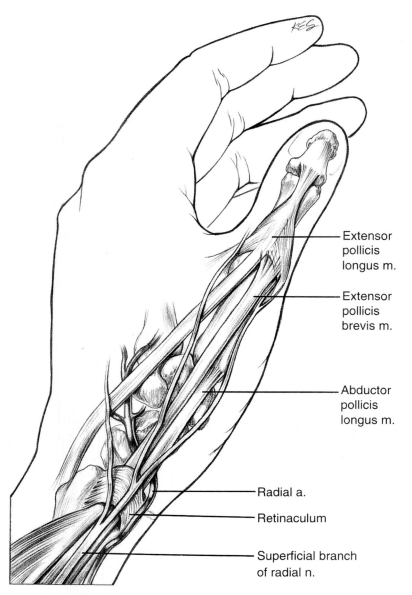

Extensor
pollicis
longus m.

Extensor
pollicis
brevis m.

Abductor
pollicis
longus m.

Radial a.

Retinaculum

Superficial branch
of radial n.

**FIGURE 2.** Anatomy of the first dorsal extensor compartment and related structures.

draping are standard. An Esmarch bandage is applied to the arm. Four wraps of the hand are made with the Esmarch and then progressed proximally to cuff (Fig. 3). The tourniquet is inflated to 250 mm Hg and the Esmarch is removed. Landmarks are carefully palpated (Fig. 4).

### Technique

The radial styloid and skin incision are marked with methylene blue skin marker (Fig. 5). A 2-cm transverse skin incision is drawn 1 cm proximal to the radial styloid process, directly over the first dorsal compartment. The skin and subcutaneous tissues are infiltrated with 1% lidocaine without epinephrine (Fig. 6). The skin is incised with a #15 scalpel along the predrawn line (Fig. 7). Subcutaneous dissection is carried out with blunt-tipped scissors down to the level of the extensor retinaculum (Fig. 8). Branches of the radial sensory nerve are identified and protected (Fig. 9). The sheath overlying the EPB and APL is incised in a longitudinal fashion at its

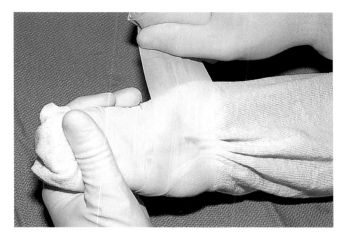

FIGURE 3. Application of the Esmarch bandage.

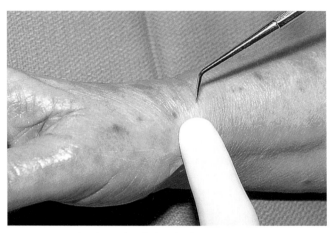

FIGURE 4. Palpation of radial styloid.

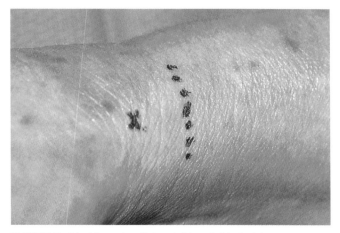

FIGURE 5. Marking of radial styloid and skin incision.

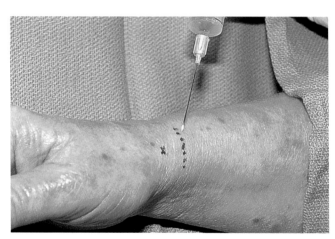

FIGURE 6. Infiltration of skin and subcutaneous tissues with local anesthetic.

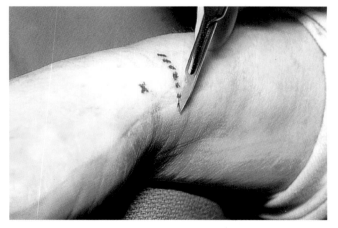

FIGURE 7. Skin incision.

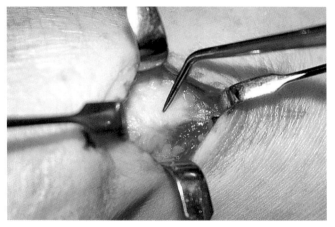

FIGURE 8. Subcutaneous dissection to the level of the extensor retinaculum.

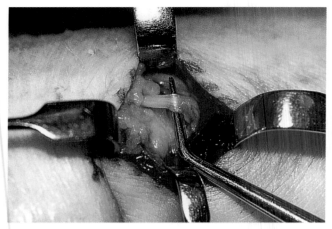

**FIGURE 9.** Identification of branches of the radial sensory nerve crossing the incision.

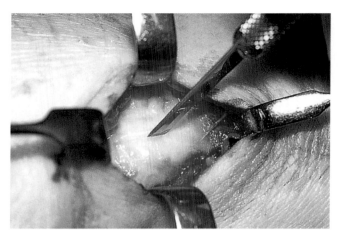

**FIGURE 10.** Incision of the sheath overlying the extensor pollicis brevis at its dorsal margin.

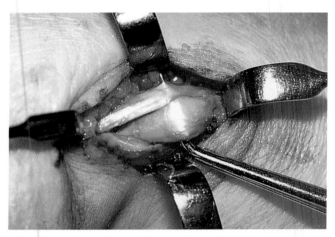

**FIGURE 11.** Inspection of the contents of the first dorsal compartment.

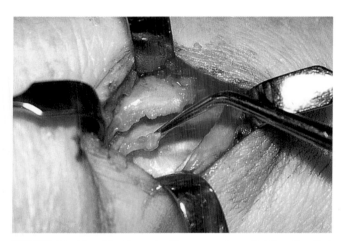

**FIGURE 12.** Identification of a fibrous septum dividing the first dorsal compartment.

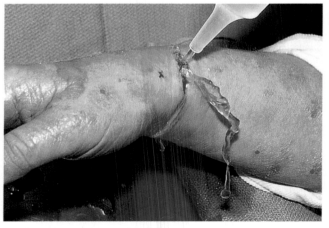

**FIGURE 13.** Irrigation of the wound with normal saline.

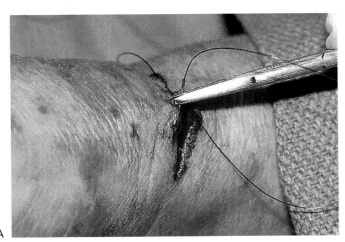
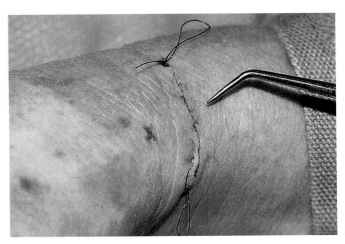

**FIGURE 14.** **A** and **B:** Closing the wound with a subcuticular 3–0 Prolene suture.

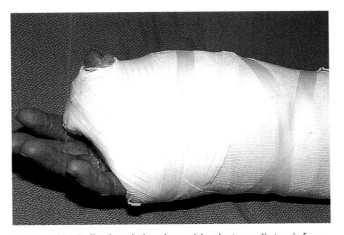

**FIGURE 15.** Bulky hand dressing with plaster splint reinforcement.

dorsal margin (Fig. 10). This leaves a palmarly based flap of retinaculum to prevent palmar subluxation of the tendons with wrist flexion (12). The first dorsal compartment is inspected for anatomic variations, including the presence of multiple APL tendons and a septum separating the APL from the EPB (Fig. 11). The EPB is lying dorsal to the APL, and having a more distally located muscle belly, is identified specifically in each case. Any constricting sheaths are released from the tendons contained within the first dorsal compartment. In the case illustrated here a fibrous septum dividing the compartment is identified (Fig. 12). The tourniquet is then released and hemostasis is obtained with electrocautery. The wound is irrigated with normal saline (Fig. 13) and is closed with a subcuticular pullout 3–0 Prolene suture (Fig. 14). A bulky hand dressing is then applied with plaster splint reinforcement (Fig. 15). The patient is taken to the recovery room and discharged to home later in the day. The patient is normally given a prescription for ten acetaminophen (Tylenol) with Codeine #3 tablets for postoperative analgesia.

## POSTOPERATIVE MANAGEMENT

At the first postoperative visit, 8 to 10 days after surgery, the bulky hand dressing is removed. The wound is inspected, and the pullout Prolene suture is removed. The patient is then given a polyethylene thumb spica splint to be worn for 2 weeks. Supervised hand therapy has not been found to be necessary. Patients are encouraged to use the hand without restrictions following removal of the splint. Prognosis for recovery is excellent. In a recent study published by one of us (RHG) all 30 patients with de Quervain's tenosynovitis who failed conservative management were afforded relief of symptoms by operative release (13).

## COMPLICATIONS

Complications following operative management of de Quervain's disease include: (a) sensory deficit and/or painful neuroma formation in the distribution of the superficial radial nerve; (b) palmar subluxation of the APL and EPB tendons; (c) incomplete release of the first dorsal compartment, including failure to recognize and release a separate compartment within or not recognizing multiple tendinous slips; and (d) scar adherence to the underlying APL and EPB. By recognizing the presence of each of these complications, measures may be enacted to prevent their occurrences.

By dissection in a bloodless field, the branches of the superficial radial nerve are identified where they cross the incision. The nerve may be transected or injured by vigorous traction. Management of a transected nerve consists of repair of the nerve in order to prevent neuroma formation and to increase the likelihood of reinnervation (4).

Palmar subluxation of the contents of the first dorsal compartment is a well-recognized complication described in detail by White and Weiland (12) in 1984. This complication is preventable by incising the sheath rather than totally excising it. We recommend incising the sheath over the EPB at its dorsal margin and completely incising all septa. By adhering to this technique a palmar-based flap of retinaculum acts to prevent the palmar subluxation of first compartment tendons. Alegado and Meals (1) reported an additional complication of this technique, however, in which the tendons were noted to glide dorsally on the fibrous remnant of the incised sheath, irritating the superficial branch of the radial nerve. If symptomatic palmar subluxation of the APL and EPB occurs postoperatively, a radially based flap of extensor retinaculum is used to restrain the tendons (12).

Inadequate operative release has resulted from failure to recognize separate compartments or multiple tendinous slips within the first dorsal compartment. This complication is avoidable by thorough inspection of the compartment at the time of operative release.

Adherence of the flexor tendons to the scar is an infrequent complication and is best avoided by early motion of the thumb and wrist. It is also avoided through the use of a transverse incision.

## ILLUSTRATIVE CASE FOR TECHNIQUE

A 49-year-old female pathologist presented with a 1-year history of pain and swelling over the radial dorsal aspect of her wrist. She described pain with pinch and grasp while manipulating slides on the stage of a microscope. She described the problem as episodic, with the most recent exacerbation beginning 1 month prior to presentation. She had noticed increasing pain over the past several weeks and had been taking 200 mg of ibuprofen for pain with minimal improvement in symptoms. She denied any significant past medical history.

Physical examination demonstrated marked tenderness over the first dorsal compartment of the wrist. Finkelstein's test caused considerable discomfort. The remainder of the physical examination was within normal limits. Specifically, the basal joint grind test was negative as was direct palpation of the triscaphoid joint.

Neurologic testing was normal. Radiographs of the patient's wrist were obtained, which showed no abnormalities.

With a diagnosis of de Quervain's disease formulated, a trial of injection and splinting was elected. The first dorsal compartment was injected with 40 mg of methylprednisolone acetate and 1% solution of lidocaine. Filling within the sheath of the first dorsal compartment was noted. The patient reported a significant reduction in pain following injection. Her wrist was fitted with a short thumb spica splint that was worn for 3 weeks.

The patient returned 6 weeks later stating that the initial improvement in discomfort lasted for several weeks, with a gradual return of pain. An operative release of the first dorsal compartment was then elected. During the procedure, a septum was encountered within the first dorsal compartment separating the EPB and APL tendons. All points of constriction were identified and released. A palmarly based flap of retinaculum was created to prevent palmar subluxation of the tendons with wrist flexion.

The patient returned to work 2 weeks postoperatively, wearing a polyethylene thumb spica splint. She noted moderate incisional pain that gradually resolved over 4 weeks. Four months following surgical release of the first dorsal compartment, she was pain free, performing all activities without restriction.

## RECOMMENDED READING

 1. Alegado, R. B., Meals, R. A.: An unusual complication following surgical treatment of de Quervain's disease. *J. Hand Surg.*, 4: 185–186, 1979.
 2. Arons, M. S.: de Quervain's release in working women: a report of failures, complications, and associated diagnoses. *J. Hand Surg.*, 12A(4): 540–544, 1987.
 3. Finkelstein, H.: Stenosing tendovaginitis at the radial styloid process. *J. Bone Joint Surg.*, 12: 509–540, 1930.
 4. Froimson, A. I.: Tenosynovitis and tennis elbow. In: *Operative Hand Surgery*, vol. 2, edited by D. P. Green, Churchill Livingstone, New York, 1988.
 5. Giles, K. W.: Anatomical variations affecting the surgery of De Quervain's disease. *J. Bone Joint Surg.*, 42B(2): 352–355, 1960.
 6. Harvey, F. J., Harvey, P. M., Horsley, M. W.: De Quervain's disease: surgical or nonsurgical treatment. *J. Hand Surg.*, 15A(1): 83–87, 1990.
 7. Hollinshead, W. H.: *Anatomy for Surgeons*, vol. 3, 3rd ed., Harper & Row, New York, pp. 420–426, 1982.
 8. Lacey, T. II, Goldstein, L. A., Tobin, C. E.: Anatomical and clinical study of the variations in the insertions of the abductor pollicis longus tendon, associated with stenosing tendovaginitis. *J. Bone Joint Surg.*, 33A(2): 347–350, 1951.
 9. Leao, L.: de Quervain's disease. A clinical and anatomical study. *J. Bone Joint Surg.*, A(5): 1063–1070, 1958.
10. Leslie, B. M., Ericson, W. B., Morehead, J. R.: Incidence of a septum within the first dorsal compartment of the wrist. *J. Hand Surg.*, 15A(1): 88–91, 1990.
11. Loomis, L. K.: Variations of stenosing tenosynovitis at the radial styloid process. *J. Bone Joint Surg.*, 33A(2): 340–346, 1951.
12. White, G. M., Weiland, A. J.: Symptomatic palmar tendon subluxation after surgical release for de Quervain's disease: a case report. *J. Hand Surg.*, 9: 704–706, 1984.
13. Witt, J., Pess, G., Gelberman, R. H.: Treatment of de Quervain tenosynovitis. A prospective study of the results of injection of steroids and immobilization in a splint. *J. Bone Joint Surg.*, 73A(2): 219–221, 1991.

# 35

# Ganglion Excision

Michael J. Botte

## INDICATIONS AND CONTRAINDICATIONS

Operative excision of a carpal ganglion is indicated when the cystic mass is painful, interferes with function, or causes signs or symptoms consistent with nerve compression. A ganglion is also excised when histologic tissue is needed for definitive diagnosis of a mass lesion. Excision is recommended in general for the lesion that causes symptoms when nonoperative methods (rest, activity modification, antiinflammatory medication, splinting, aspiration, cyst wall needle puncture, steroid injection, and patient reassurance) have proven inadequate (1,9,14–16). Symptomatic ganglia that warrant excision cause pain, tenderness, loss of wrist motion, weakness, and numbness or paresthesias (2,3,11,16,17).

Lesions that encroach on neurovascular structures and result in carpal tunnel syndrome, ulnar tunnel syndrome, compression of the superficial branch of the radial nerve, or radial artery compression are excised (8,10), including ganglia encountered incidentally during decompression of the carpal tunnel or Guyon's canal. Small occult ganglia are also excised if encountered incidentally during operative exploration in the patient with chronic wrist pain (16,18). Although rare, ganglia that cause unusual symptoms such as tendon triggering or loss of wrist motion should usually be excised.

Relative contraindications to excision include poor medical status or an allergy history that precludes use of general, regional, or local anesthesia; the presence of infection, open wounds, or abrasions; or chronically contaminated inflammatory skin conditions (such as severe psoriasis).

## PREOPERATIVE PLANNING

Preoperative planning includes medical history, physical examination (including transillumination of the cyst), roentgenograms, and diagnostic or therapeutic aspiration. Occasionally, additional tests such as ultrasound or magnetic resonance imaging (MRI) are indicated for further evaluation (4,5,13,18). It is important to inform patients of the possible need for postoperative hand therapy to regain motion and strength.

## Medical History

Salient medical history that aids diagnosis includes the circumstances of the mass and its origin (spontaneous or following trauma); length of time the mass has been present; changes in size, shape, or consistency; and the nature, degree, and fluctuations of related symptoms. Information relevant to treatment decisions includes the degree of discomfort or dysfunction (such as night pain and pain that interferes with work or activities of daily living) and any related symptoms of nerve compression or carpal instability. A history of previous treatment such as aspiration or excision is important.

Because ganglia are somewhat unique in their ability to change in size and associated symptoms, such characteristics are key aspects in diagnosing the lesion. Ganglia often enlarge or become more symptomatic after activity. The lesions can regress in size or resolve, spontaneously or after direct and sudden applied pressure or trauma. Other lesions, neoplasms, and infections rarely change or regress as readily.

A history of a previous puncture wound in the presence of a wrist mass that resembles a ganglion raises additional diagnostic considerations of an inclusion cyst, foreign body granuloma, or infectious granuloma. A history of inflammatory arthritis or crystalline arthropathy is significant, because synovitis, tenosynovitis, rheumatoid nodules, gouty tophi, or joint effusions can resemble ganglia.

The occurrence of previous trauma may be relevant if the patient has concomitant carpal instability or arthritis that may be related to the cause of the ganglion. These other problems may warrant treatment as well.

Patient history concerning occupation and handedness aides little in diagnosis of the lesion, since there has been no demonstrated correlation of these factors with the presence of ganglia (2,3,11). Ganglia have been shown to be slightly more prevalent in women, occurring most often in the second, third, and fourth decades (2,3,6,11).

## Physical Examination

Examine the mass as to location, size, extension, and presence of adjacent satellite lesions or loculations. Palpate for tenderness, consistency, fluctuance, and adherence to other structures. Digital compression or ballottement of the mass may help reveal the lesion's extent and the direction of the pedicle.

Ganglia on the dorsum of the wrist (70% of all hand and wrist ganglia [2,3,6,11]) usually are located mid-dorsally, originating most often from the scapholunate joint (Fig. 1A–D). Palmar flexion of the wrist accentuates the boundaries of the dorsal ganglion and may reveal an occult ganglion. Palpate multiloculated lesions to assess extent and origin of the pedicle (Fig. 1E). Palpation helps distinguish ganglions from extensor tenosynovitis, dorsal carpal synovitis, carpal effusion, rheumatoid nodules, gouty tophi, or a carpal boss.

Perform preoperative functional hand and wrist evaluations, including active and passive motion, manual muscle testing, grip and pinch strength, and sensibility evaluation with two-point discrimination and monofilament testing. Perform standard vascular examination (noting skin temperature, color, capillary refill, and turgor), palpation of pulses, and Allen's testing (to demonstrate possible arterial compromise, especially with palmar ganglia located adjacent to the radial artery). Examine for carpal instability with palpation for wrist clicks during active or passive motion, and perform the scaphoid shift test on the affected and unaffected sides to determine scaphoid instability (7). Examine digital and wrist motion for mechanical block or tendon triggering, which can occur if ganglia are near the

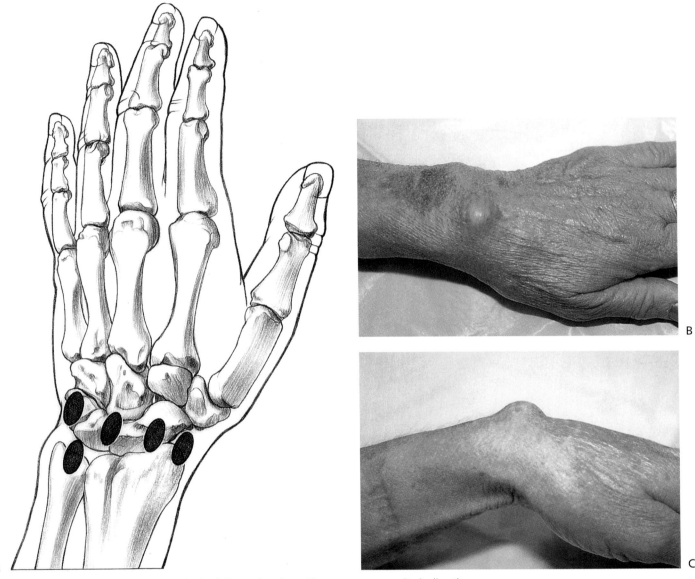

**FIGURE 1.    A:** Dorsal ganglia can arise in different locations. The most common site is directly over the scapholunate ligament. The other sites may be connected to the scapholunate ligament through an elongated pedicle. (Redrawn from Angelides, A. C.: Ganglions of the hand and wrist. In: *Green's Operative Hand Surgery,* 4th ed., edited by D. P. Green, R. N. Hotchkiss, and W. C. Pederson, Churchill-Livingstone, New York, pp. 2171–2183, 1999, with permission.) **B:** Typically, a dorsal ganglion is located over the mid-dorsal carpal area and originates from the scapholunate ligament and overlying capsule. **C:** Palmar wrist flexion accentuates the size and shape of the ganglion. (*continued.*)

extensor retinaculum or within the carpal canal. Gently percuss the lesion to elicit Tinel's sign, which indicates peripheral nerve encroachment.

Ganglia on the palmar aspect of the wrist usually are located near the radial artery or flexor carpi radialis tendon, and originate from the scaphotrapeziotrapezoid joint, radiocarpal joint, or trapeziometacarpal joint (Fig. 1F–J) (6,10,19). Dorsiflexion of the wrist may accentuate the boundaries of a small or occult palmar ganglion (Fig. 1I). Obtain a functional examination as described above, including assessment of the relative location and function of the radial artery, flexor carpi radialis tendon, brachioradialis tendon, and palmar cutaneous branch of the median nerve. Test patency of the radial artery by palpation, Allen's testing, and, if needed, Doppler evaluation.

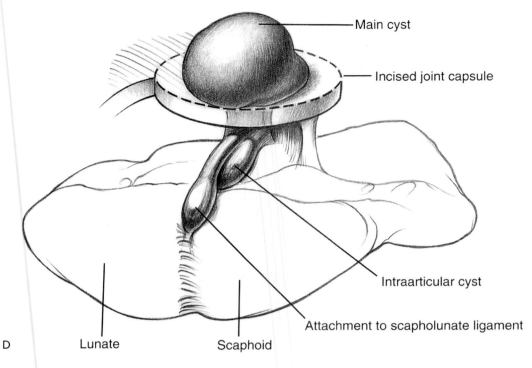

Main cyst

Incised joint capsule

Intraarticular cyst

Attachment to scapholunate ligament

D     Lunate     Scaphoid

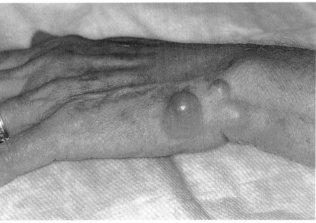

E

**FIGURE 1.** (*continued.*) **D:** Schematic representation of the ganglion *in situ*, with attachments to the scapholunate ligament visualized. (Redrawn from Angelides, A. C.: Ganglions of the hand and wrist. In: *Green's Operative Hand Surgery*, 4th ed., edited by D. P. Green, R. N. Hotchkiss, and W. C. Pederson, Churchill-Livingstone, New York, pp. 2171–2183, 1999, with permission.) **E:** Some ganglia exhibit multiple adjacent or loculated satellite lesions, which should be sought by careful palpation. (*continued.*)

Palpate the radial artery with and without manual occlusion of the ulnar artery to eliminate retrograde pulsation. Evaluate sensibility on the dorsoradial aspect of the hand and the base of the thenar eminence to reveal compression of the superficial branches of the radial nerve and the palmar cutaneous branch of the median nerve, respectively. Ganglia on the ulnar side of the wrist warrant similar evaluation of ulnar nerve and artery function.

### Transillumination

Place a small light against the lesion to transilluminate it; the passage of light through a cystic lesion confirms the diagnosis (Fig. 2) and can establish the extent of the boundaries of the lesion. Superficial lesions that do not allow light to pass through raise the suspicion of solid masses (such as a carpal boss, rheumatoid nodule, gouty tophus, or a neoplasm such as a benign fibrous histiocytoma or epithelioid sarcoma).

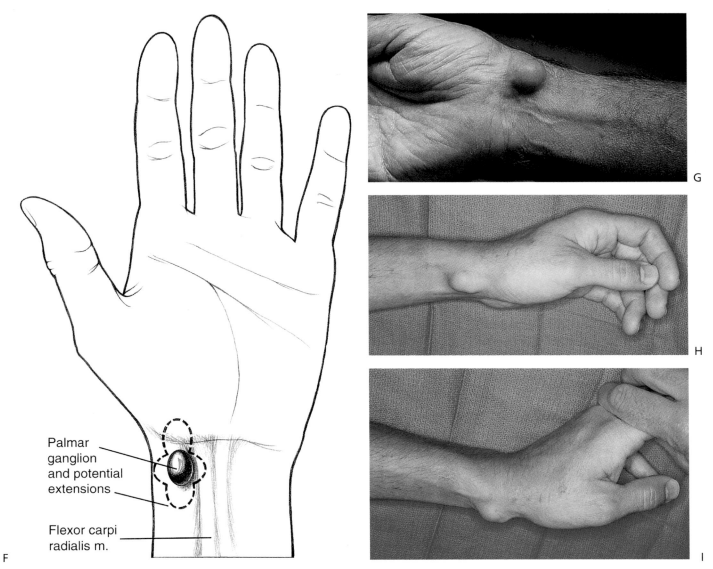

**FIGURE 1.** (*continued.*) **F:** A typical palmar ganglion on the radial side of the wrist. Possible subcutaneous extensions (*dotted lines*) are often palpable. (Redrawn from Angelides, A. C.: Ganglions of the hand and wrist. In: *Green's Operative Hand Surgery,* 4th ed., edited by D. P. Green, R. N. Hotchkiss, and W. C. Pederson, Churchill-Livingstone, New York, pp. 2171–2183, 1999, with permission.) **G:** A typical palmar carpal ganglion on the radial side of the wrist may extend between the tendons of the flexor carpi radialis and brachioradialis, usually in the vicinity of the radial artery. **H:** The ganglion usually originates from the scaphotrapezial, trapeziometacarpal, or radiocarpal ligaments and overlying capsule; it can extend along the tendon sheath of the flexor carpi radialis. **I:** Dorsiflexion of the wrist aids in the detection of small or occult palmar ganglia and ganglion boundaries. (*continued.*)

## Roentgenograms and Related Imaging Studies

Standard roentgenograms may show a soft tissue shadow that further documents the presence and location of the lesion. Roentgenograms also may demonstrate abnormalities associated with or related to the development of the ganglion, including arthritis or carpal instability.

The diagnosis may not be clear in the case of a thick-walled, firm, deeply seated, or small-sized lesion (13,16). Additional helpful diagnostic tests are ultrasound and MRI (Fig. 3) (4,5,13,18). Ultrasound determines the cystic nature of a lesion and assesses the proximity and the patency of the radial artery to a palmar carpal ganglion (Fig. 3 A, B). MRI is helpful in establishing the diagnosis in deep-

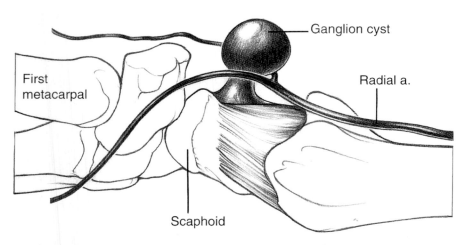

J

**FIGURE 1. (*continued*.) J:** As illustrated, the palmar ganglion is very close to the radial artery. (Redrawn from Angelides, A. C.: Ganglions of the hand and wrist. In: *Green's Operative Hand Surgery,* 4th ed., edited by D. P. Green, R. N. Hotchkiss, and W. C. Pederson, Churchill-Livingstone, New York, pp. 2171–2183, 1999, with permission.)

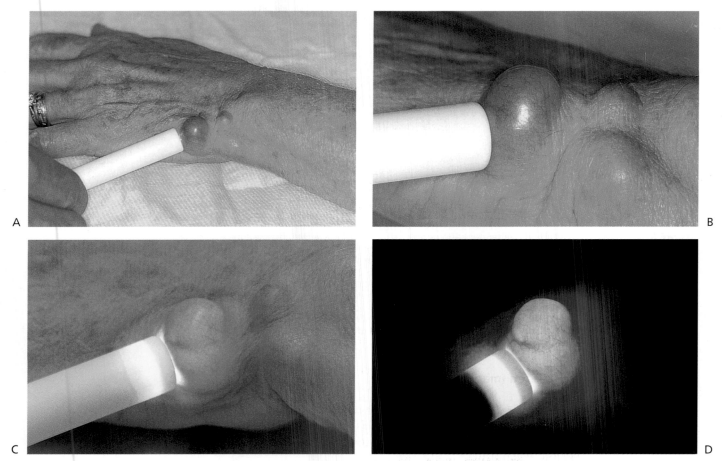

**FIGURE 2.** Transillumination of the dorsoulnar ganglion seen in Figure 1E. **A** and **B:** Place a small penlight or otoscope light gently against the ganglion, and **(C)** illuminate it to confirm the cystic nature of the lesion. **D:** Darkening the overhead room lights aids in transillumination.

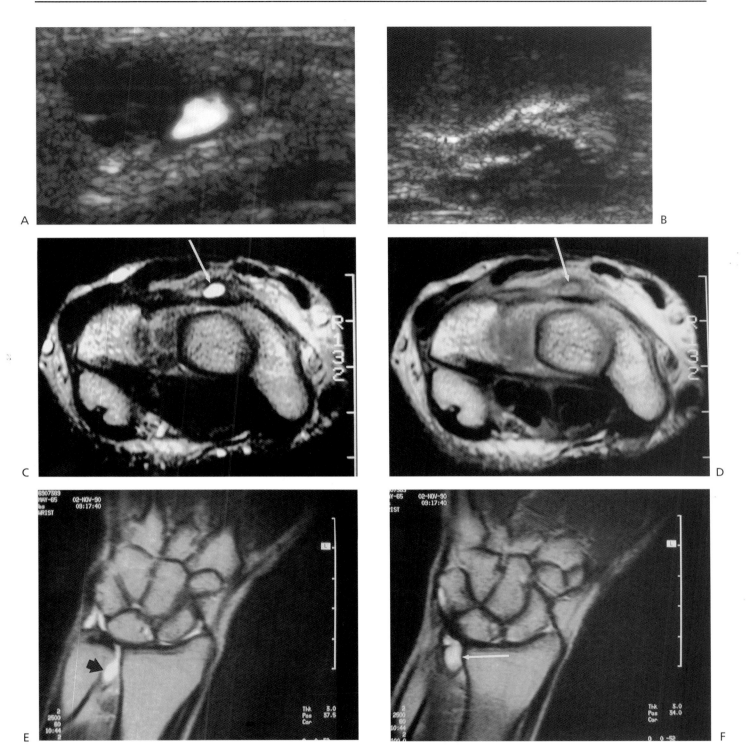

**FIGURE 3.** **A** and **B:** Photographs of ultrasound and **(C)** to **(G)** magnetic resonance imaging of carpal ganglia. **A:** A transverse sonogram with power Doppler imaging demonstrates a palmar ganglion with an adjacent radial artery. The bright white central form represents the radial artery; the ganglion is the large dark shadow area to the left of the artery. The dark (anechoic) image of the ganglion shows no blood flow within the ganglion. **B:** A transverse sonogram demonstrates a hypoechoic/anechoic ganglion (*central dark area*) with a pedicle extending toward the radiocarpal joint. The ultrasound images usually are viewed more easily and interpreted in real time as opposed to static photographs. Ultrasound allows the examiner to manipulate the angles of view for clarification and observe movement such as pulsations of the radial artery for orientation. **C** and **D:** Magnetic resonance images of the wrist of a 30-year-old man with chronic wrist pain and an associated occult dorsal wrist ganglion. **C:** In this T2-weighted image, the ganglion appears as the bright white spot (*arrow*), dorsal to the radius. **D:** In this proton-weighted image, the ganglion can be seen in finer detail (*arrow*) but is less brightly illuminated. **E** and **F:** Magnetic resonance images of the wrist in the frontal plane demonstrate a small occult ganglion (*arrow*) from the distal radioulnar joint (T2-weighted images). (*continued.*)

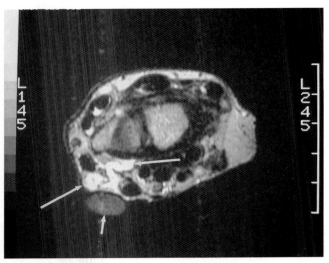

G

**FIGURE 3.** (*continued.*) **G:** T2-weighted scan shows a palmar ganglion on the ulnar side of the wrist. The ganglion appears as the white tortuous image (*long arrows*), with a winding stalk that extends to the underlying carpal joint. The circular object (*short arrow*) is a marker placed on the skin to identify the area of interest for imaging. (Photographs 3A and 3B courtesy of David Fessell, M. D., Department of Radiology, University of Michigan Hospitals, Ann Arbor, Michigan. Photographs 3C–G courtesy of Christine B. Chung, M. D. and Donald L. Resnick, M. D., Department of Radiology, San Diego Veterans Affairs Health Care System, and University of California, San Diego.)

seated or occult ganglia, such as those within the carpal canal or within Guyon's canal (Fig. 3 C–G). Both ultrasound and MRI are effective diagnostic methods if an occult ganglion is suspected, but ultrasound costs less and has fewer contraindications. Ultrasound thus is more suitable for establishing the diagnosis of an occult ganglion when clinical findings are inconclusive (4).

Although arthrograms of the wrist have demonstrated the "one-way" valve mechanism and connection of the pedicle to the main cyst, the routine use of arthrograms is not warranted (11,20). Similarly, arteriograms can assess the patency of the radial artery with adjacent palmar ganglia and have been used to diagnose ganglion-related thromboses. Routine use of arteriograms for palmar ganglia, however, is not indicated because less invasive, accurate techniques such as careful palpation, Allen's testing, Doppler evaluation, and ultrasound are available.

The differential diagnosis of the carpal ganglion includes inclusion cysts, inflammatory (rheumatoid) or infectious (tuberculous) synovitis, tenosynovitis, rheumatoid nodules, and gouty tophi. Other conditions that must be considered include foreign-body granulomas, giant-cell tumors of tendon sheath, lipomas, fibromas, neurilemomas, neurofibromas, carpal bosses, osteochondromas, and, less commonly, lymphangiomas, aneurysms, arteriovenous malformations, leiomyomas, aberrant muscle bellies, and chronic abscesses.

## Diagnostic and Therapeutic Aspiration

Although aspiration was established as a method of treatment, it is also useful as a diagnostic procedure (Fig. 4). Under sterile conditions, anesthetize the skin with 1% lidocaine without epinephrine. Use a large-bore needle to aspirate the lesion; mucinous material is usually diagnostic for a ganglion.

If aspiration is performed for treatment as well, place multiple punctures in the cyst wall, using digital palpation to direct the needle and decompress the mass.

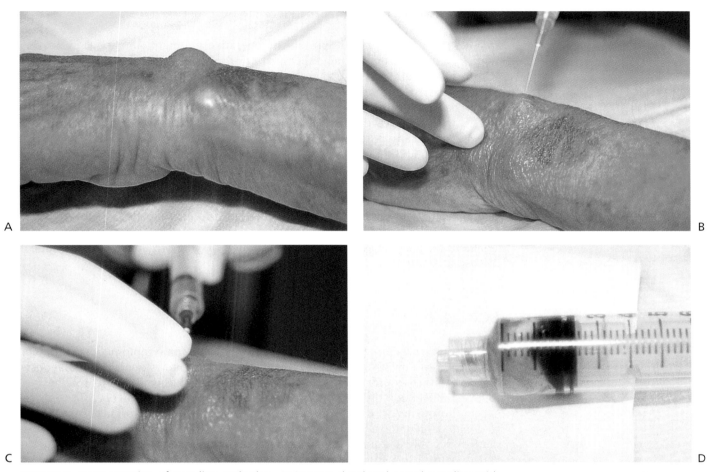

**FIGURE 4.** Demonstration of ganglion aspiration. **A:** Prepare the dorsal carpal ganglion with povidone-iodine solution. **B:** Anesthetize the skin with 1% lidocaine without epinephrine. **C:** Use a 15- to 18-gauge needle to aspirate the lesion. Place multiple cyst wall punctures using digital palpation to direct the needle and decompress the mass. **D:** Thick, mucoid or gel-like material obtained from aspiration aids definitive diagnosis. The carpus is immobilized for 3 weeks following aspiration in a plaster cast or thermoplast splint, with the wrist in 10° extension. The technique is described by Richman et al. (15).

Take care during aspiration of palmar carpal ganglia to avoid injury to the radial or ulnar arteries. Following aspiration, immobilize the carpus, with the wrist in 10° extension; immobilization should last 3 weeks (15).

From a therapeutic standpoint, aspiration, cyst wall puncture, injection of a steroid solution, or combinations thereof have been shown to be an effective method of treatment, especially for a dorsal ganglion (2,8,9,11). The additional use of hyaluronidase as a potential adjuvant to aspiration has been investigated recently (14).

With aspiration and cyst wall puncture, successful outcomes for dorsal carpal ganglia have been reported in 27% to 48% of cases (9,15,17). For palmar carpal ganglia, successful outcomes have been achieved in 13% to 48% of cases (9,19). Immobilization following aspiration has been shown to improve results of dorsal carpal ganglion aspiration, with 40% of those immobilized for 3 weeks having no recurrence, compared with only 13% of those mobilized early (15). Although the role of immobilization has been questioned recently (9), immobilization following aspiration and cyst wall puncture of most carpal ganglia seems warranted for patient comfort as well as to minimize the possibility of recurrences (15).

Because of the relatively high recurrence rate following aspiration of palmar carpal ganglia, excision instead of aspiration has been suggested as the primary definitive treatment (19).

### Patient Discussion and Therapy Planning

When loss of function is present preoperatively, obtain functional evaluation and consultation from the hand therapist prior to surgery.

Inform the patient before surgery of the benefit of postoperative hand therapy; indicate that such therapy may be needed to regain strength and motion (especially palmar flexion motion following excision of a dorsal carpal ganglion). Such a preoperative discussion alleviates many patient concerns, especially if prolonged therapy is required later. It is common for workers to require several weeks of rehabilitation before they return to heavy or repetitive work (2,3); therefore, it is necessary to inform patients of the potential length of the recovery period.

When a palmar ganglion is present, the surgeon should discuss and obtain preoperative surgical consent for carpal tunnel release, because the pedicle may originate from within the carpal tunnel and require transection of the transverse carpal ligament for adequate exposure. Rehabilitation may be prolonged if carpal tunnel release is required.

## SURGERY

Operative excision remains the treatment of choice for symptomatic ganglia not responsive to conservative management, or when tissue is needed for diagnosis (Fig. 5). Arthroscopic management has been presented as well, but its role has yet to be established in the standard treatment of the carpal ganglion (12,17).

Ganglion excision usually is performed in the outpatient surgical suite under regional or general anesthesia. Local anesthesia is not recommended, because deep dissection is required to isolate and excise the associated pedicle.

It is helpful to verify the presence and location of the ganglion on the day of surgery before administering anesthesia. Occasionally, in the interval between the preoperative clinic visit and the day of surgery, a ganglion can decompress spontaneously, making identification at surgery difficult.

### Technique: Dorsal Carpal Ganglion Excision

Position the patient supine with the upper extremity placed on an arm board in 90° abduction (Fig. 5A–C). Position two overhead lights in line with the arm board with their rims touching. Clip roentgenograms to the lighted film box. Wrap a pneumatic tourniquet over a layer of cast padding on the proximal arm.

Have the extremity prepared with povidone-iodine solution from above the elbow distally. Place a sterile towel around the tourniquet. Drape in standard fashion, with at least two layers of sterile drape covering the arm board and all parts of the patient's body. I prefer split sheets or special upper-extremity drapes with a hole for the extremity. Connect suction and electrocautery (Fig. 5B, C).

The surgeon sits on the axillary side of the extremity and the assistant on the cephalad side. Pronate the forearm for a dorsal ganglion and supinate it for a palmar ganglion. Place a small pad of folded towels under the hand. Use the standard hand surgical instrument set.

Sketch the incision on the skin before inflating the tourniquet, using a sterile marking pen (Fig. 5D, E). Wrap an Esmarch bandage firmly but gently to exsanguinate the extremity before inflating the tourniquet, taking care to avoid ganglion rupture (Fig. 5F). If the diagnosis of the mass is in question, with suspicion of a neoplasm or infection, avoid exsanguination with the Esmarch and perform gravity exsanguination via extremity elevation.

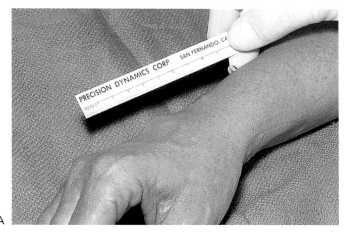

A

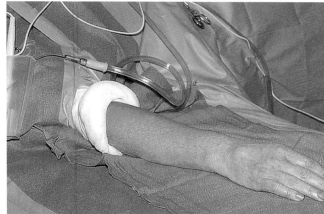

B

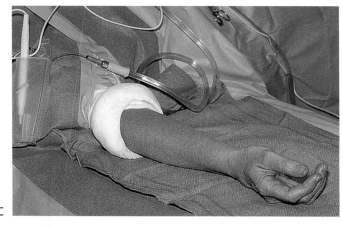

C

**FIGURE 5.** Step-by-step demonstration of carpal ganglion excision. **A:** A dorsal carpal ganglion is present on the right wrist of a 40-year-old woman. **B:** Prepare and drape the upper extremity in the usual fashion for hand surgery with cauterization and suction available. The forearm is pronated for this dorsal carpal ganglion or **(C)** supinated for a palmar ganglion. (*continued.*)

Undertake surgery with loupe surgical telescopes of 2.5× or 3.5× magnification. I do not give preoperative antibiotics unless the risk of infection is high (e.g., patients with diabetes, peripheral vascular disease, or those taking steroid medications).

To help prevent scar contracture over the wrist crease, it is generally preferable to make a transverse incision along Langer's lines of the wrist for an uncomplicated dorsal carpal ganglion. For extensive multiloculated lesions or those with multiple satellite lesions, a longitudinal incision will aid a more extensile exposure (Fig. 6). If lesions are located a few centimeters proximal or distal to the wrist, bear in mind that most dorsal ganglia arise from the scapholunate articulation, and a long pedicle may be present. The incision should allow access to the ganglion, its pedicle, and its intracarpal origin. Multiple smaller incisions may be used as an alternative to a longitudinal incision.

Incise the skin using a #15 scalpel (Fig. 5G). Place skin hooks or retraction sutures along the skin margins (using 3–0 nylon or silk) (Fig. 5H), and dissect the subcutaneous layer using a small dissection scissors and an Adson forceps (Fig. 5I). Small Storz (Storz, St. Louis, MO) or Iris scissors are useful; their small size aids control. The semiblunt tips of the Storz scissors provide some safety against inadvertent ganglion wall penetration.

Identify and mobilize the lesion in a circumferential fashion (Fig. 5J–M). Protect cutaneous nerves such as the dorsal branches of the ulnar nerve or the superficial branches of the radial nerve. Obtain hemostasis by cauterization. The distal edge of the extensor retinaculum can be incised or a portion excised if needed.

Ganglia often penetrate between the tendons of the fourth dorsal compartment or between compartments (Fig. 5J–L). Retract the tendons and continue dissec-

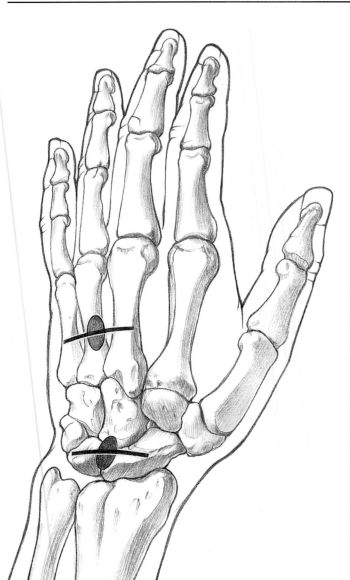

D

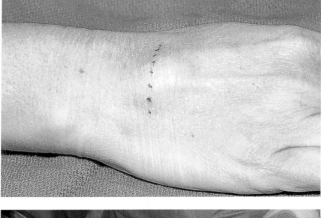

E

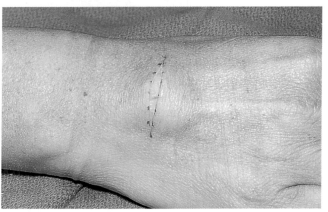

F

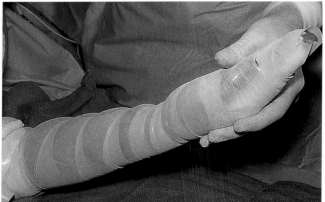

G

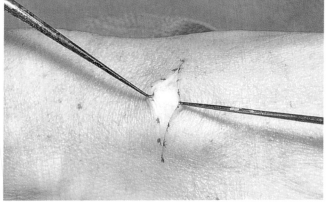

H

**FIGURE 5.** (*continued.*) **D** and **E:** Use a transverse incision for most dorsal ganglia (longitudinal incisions are used for most palmar ganglia). (**D** redrawn from Angelides, A. C.: Ganglions of the hand and wrist. In: *Green's Operative Hand Surgery,* 4th ed., edited by D. P. Green, R. N. Hotchkiss, and W. C. Pederson, Churchill-Livingstone, New York, pp. 2171–2183, 1999, with permission.) Sketch the incision on the skin before inflating the tourniquet. **F:** Gently exsanguinate the extremity and inflate the tourniquet. **G:** Make the incision through the full thickness of skin with a #15 scalpel, and (**H**) position skin hooks or retraction sutures. **I:** Use Storz (Storz, St. Louis, MO) scissors or small tenotomy scissors to dissect through the subcutaneous tissues. Use electrocautery for hemostasis of small veins. **J:** Continue dissection through the subcutaneous tissues to isolate the lesion. Put small right-angle retractors (Ragnell or Senn) in place. **K:** Identify the extensor tendons. In this patient, the ganglion is located between the extensor digitorum communis of the index finger and extensor indicis proprius on the radial side, and the remaining extensor digitorum communis tendons on the ulnar side of the lesion. **L:** The ganglion between the third and fourth dorsal compartments. EDC, extensor digitorum communis; EIP, extensor indicis proprius; EPL, extensor pollicis longus. (Redrawn from Angelides, A. C.: Ganglions of the hand and wrist. In: *Green's Operative Hand Surgery,* 4th ed., edited by D. P. Green, R. N. Hotchkiss, and W. C. Pederson, Churchill-Livingstone, New York, pp. 2171–2183, 1999, with permission.) (*continued.*)

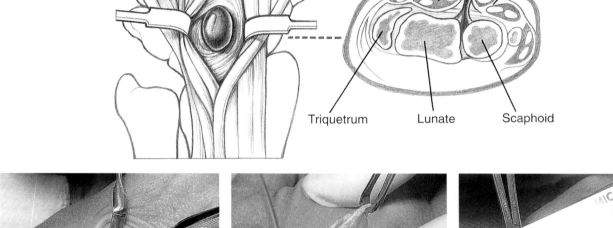

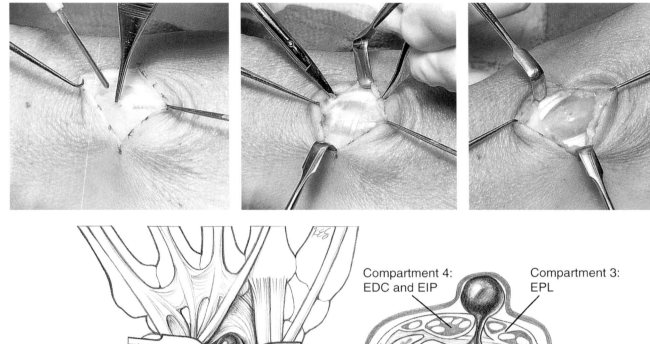

Compartment 4:
EDC and EIP

Compartment 3:
EPL

Triquetrum          Lunate          Scaphoid

L

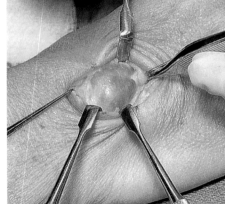

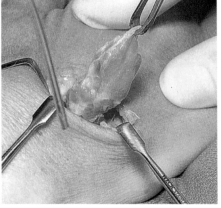

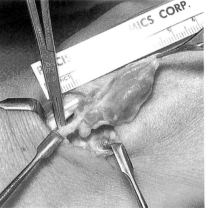

M

N,O

**FIGURE 5.** (*continued.*) **M:** Incise or partially excise the distal portion of the extensor retinaculum if needed. Retract the tendons and continue dissection in a circumferential fashion. **N:** Mobilization of the ganglion is aided by grasping the lesion with an Allis forceps. **O:** Identify the pedicle and trace it to its origin. (The tip of the scissors is identifying the pedicle.) In most cases, dorsal ganglia originate from the scapholunate ligament and overlying capsule. In this case, the relatively large ganglion and pedicle involved the capitohamate joint as well. (*continued.*)

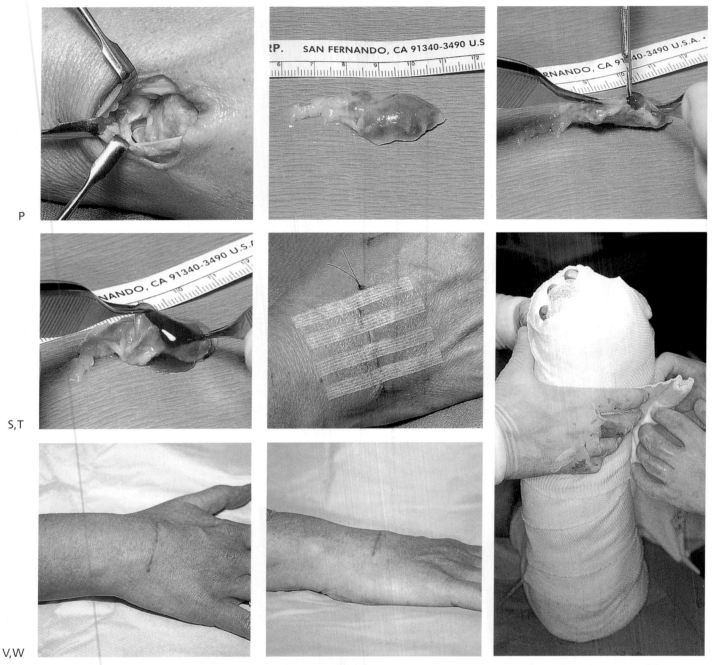

**FIGURE 5.** (*continued.*) Remove the pedicle with a portion of capsule and ligament, **(P)** thus creating a window arthrotomy with joint surfaces visible. **Q:** Examine and measure the excised lesion. **R** and **S:** We prefer to open the lesion with a scalpel on the surgical field to confirm the diagnosis at the time of surgery. The presence of mucoid fluid helps confirm the diagnosis. Copiously irrigate the wound, and remove all remaining suspicious or glistening tissue, using synovial rongeurs. Deflate the tourniquet, obtain hemostasis, and **(T)** close the skin with either 5–0 or 6–0 nylon interrupted horizontal mattress sutures or a running 3–0 Prolene subcuticular suture. The dorsal capsule is not closed. Place Steri-strips when a subcuticular suture is used. **U:** Apply a bulky hand dressing with dorsal and plaster splints, placing the wrist in 30° dorsiflexion. Place the metacarpophalangeal joints in 80° flexion and the proximal interphalangeal joints in 10° flexion. **V** and **W:** The incision has healed at 4 weeks postsurgery.

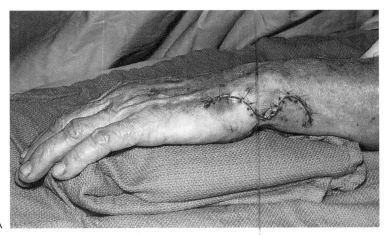

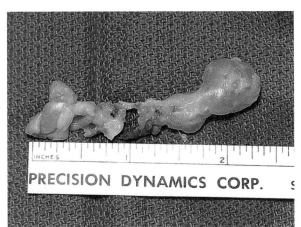

A                                                                                                                    B

**FIGURE 6. A:** Although most dorsal ganglia are excised with a transverse incision, extensive lesions such as the one transilluminated in Figure 2 can be removed easier with longitudinal curved incisions. **B:** The excised lesion had multiple loculations and satellite lesions.

tion to identify the pedicle (Fig. 5M–O). Gently place an Allis forceps on the ganglion (Fig. 5N) to aid mobilization for circumferential dissection. Carefully isolate the pedicle and continue dissection to its origin from the associated carpal joint (Fig. 5O).

The pedicle penetrates the joint capsule and usually originates from the scapholunate ligament and overlying capsule. Remove the ganglion and pedicle in its entirety as one specimen of tissue. Take a portion of associated dorsal wrist capsule and a small portion of the scapholunate ligament to ensure thorough removal of the pedicle. Usually, a section of capsule 5 mm × 5 mm is removed, creating a window in the dorsal wrist capsule that allows visualization of the associated articular surfaces (Fig. 5P). Carefully inspect the dorsal capsule for glistening cystic wall tissue or small additional lesions and excise any remaining pathological tissue. Inspect the normal joint synovium and visible carpal contents through the window created in the capsule.

If a dorsal ganglion becomes ruptured or deflated before it is removed, or a long pedicle cannot be traced adequately to its origin, explore the scapholunate ligament. Perform limited excision of the capsular attachment if it appears to be the site of origin of the pedicle (2).

Because of the defect left by removal of a portion of capsule, capsular closure is neither possible nor recommended (2). Inspect the excised lesion, measure it, and open it on the back surgical table to verify correct diagnosis (Fig. 5Q–S).

Send tissue to pathology for definitive histologic analysis. Irrigate the wound, deflate the tourniquet, and obtain hemostasis. Close the skin using a 3–0 absorbable (Vicryl) interrupted subcutaneous closure combined with a 3–0 Prolene running subcuticular suture (Fig. 5T) or with a 4–0 or 5–0 nylon suture in an interrupted horizontal mattress fashion. A surgical drain is not used. Infiltrate the wound with 5-cc 0.05% bupivacaine without epinephrine for pain relief in the immediate postoperative period.

Apply a sterile dressing followed by fabrication of a bulky below-elbow compressive hand dressing with dorsal and palmar plaster splints (Fig. 5U). Position the wrist in 30° extension. Place the metacarpophalangeal joints in 80° flexion and the proximal interphalangeal joints in 10° flexion. The patient usually is discharged from the surgical suite the same day. Outpatient analgesia is accomplished with oral narcotic medication such as Tylenol with codeine or Vicodin. The healing incision at 4 weeks is shown in Figure 5V and W.

### Technique: Palmar Carpal Ganglion Excision

Figure 7 illustrates the salient surgical anatomy and operative technique for the typical palmar ganglion excision. As for a dorsal carpal ganglion, begin by sketching the incision on the skin before inflating the tourniquet (Fig. 7A–C, L). The cyst is often situated between the radial artery and the flexor carpi radialis tendon or the brachioradialis tendon (Fig. 7M). Although transverse incisions are usually preferred for the dorsal carpal ganglion, a longitudinal incision is optimal for the palmar ganglion, because the pedicle commonly originates from the scaphotrapeziotrapezoid, radiocarpal, or trapeziometacarpal joint and may track the flexor carpi radialis tendon sheath longitudinally to surface near or adjacent to the radial artery (3,6,10,19). A curved or zigzag incision allows greater extensile exposure and access to multiple joints, and can facilitate exploration of the flexor carpi radialis tendon and the radial artery as well as carpal tunnel release, if necessary. Use of this incision avoids crossing the wrist crease at 90° (using a curved or zigzag component), minimizing skin scar contracture (Fig. 7A–D).

Incise the skin with a #15 scalpel (Fig. 7D). Place skin hooks or retraction sutures (of 3–0 nylon or silk) and dissect the subcutaneous tissue using a small dissection scissors and an Adson forceps. Divide the deep fascia of the forearm longitudinally (Fig. 7D), and note the position of the ganglion relative to neighboring structures. Identify the radial artery and flexor carpi radialis tendon (Fig. 7D–F). Tag these structures with a rubber dam, and protect them. It is usually preferable to identify the radial artery proximal to the ganglion and trace it distally. It may be found adherent to the wall of the ganglion, and careful dissection may be required to separate it from the cyst wall.

A bilobular palmar ganglion in the vicinity of the radial artery may involve the radial artery running across the body of the cyst, thus dividing it into two lobules. The artery may not be readily apparent and, if adherent to the ganglion wall, may appear as a septum. Careful identification of the artery proximal to the cyst and dissection in a proximal-to-distal direction across the ganglion help avoid injury to the artery. Identify the small superficial palmar branch of the radial artery (Fig. 7F) as it crosses the palmar surface of the scaphoid, and preserve it if possible.

The ganglion often will be located in the interval between the flexor carpi radialis tendon, the radial artery, and the superficial palmar branch of the radial artery (Fig. 7G). If the ganglion is located ulnar to the flexor carpi radialis tendon, identify the median nerve and the palmar cutaneous branch of the median nerve, tag them with a rubber dam, isolate them in a proximal-to-distal direction, and protect them along their course. Identify the neighboring tendons along with these neurovascular structures.

Dissect the ganglion in a circumferential fashion as described for the dorsal ganglion. Gently place an Allis forceps on the lesion for mobilization and circumferential dissection. Trace the pedicle of the ganglion to its origin from the associated palmar carpal joint (Fig. 7H–J). Because the flexor carpi radialis tendon dives deep within a fibroosseous tunnel to reach its insertion at the base of the index and long finger metacarpals, it may be necessary to open this tunnel to achieve adequate exposure of the pedicle. Retraction of the adjacent flexor pollicis longus tendon may be necessary as well (Fig. 7K).

Tendon retraction and deep dissection usually reveal the origin of the pedicle to be the scaphotrapeziotrapezoid, radiocarpal, or trapeziometacarpal. To facilitate exposure further, partially detach the base or proximal margin of the thenar muscles from the transverse carpal ligament, scaphoid, or trapezium, using a #15 scalpel. This detachment is helpful if the ganglion tracks distally to the scaphotrapezial joint. An appreciation of this deep anatomy is necessary for adequate ganglion pedicle excision (Fig. 7J, K).

Rarely, the pedicle of a palmar ganglion originates from the scapholunate joint and dissection is carried out accordingly (Fig. 7H, K, P). Remove the pedicle of

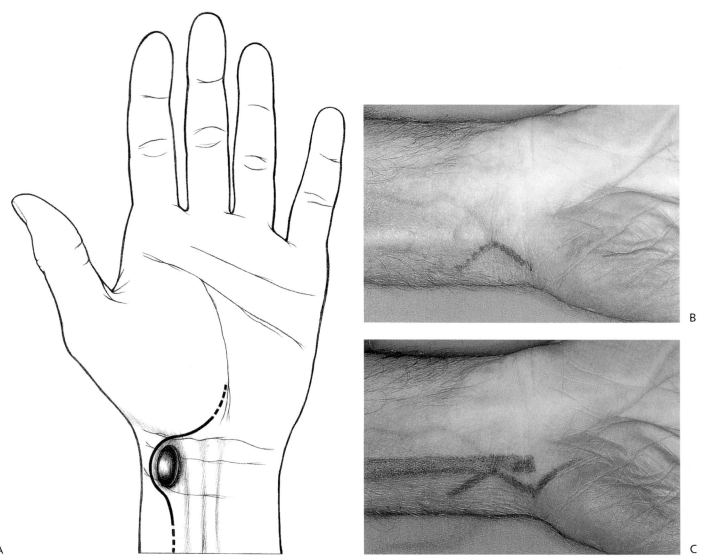

A

B

C

**FIGURE 7. A:** Curved incision used for the typical palmar ganglion located on the radial side of the wrist. (Redrawn from Angelides, A. C.: Ganglions of the hand and wrist. In: *Green's Operative Hand Surgery,* 4th ed., edited by D. P. Green, R. N. Hotchkiss, and W. C. Pederson, Churchill-Livingstone, New York, pp. 2171–2183, 1999, with permission.) **B** to **K:** Figures (cadaver specimen) demonstrate salient anatomy and operative approach in the area of the typical palmar ganglion. **A** to **C:** Sketch the incision on the skin before inflating the tourniquet; **(B)** mark the flexor carpi radialis tendon in solid ink on the skin for identification. The cyst often is situated adjacent to the flexor carpi radialis tendon or radial artery. A longitudinal incision is preferable for a palmar ganglion, whose pedicle usually originates from scaphotrapezial, trapeziometacarpal, or radiocarpal joint and tracks the flexor carpi radialis tendon. The ganglion also may originate from the palmar scapholunate joint. A zigzag or curved incision allows for greater extensile exposure. The incision avoids crossing the wrist crease at 90° (using a zigzag or curved component) to minimize skin scar contracture, and is extended proximally as needed from **(A)** to **(C)**. Open the deep fascia of the forearm in a longitudinal fashion and note the position of the ganglion relative to neighboring structures. (*continued.*)

the ganglion with a portion of normal tissue, usually a 5 mm × 5-mm portion of joint capsule. Further inspection or digital compression of surrounding tissues may help identify further mucin-filled sacs, which should be excised as well.

After palmar ganglion excision, irrigate wounds, deflate the tourniquet, obtain hemostasis, and close the skin with either 4–0 or 5–0 nylon using interrupted horizontal mattress sutures or with a 3–0 Prolene suture using a subcuticular closure. Surgical drains are not used routinely. Infiltrate the wound with 5 cc of 0.05% bupivacaine without epinephrine.

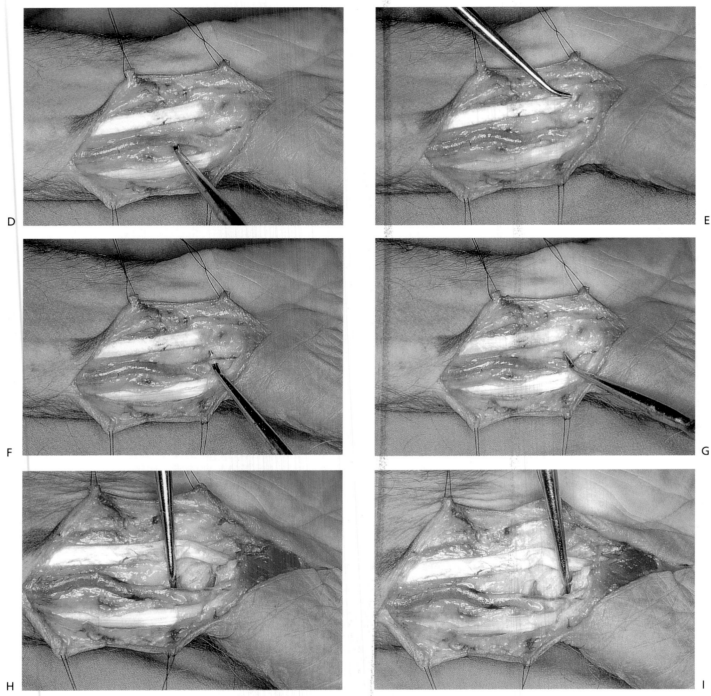

**FIGURE 7. (continued.) D:** The probe identifies the radial artery, **(E)** the flexor carpi radialis tendon, and **(F)** the superficial palmar branch of the radial artery located **(G)** in the interval between the flexor carpi radialis and radial artery. **H:** The pedicle may originate from the radiocarpal joint or **(I)** from the scaphotrapezial joint and extends along the tendon sheath of the flexor carpi radialis. *(continued.)*

After application of a sterile dressing, fabricate a bulky below-elbow compressive hand dressing with dorsal and palmar plaster splints (Fig. 5U). Place the wrist in neutral position to allow for palmar capsule healing. Place the metacarpophalangeal joints in 80° flexion and the proximal interphalangeal joints in 10° flexion. The patient usually is discharged from the outpatient surgical suite on the same day.

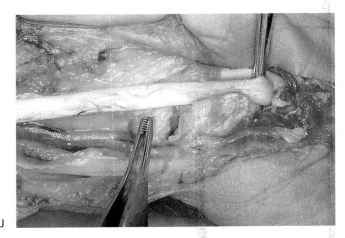

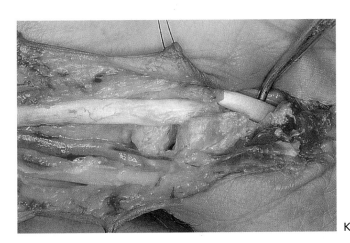

J

K

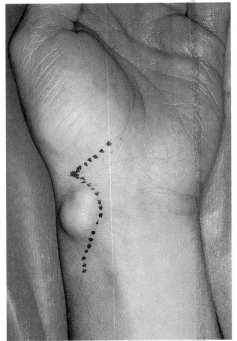

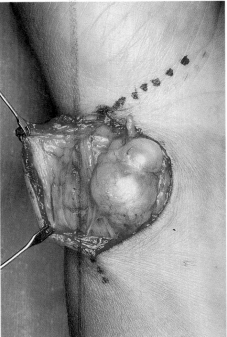

L

M

**FIGURE 7.** (*continued.*) **J**: Once the most proximal margin of the thenar muscles has been released, open the fibroosseous tunnel that contains the flexor carpi radialis to facilitate exposure (sometimes necessary for adequate excision of the pedicle). The probe identifies the flexor carpi radialis, the forceps identifies the scaphoid tubercle, and the radiocarpal joint is visible proximal to the scaphoid tubercle. The scaphotrapezial joint is visible just distal to the scaphoid tubercle. **K**: The carpal tunnel has been opened partially, and the probe identifies the flexor pollicis longus tendon. **L**: Large palmar carpal ganglion with incision sketched for excision. **M**: The ganglion is located radial to the flexor carpi radialis. The incision is placed and ganglion identified. (*continued.*)

Ganglia from the palmar aspect of the wrist are known causes of median and ulnar nerve compression. Routinely inspect the canal contents following open carpal tunnel or ulnar tunnel decompression to rule out an occult ganglion or other space-occupying lesion as a cause of the nerve compression syndrome.

## POSTOPERATIVE MANAGEMENT

Continue postoperative elevation of the extremity for the first week, or as indicated for comfort and swelling. On the fifth to seventh postoperative day, remove the bulky dressing and inspect the wound. Immobilize the wrist with a splint,

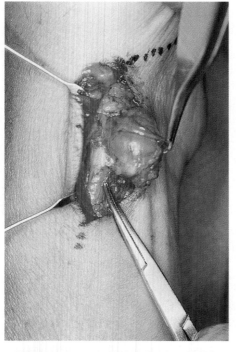

N

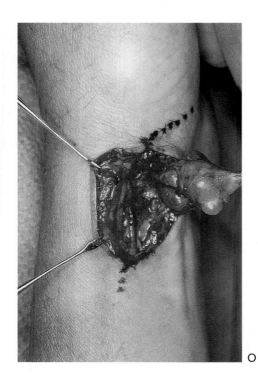

O

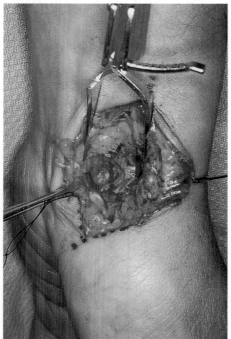

P

**FIGURE 7.** (*continued.*) **N:** The radial artery is located radial to the ganglion, identified with forceps. **O:** The ganglion is mobilized circumferentially, preserving the stalk to the underlying carpal joint. **P:** The ganglion has been excised and the origin identified as the radiocarpal joint. The manual retractor holds the flexor carpi radialis tendon. (Special thanks to Kirk F. Granlund, M. D., San Diego, California, for assistance with surgery and photographs 7L–P.)

maintaining the wrist in 30° extension for the dorsal ganglion and in neutral wrist position for the palmar ganglion. The digits and elbow are not immobilized. Encourage the patient to initiate active digital motion while the wrist is immobilized. Sutures usually are removed in 7 to 14 days.

Wrist immobilization is maintained for 2 to 3 weeks. Following this period, have the patient initiate progressive wrist active range-of-motion exercises. Provide hand therapy to regain range of motion and strength or to control edema.

## COMPLICATIONS

### Dorsal Carpal Ganglion

Complications following dorsal carpal ganglion excision include recurrence, continued pain or tenderness, wrist stiffness or weakness, neuroma formation, wound infection, and scar contracture or keloid formation. Carpal instability (including scapholunate dissociation), although possible, does not seem to be a common problem despite the fact that a portion of capsule has been removed surgically. Conversely, recent evidence indicates that dorsal wrist ganglia frequently are associated with a positive scaphoid shift test preoperatively and that excision of the ganglion followed by 2 weeks' immobilization may lead to resolution of the signs and symptoms of instability, at least in the short term (7). Avascular necrosis of the scaphoid or lunate has been mentioned as a possible complication, but it is not common (1).

Early recurrence is one of the most common complications and may be due to inadequate resection. This complication is avoided best by adequate resection of the pedicle to the level of the scapholunate ligaments and a portion of adjacent normal-appearing capsule to ensure removal of all involved tissue. When tissue is excised in this manner, the reported recurrence rate has been between 1% and 24% (2,3,11,17). When only the main cyst was excised without adequate pedicle or capsular resection, recurrence rates were between 30% and 40% (2).

A cluster of small ganglia is often present at the base of the pedicle; if they are not removed, they can form an additional new ganglion. Once formed, a recurrent ganglion can be more difficult to manage because of the additional scar adhesions from the previous excision as well as the patient's decreased confidence. Initial repeat aspiration/steroid injection can be performed, though repeat excision is often required. Dissection is carried out in a similar manner as described. Increased scarring and adhesions usually make repeat surgery more difficult.

Reappearance of ganglia at the same site years later indicates the formation of new ganglia (1,2). Management is similar to that for the initial ganglion.

Continued pain or discomfort in the area of excision can be caused by formation of a painful scar, contracture, adhesions of neighboring structures, small neuromata, incomplete ganglion excision, or occult underlying carpal instability. Painful scars or adhesions are treated symptomatically with oral nonsteroidal antiinflammatory medication, hand therapy for desensitization, heat, and rest, followed by mobilization and intermittent splinting as needed. Hand therapy is indicated for gentle mobilization of painful contractures. Observation for early signs of reflex sympathetic dystrophy and appropriate treatment is warranted.

Continued wrist pain following ganglion excision may be secondary to underlying scaphoid instability. Evaluation for static or dynamic instability is performed using the scaphoid shift maneuver, standard roentgenograms, and provocative roentgenograms with the carpus in ulnar and radial deviation, and with the fist clenched.

After dorsal carpal ganglion excision, loss of wrist palmar flexion has been reported to occur in 1% of cases (2). Carpal stiffness is avoided by early active mobilization following the initial period of postoperative immobilization. Treat residual weakness of the hand and wrist by hand therapy for strengthening and work hardening.

Neuroma formation is avoided by identification and protection of sensory nerves during dissection. Branches of the superficial branch of the radial nerve and of the dorsal branch of the ulnar nerve are at risk. Injury to these nerves is minimized by an appreciation of their anatomic course combined with careful dissection aided by loupe magnification (2,3). Once formed, a painful neuroma is a difficult management problem. Steroid/lidocaine injection, antiinflammatory medication, protective splinting, and hand therapy for desensitization can be initiated. For refractory neuromata, consider operative exploration and neuroma excision. For terminal neuromata, sharply dissect the lesion and place the nerve end in a protected environment. A neuroma-in-continuity can be treated with resection and neurorrhaphy or placement of the nerve end in protective soft tissue.

### Palmar Carpal Ganglion

Complications following palmar carpal ganglion excision are similar to those of the dorsal ganglion, with the additional potential for injury to the radial or ulnar artery or to the palmar cutaneous branch of the median nerve. The postoperative recurrence rate is slightly higher and more variable for palmar ganglia, with recurrence rates reported at 7% (6), 19% (19), and 30% to 33% (1,2). The difference in recurrence is thought to be due to the more variable sites of origin of palmar ganglia (2,6).

Avoid injury to the radial and (less commonly) ulnar artery and palmar cutaneous branch of the medial nerve by appreciation of the proximity of these structures to palmar ganglia (2,3). Preoperative Allen's testing for radial and ulnar artery patency is important inasmuch as these arteries can be adherent to the ganglion wall (3,10). Ultrasound can show the relationships of these structures to each other, as well as demonstrate arterial patency. At surgery these neurovascular structures should be identified proximal to the ganglion, and dissection carried out in a proximal-to-distal direction.

Because many of the palmar carpal ganglia arise from the scaphotrapezial, radiocarpal, or trapeziometacarpal joints and track the sheath of the flexor carpi radialis, dissection along the flexor carpi radialis can lead to tendon adhesions and carpal stiffness. Early gentle mobilization of the wrist and the use of hand therapy as needed minimize this problem.

## ACKNOWLEDGMENTS

The author would like to thank the following physicians for their contributions and assistance with photographs or imaging studies: Kirk F. Granlund, M. D., Department of Orthopaedic Surgery, University of California, San Diego; David Fessell, M. D., Department of Radiology, University of Michigan Hospitals, Ann Arbor, Michigan; Christine B. Chung, M. D. and Donald Resnick, M. D., Department of Radiology, San Diego Veterans Affairs Health Care System, and the University of California, San Diego.

## RECOMMENDED READING

1. Angelides, A. C.: Ganglions of the hand and wrist. In: *Green's Operative Hand Surgery,* 4th ed., edited by D. P. Green, R. N. Hotchkiss, W. C. Pederson, Churchill-Livingstone, New York, pp. 2171–2183, 1999.
2. Angelides, A. C., Wallace, P. F.: The dorsal ganglion of the wrist: its pathogenesis, gross and microscopic anatomy, and surgical treatment. *J. Hand Surg.,* 1: 228–235, 1976.
3. Barnes, W. E., Larsen, R. D., Posch, J. L.: Review of ganglia of the hand and wrist with analysis of surgical treatment. *Plast. Reconstr. Surg.,* 34: 570–577, 1964.
4. Blam, O., Bindra, R., Middleton, W., Gelberman, R. H.: The occult dorsal carpal ganglion: usefulness of magnetic resonance imaging and ultrasound in diagnosis. *Am. J. Orthop.,* 27(2): 107–110, 1998.
5. Cardinal, E., Buckwalter, D. A., Braunstein, E. M., Mih, A. D.: Occult dorsal carpal ganglion: comparison of US and MR imaging. *Radiology,* 193(1): 259–262, 1994.
6. Greendyke, S. D., Wilson, J., Shepler, T. R.: Anterior wrist ganglia from the scaphotrapezial joint. *J. Hand Surg.,* 17A: 487–490, 1992.

7. Hwang, J. J., Goldfarb, C. A., Gelberman, R. H., Boyer, M. I.: The effect of dorsal carpal ganglion excision on the scaphoid shift test. *J. Hand Surg.*, 24B(1): 106–108, 1999.

8. Kerrigan, J. J., Bertoni, J. M., Jaeger, S. H.: Ganglion cysts and carpal tunnel syndrome. *J. Hand Surg.*, 13A: 763–765, 1988.

9. Korman, J., Pearl, R., Hentz, V. R.: Efficacy of immobilization following aspiration of carpal and digital ganglions. *J. Hand Surg.*, 17A: 1097–1099, 1992.

10. Lister, G., Smith, R.: Protection of the radial artery in the resection of adherent ganglions of the wrist. *Plast. Reconstr. Surg.*, 61: 127–129, 1978.

11. Nelson, C. L., Sawmiller, S., Phalen, G. S.: Ganglions of the wrist and hand. *J. Bone Joint Surg.*, 54A: 1459–1464, 1972.

12. Osterman, A. L., Raphael, J.: Arthroscopic resection of dorsal ganglion of the wrist. *Hand Clin.*, 11(1): 7–12, 1995.

13. Osterwalder, J. J., Widrig, R., Stober, R., Gachter, A.: Diagnostic validity of ultrasound in patients with persistent wrist pain and suspected occult ganglion. *J. Hand Surg.*, 22A(6): 1034–1040, 1997.

14. Paul, A. S., Sochart, D. H.: Improving the results of ganglion aspiration by the use of hyaluronidase. *J. Hand Surg.*, 22B: 219–221, 1997.

15. Richman, J. A., Gelberman, R. H., Engber, W. D., Salamon, P. B., Bean, D. J.: Ganglions of the wrist and digits: results of treatment by aspiration and cyst wall puncture. *J. Hand Surg.*, 21A: 1041–1043, 1987.

16. Steinberg, B. D., Kleinman, W. B.: Occult scapholunate ganglion: a cause of dorsal radial wrist pain. *J. Hand Surg.*, 24A(2): 225–231, 1999.

17. Thornburg, L. E.: Ganglions of the hand and wrist. *J. Am. Acad. Orthop. Surg.*, 7(4): 231–238, 1999.

18. Vo, P., Wright, T., Hayden, F., Dell, P., Chidgey, L.: Evaluating dorsal wrist pain: MRI diagnosis of occult dorsal wrist ganglion. *J. Hand Surg.*, 20A(4): 667–670, 1995.

19. Wright, T. W., Cooney, W. P., Ilstrup, D. M.: Anterior wrist ganglion. *J. Hand Surg.*, 19A(6): 954–958, 1994.

20. Ziegler, L., Kuffer, G., Euler, E., Wilhelm, K.: Arthrographic imaging of ganglions of the hand. *Rofo Fortschr. Geb. Rontgenstr. Neuen Bildgeb. Verfahr.*, 153(2): 143–146, 1990.

# Subject Index